Targeting the Positive with Behaviours that Challenge

of related interest

Understanding Behaviour in Dementia that Challenges, Second Edition
A Guide to Assessment and Treatment
Ian Andrew James and Louisa Jackman
ISBN 978 1 78592 264 0
eISBN 978 1 78450 551 6

Supporting Positive Behaviour in Intellectual Disabilities and Autism
Practical Strategies for Addressing Challenging Behaviour
Tony Osgood
ISBN 978 1 78775 132 3
eISBN 978 1 78775 133 0

Supporting Positive Behaviour
A Workbook for Social Care Workers
Suzan Collins
ISBN 978 1 84905 073 9
eISBN 978 0 85700 267 9

Confused, Angry, Anxious?
Why Working with Older People in Care Really Can Be Difficult, and What to Do About It
Bo Hejlskov Elven, Charlotte Agger and Iben Ljungmann
ISBN 978 1 78592 215 2
eISBN 978 1 78450 494 6

TARGETING THE POSITIVE WITH BEHAVIOURS THAT CHALLENGE

Empathic Strategies for Working with Children and Adults

ANDY BAKER

Jessica Kingsley Publishers
London and Philadelphia

First published in Great Britain in 2025 by Jessica Kingsley Publishers
An imprint of John Murray Press

2

A CIP catalogue record for this title is available from the British Library and the Library of Congress

ISBN 978 1 83997 900 2
eISBN 978 1 83997 901 9

Printed and bound in in the United States by Integrated Books International

Jessica Kingsley Publishers' policy is to use papers that are natural, renewable and recyclable products and made from wood grown in sustainable forests. The logging and manufacturing processes are expected to conform to the environmental regulations of the country of origin.

Jessica Kingsley Publishers
Carmelite House
50 Victoria Embankment
London EC4Y 0DZ

www.jkp.com

John Murray Press
Part of Hodder & Stoughton Ltd
An Hachette Company

The authorised representative in the EEA is Hachette Ireland, 8 Castlecourt Centre, Castleknock Road, Castleknock, Dublin 15, D15 YF6A, Ireland

Contents

Part 5: The 6-Stage Target Model Stage 3: Proactive Planning

Part 6: The 6-Stage Target Model Stage 4: Recognise Escalation

Part 7: The 6-Stage Target Model Stage 5: Respond Appropriately

Part 8: The 6-Stage Target Model Stage 6: Learn from Incident

Preface

This book has been in development for over 26 years, since I first started my journey of trying to understand human behaviour. My interest in human behaviour began after a life event triggered a desire to better understand myself and my reactions to stimulus. I was robbed at knifepoint. This event had a profound impact on me. Rather than feeling fear, as expected, I found it made me want to better understand my reaction to the aggression and also the behaviour of the aggressor. This began my tumble down the rabbit hole that is the nature of behaviour. People are wonderful, diverse and interesting, but they are complex, and every single one of them contains at their core the most complex structure in the known universe – the human brain.

> *It produces our every thought, action, memory, feeling and experience of the world. This jelly-like mass of tissue, weighing in at around 1.4 kilograms, contains a staggering one hundred billion nerve cells, or neurons.*[1]

I very quickly realised this was not going to be a short journey but one I would continue for the rest of my life as I began to study the exciting world of psychology.

I have worked in many different settings, including hospitality, retail, sales, and health and social care. Each one demonstrated to me that understanding people to some greater degree than I already did would benefit my interactions and outcomes, and my relationships as a result. When I combined teaching with the mix, I discovered the joy of sharing what I was learning with others.

I started my training company in 2014, with a focus on delivering courses in subjects about understanding people and behaviours that the environments found challenging. We would receive requests for training from organisations in many different settings such as care homes, foster care, schools, retail, security and so on. Often, the request would ask for a special focus on a certain set of requirements or certain difficulties that were being experienced.

After a while, I realised that although each setting was different and each circumstance unique, there were certain 'golden rules' or principles that could be applied generally. So, standing on the shoulders of giants, I started to combine the disciplines I had studied and trained in to develop my own model. A model to work from that would allow others to have a simple system to use to both proactively and dynamically understand, respond to, manage and potentially change behaviours that challenge.

The ABLE Target System® and the 6-Stage Target Model (6STM) were developed.

The system includes principles of positive behaviour support, trauma-informed care, therapeutic parenting, cognitive behaviour therapy and more, with the target being positive outcomes for all. It is an analytical model for use within a setting to evaluate, assess and plan for behaviours in line with the setting's care planning or behavioural management plans. Or it can be used by caregivers as a dynamic system on a day-to-day basis to manage behaviours as they arise.

The positive outcomes include:

- improved quality of life
- reduction of behavioural challenges
- reduction in the use of restrictive practice
- improved morale and relationships
- improved service reputation and lower costs.

Why would we want to or need to manage or change any person's behaviour? Answer: to improve their outcomes, to promote equality of opportunity, to raise self-esteem and a sense of worth and to encourage feelings of inclusivity and connection that are appropriate to the person themselves. All of these increase wellbeing; and increasing wellbeing for one person has a domino effect of increasing wellbeing for all others in the setting.

Note especially 'all others'.

I sometimes saw that the focus of certain settings was solely on the outcomes of those being supported or using a service. I often felt there was something missing, *that the wellbeing of the people doing the training or providing the service was neglected.* And this neglect happened without the realisation that both caregivers and individuals are directly connected, and this connection impacts on the setting, the business, the overheads, the costs and so much more!

Caregivers are often undersupported. I saw caregivers being assaulted and abused, getting hurt, being at the end of their tether but not knowing how to deal with certain behaviours that challenge, resulting in placement breakdowns, high staff turnovers and stressed staff... As well as the direct impact they had on the staff, these issues indirectly impacted the individuals being supported.

I want to give people the tools that I discovered during my journey from the crime I was involved in as a 16-year-old.

Tools such as an understanding and empathy towards the perpetrator (mugger), an awareness of and resilience to our own responses and reactions, and tools to reduce the chances of incidents occurring at all.

Therefore, my goal is, through knowledge, to increase competency, confidence, resilience and empathy, so that caregivers feel more assured and settled about what they do.

It is my greatest hope that this book will help all levels of caregivers within the care industry, parents and teachers to gain a better insight into why the individuals they support behave as they do and to embrace techniques for how to deal with behaviours that challenge.

I would humbly like to assert that I do not consider myself an expert, only a student of behaviour with a passion to share what I have learned. I have read, listened to and engaged with the experience and teachings of so many people with amazing insights and understandings; these I have taken and adopted into my own understanding. I have not been able to reference them all, as I do not remember the source of many, but I thank every person who over the years has been part of my education, including those individuals with whom I have been involved in changing their outcomes through my work. The caregivers and the individuals we support teach the greatest lessons of all.

All of the case studies in this book are based on real situations or are adapted from real circumstances. Names and details have been changed for discretion, but thank you to everyone who made this book a reality.

There are bonus chapters available for download at https://library.jkp.com/redeem using the code ESGBAKQ, covering risk assessments, aspects of communication and practical examples of behavioural plans. You will find references to these at the relevant sections in the book.

I would like to thank my parents Philip and Cathrine, my son Josh and all my friends who've supported me. Cheers to Fran and Chris, my sister and brother-in-law, for letting me hibernate in your caravan to write some of this. Thank you Keith Ougden, my copywriter, for challenging me and all of your help. Thanks to all my staff team at Able Training – you are amazing, and I love you all. Special thanks to Karen Hayes, my absolute rock. To all the people I have worked with over the years, I have learnt more than I have taught and I couldn't have written this without you.

INTRODUCTION

An ounce of prevention is worth a pound of cure.

BENJAMIN FRANKLIN

The goal of this book is to enable and encourage those who support, care for or engage with individuals who may have behavioural, emotional and cognitive challenges to focus on *understanding, planning, preventing and responding* – not reacting.

The target is positive outcomes for all!

DEFINITIONS: 'CAREGIVER' AND 'INDIVIDUAL'

Throughout this book the following terms are used:

Caregiver: This general term is used to describe anyone who has a duty of care to another. This can include parents, foster carers, schoolteachers, carers in care homes, home carers, nurses and so on.

It is especially important to appreciate that the term 'caregiver' in this book also includes those who manage caregivers; in organisations, it is management's responsibility to improve the organisation by implementing the proposals contained in this book.

Individual: There are many terms, like customer, individual, young person and resident, but the general term of 'individual' will be used for anyone who is being supported and cared for by another. This can include children, elderly people, patients and so on.

GENERAL TERMINOLOGY

Throughout the book we will try to use the most appropriate and well-known terms to aid understanding and standardisation. There are some terms that may change over time as people's perspectives and feelings change. Any future revisions of the book will always aim to pick these up and move forwards with the changing terminology status quo.

BACKGROUND AND GOAL

This book has been developed in line with the ABLE Target System®, a full training syllabus taught by ABLE Training Support Ltd in a variety of care and education settings. The programme is recognised by the Institute of Conflict Management and the British Institute of Learning Disabilities.

The total content of this book explains the ABLE Target System®. This *system* covers aspects of the caring environment as a whole, especially as described in Part 1.

Parts 2–8 deal specifically with the 6-Stage Target Model (6STM). This *model* is part of the ABLE Target *System*® and describes a process that is designed to help caregivers, care managers, parents and teachers to manage behaviours that challenge *shown by an individual.*

The goal of this book is for the reader to:

- understand the causes and functions of behaviours that challenge
- identify the difference between preventative, proactive and responsive strategies for handling such behaviours
- understand how the environment, culture, language and relationships can impact on behaviour
- understand the six stages of the 6STM and explain how each stage is implemented
- recognise the importance of proactive as well as responsive strategies
- explore factors and conditions that change behaviour
- understand the effects of trauma and how it affects behaviour
- recognise stages of escalation and understand appropriate response methods
- develop strategies to manage individual needs based on planning and response
- develop situation awareness and assess risk
- practise the principles of signalling non-aggression and positive communication
- implement an appropriate debrief and reflection process after an incident.

Part 1 focuses on the care setting itself. It includes a definition of the term 'behaviour that challenges' and an introduction to the law concerning aggressive behaviour. It goes on to describe primary, secondary and tertiary strategies for handling such behaviours, with the emphasis on being PRO-active, not RE-active.

Part 2 is an introduction to the 6STM itself, which is a six-stage process designed to assist caregivers in subjects covered by Parts 3 to 8:

- **Part 3**: Identifying behaviours that challenge.
- **Part 4**: Understanding *why* the behaviour is occurring and empathising with the individual. This section includes an explanation of the physiological and psychological causes that can underlie behaviours that challenge. Causes are categorised as 'Reflex', 'Reactive' and 'Intentional'.
- **Part 5**: Proactive planning to avoid such behaviours rather than tackling them as they occur.
- **Part 6**: Recognising when escalation of behaviour is about to happen.
- **Part 7**: Planning to respond appropriately.
- **Part 8**: Learning from each incident.

The book is aimed at understanding people regardless of the setting, and it can be used in elderly care, adult and child health and social care, schools and foster care, and much of it can be beneficial for parents. Some sections may feel more relevant to some settings than others but there are nuggets of useful information in every chapter.

The overall aim of dealing with behaviours that challenge is: *positive outcomes for all.*

PART 1

THE ENVIRONMENT

CHAPTER 1

WHAT IS 'BEHAVIOUR THAT CHALLENGES'?

CASE STUDY 1.1 WHO CAN BE A CHALLENGE?!

Many individuals in care receive the label of 'challenging', 'complex' or 'difficult', but think of the people you have cared for in your life. Have some been more 'challenging' than others?

Were those who were more 'challenging' always challenging, or were they sometimes easier to interact with than at other times?

It is extremely unlikely, if not impossible, that anyone is 100% challenging 100% of the time with 100% of people in 100% of environments.

Now, if we surveyed everyone who has been labelled as challenging in care settings and asked them the following questions, the answers would almost inevitably be 'yes'!

1. Have you ever found any of the caregivers in your life challenging?
2. Have you found some caregivers easier to interact with than other caregivers?
3. For those caregivers that you find more challenging – is it true that they weren't always challenging and they were easier to interact with at some times than at other times?

Commentary: We can all be challenging to somebody at some point. If you were asked whether you ever find your own parents, partner, children, siblings or the cashier at the post office 'challenging', we could make a confident prediction of the answer: 'yes'.

We deal with behaviour that challenges every day, often without awareness, but sometimes the behaviour goes past what our knowledge, skills or the environment can manage, and we need additional support, facilities, guidance or ideas to feel better able to provide positive outcomes for ourselves and those we support. This book and the 6STM aim to meet exactly those needs.

The *Oxford English Dictionary* definition of behaviour is: 'The way in which an animal or person behaves in response to a particular situation or stimulus.'

When working with or supporting people, there is always the possibility that certain behaviours may be perceived by others as inappropriate or maladaptive, either for the individual themselves or the impact of the behaviour on others. These (at least perceived) detrimental behaviours have been, and are, referred to using many different terms – some derogatory generalisations, others empathic, indicating a willingness to understand and explore.

Trends towards preferred terms when exploring behaviours come and go, with many different opinions and perspectives.

'Behaviours of concern' and 'distressed behaviour' are two terms used by different settings and are often considered positive terms by some groups, but they may not correctly describe some behaviours. 'Concerning' may not appropriately address the urgency, intensity or risk of a behaviour, and some behaviours are not triggered purely by distress – they may be a conditioned response to meet a need; for example, stealing.

'Hazardous behaviour' is a good term to cover a particular set of behaviours that carry significant risk to the individual or others. This term will be used in the book but only in some instances.

One term that has fallen out of favour and will not be used in this book is 'challenging behaviour'. This book will use the term 'behaviour that challenges' for all behaviour that caregivers in all settings may experience as difficult or concerning.

The simple addition of the word 'that' shifts the focus from the individual to the caregiver's perspective of the behaviour. 'I find this behaviour challenging but maybe that's my problem not theirs, let's explore.' It also conveys the message that many behaviours that challenge are a challenge for the individual who is displaying the behaviour as well as those around them whose quality of life and wellbeing may be affected.

The word 'challenges' has some positive undertones. To overcome a challenge – a task or situation that tests someone's abilities – is something to work towards. It promotes the notion that additional skills or understanding may be required to:

- manage the behaviour itself
- manage our reactions to it
- review our beliefs and thoughts about it
- support an individual to overcome their own challenges.

Engaging in 'behaviours that challenge' is not specific to individuals in care or education, as discussed at the start of this chapter. If we think of a time when we felt anxious or frustrated by something, did we potentially act in a way that, with hindsight, when calm, we could recognise as being not the most logical way to behave and even detrimental to ourselves or others? However, in that moment, it felt like the right thing to do, despite the potential negative impact. For example, avoiding something that you wanted to do because it felt scary; getting angry and saying something you wish you hadn't; driving faster than the speed limit as you were worried about being late. These are all examples of times when we felt emotionally challenged and acted in a way that was potentially *behaviour that challenged.*

The behaviours from individuals we support may be more extreme, more repetitive or more detrimental than the above day-to-day examples, which may mean we need additional time, skills and abilities to support or manage them. But the individual should be seen not as a problem to solve but as a person to understand.

Here is a list of behaviours that are often described as challenging in various settings:

- Verbal, physical or passive aggression
- Bullying
- Destruction of property
- Self-sabotaging behaviours
- Self-injury
- Swearing
- Hyperactivity
- Repetitive behaviours
- Poor self-care, personal care
- Socially inappropriate, antisocial behaviour
- Emotional distress
- Resistance/defiance/refusal/demand avoidance/rule breaking
- Smearing excrement, manual evacuation or toileting issues
- Sleeping issues
- Untidiness
- Apathy, non-engagement, withdrawal
- Sexualised – inappropriate actions towards themselves or others, inappropriate place
- Lying/telling untruths
- Attention-seeking
- Allegations – malicious or misdirected
- Manipulation/emotional blackmail, controlling behaviour
- Absconding/running away
- Disruptive behaviour

This list is non-exhaustive, and although some examples such as physical aggression, self-harm and destructive behaviour may seem obviously challenging, they are all dependent on the values, beliefs, attitudes and experiences of the observer, as well as the context or situation in which the behaviour occurs. Physical aggression to defend yourself may be appropriate; self-harm is used in certain religions as a form of spiritual discipline; people pay money to use rage rooms where they can smash inanimate objects to pieces to dispel their stress. Behaviour that challenges is often a personally subjective experience and therefore not definite truth.

Let's look at an example – swearing. Swearing may be offensive to one observer, but another may just shrug it off as: 'It's only words.' So, one observer may describe the behaviour as challenging, the other may not. Their subjective attitudes are neither right nor wrong; it's what they experience as challenging. However, if one claims the behaviour needs to stop, their subjective opinion needs to be objectively assessed before they enforce change on the swearer's behaviour. A lot needs to be explored (the cost versus benefits of the behaviour, the cause or function of the behaviour and the context of the behaviour).

For example, suppose the swearer has a form of Tourette's syndrome that includes coprolalia (obscene phrases and gestures). The individual won't be *able* to change their actions, so a caregiver may have to address their own beliefs and change their own perspective, not seek to change the individual.

Let's look at one behaviour that is rarely described as challenging – submissive/passive behaviour. This is where an individual does whatever they're asked to do; they don't draw attention to themselves; they keep quiet and just comply. This may not be perceived as challenging by a caregiver; they may even see the individual as easy to manage. However, if we are genuinely concerned about 'positive outcomes' for those we care for, this behaviour is worrying. How can we meet this person's needs if we don't know what their needs are? Is this individual vulnerable to coercion or manipulation by others?

This may mean that this behaviour should be considered challenging, as it is potentially maladaptive depending on the individual's vulnerability. The target and behavioural plans may aim, over time, to raise the individual's self-esteem, reduce fear and develop assertion skills.

SOME DEFINITIONS

It is important at this point to give some additional definitions.

Behaviours that challenge are typically excess behaviours that people around the individual find difficult or concerning based on their own values, beliefs and attitudes towards the behaviour or the context in which the behaviour happens. The behaviours may or may not be detrimental to the individual, the environment, the caregivers or others in the setting; whether they are or not will depend on the frequency, context and cost-versus-benefit analysis. Behaviours that challenge, where the cost of the behaviour is greater than the benefits, then fall into two categories: maladaptive and hazardous.

Below is a brief explanation of terms that will be used throughout the book.

Behavioural deficits: Limitations that affect a person's abilities to meet their own needs or manage emotions/stress or that impact their ability to communicate in socially preferred ways. They rarely impact others or the environment. We wish to state that a behavioural deficit is not an insinuation that a person is 'less than' as a result of said deficit. For example, the medical model historically frames disability as a 'deficit', whereas the social model understands that society creates barriers that cause difficulties for people with disabilities in society. In this book, the term is used where a person's own wellbeing is negatively impacted by for example, emotional dysregulation, memory impairments and language barriers.
Excess behaviours: Behaviours a person uses to cope with stress, meet their needs or communicate. These are likely to impact on others or the environment to some extent, and the person may have some control of these behaviours. These may or may not be viewed as negative but are labelled as 'excess' by being considered non-typical or more intense examples of typical behaviours. For example, eating versus eating disorder, subtle fidgeting versus excess rocking/stimming.
Adaptive behaviours: Behaviours that are viewed as positive and seem to improve wellbeing and harmony. They may help the person to communicate, meet needs or cope with stress and are considered safe and socially and culturally acceptable.
Maladaptive behaviour: Excess behaviours that negatively impact on an individual's, or others', outcomes, wellbeing or safety. These will be contextual to the environment, the situation and the individual. The cost of these behaviours is considered higher than the benefit, and these behaviours may need to be managed or potentially changed over time.
Hazardous behaviour: Behaviours that pose an immediate risk of harm or exclusion for the individual displaying the behaviour or others in the environment; for example, fighting, arson, ligaturing.

Let's look at an example:

CASE STUDY 1.2 MANY BEHAVIOURS IN ONE PERSON

Sue lives in a residential care facility. She has come from a traumatic background. She is shy, has no self-esteem and suffers from anxiety. (Behavioural deficits)

Sue also lives with anorexia nervosa. Sue uses lots of strategies to avoid eating and feels happier having control over what she eats. (Excess behaviours)

The staff find her strategies to avoid food or lose weight very challenging. Some staff get upset that Sue is so thin from lack of food. Sue also follows staff around a lot when she is feeling anxious, and some staff get irritated with her when she does this. (Behaviours that challenge)

Sue's eating habits are maladaptive, and a full behavioural plan is created to help build Sue's self-esteem and confidence, and her sense of control and safety, as well as food management plans. The care facility also starts to give Sue other ways to cope with her anxiety.

The staff are told to support Sue when she is following them and to give her some one-to-one time, because when she is anxious she needs nurturing before redirecting (for now, and this can be addressed later).

Sue chooses gardening as a way of relaxing, self-caring and reducing anxiety; she starts really well – weeding and seeding the pots around the grounds, sometimes with staff engagement and support. Sue is engaging well with her therapy and her eating habits are beginning to settle. (Adaptive)

Unfortunately, Sue gets some bad news one day and things begin to change. Sue continues to go into the garden but rather than doing gentle planting she has started digging. Initially the staff don't perceive this behaviour as challenging; they think this may be positive as it's exercise and she is still interacting with nature.

The staff soon realise, though, that Sue is digging to the point of physical exhaustion. Sue is now using excessive exercise to control her weight after every meal.

The digging is maladaptive, and the level of the behaviour is hazardous, so all digging tools have to be removed from the site and Sue has to be supervised when she goes into the garden.

CASE STUDY 1.3 BEHAVIOUR THAT CHALLENGES... MALADAPTIVE OR NOT?

This is about Liam, a six-year-old boy with foetal alcohol spectrum disorder and autism. At night after being put to bed, Liam would usually jump on his bed for over an hour before settling down to sleep. This was clearly most disconcerting for the caregivers and disruptive to the environment.

Part of Liam's condition was sensory processing disorder (SPD), which affects an individual's ability to separate and automatically filter sensory inputs. Most people are able to automatically focus on the sense that is perceived to be important to them at the time. For example, you might be watching TV when an aeroplane passes. You can effectively block out the aeroplane noise and concentrate on the TV. But with SPD, all senses may be active at once; the filtering process does not work. Many of us have experienced this when we are trying to concentrate on something important and there are lots of external distractions – we can feel our frustration building as a result... imagine that sensation multiplied by a thousand every moment of the day!

The bed jumping was Liam's attempt to focus on one sense – the sensation of jumping. It 'drowned out the other sensory noise' and gave him space to think about his day and progress into a sleep cycle. On days when he jumped, he slept better and had a better following day as a result.

So, there were *benefits* to Liam's behaviour, and attempts to change it could cause worse problems. As Liam grows older, he will find other ways to settle.

Should we *manage* the behaviour? Well, yes – we could ensure Liam has a strong bed and maybe has an earlier bedtime.

The point here is that the *benefit* of the behaviour outweighed the *costs* of the behaviour to the boy, and so management, not change, was the aim.

POSITIVE OUTCOMES FOR ALL

It is important when trying to understand the impact of an individual's behaviour on their wellbeing to also consider the wellbeing of those who care for them. As will be explored throughout the book, it is important to recognise, acknowledge and manage the impact on everyone within a setting. Let's use the swearing example again. The observer who finds swearing upsetting or difficult should not be told to 'just get over it'. They may need support and training to better cope with the behaviour they find challenging.

There are professional caregivers who have been told that 'getting hit is just part of the job'. Although caregivers should understand that their job has risks (like every job), that doesn't mean we shouldn't always look to make things safer and offer appropriate support in the event of an incident.

Health and safety law states that our job should not cause us harm. If in the course of their work a caregiver is physically injured to the point that their wellbeing is affected, the setting has an obvious responsibility. But non-physical behaviours, such as having to put up with a day of non-stop verbal abuse or working for 12 hours with an individual who screams at the top of their voice every two minutes (due to distress or sensory needs), can cause any person to feel overwhelmed and have feelings of negativity and stress about their role, the person or their job. This could then affect their family and home life and their morale and productivity, cause them to not look forward to the next day and so on. So, the caregiver's overall wellbeing is affected. Such non-physical behaviours that challenge are still 'maladaptive' and even 'hazardous' and should be managed. The management of the behaviour may involve supporting the staff through risk assessment and control measures rather than changing the behaviour itself.

CHAPTER 2

PREVENTION STRATEGIES

The principle that 'prevention is better than cure' is understood by many but implemented by few. It can be so easy to fall into a trap of spending all resources on *reacting* to behaviours and thus leaving no time or resources to explore *preventative* and *proactive* options.

One of the underpinning themes of the 6STM is the focus on a *positive* model and a hierarchy of managing behaviours that challenge. This may require more time upfront but will ultimately result in an increase in available resources and time.

We need to look at long-term solutions rather than short-term fixes.

CASE STUDY 2.1 SIMILARITY TO FIRE

Handling behaviours that challenge is similar to the approach we take with reducing fire risk. The risks of fire are similar: fire can spread; it can affect individuals, the community and environment, in both the short term and long term.

The following 'Management Strategy Hierarchy' diagram shows the three levels of strategies that could well be in place for handling fire risk.

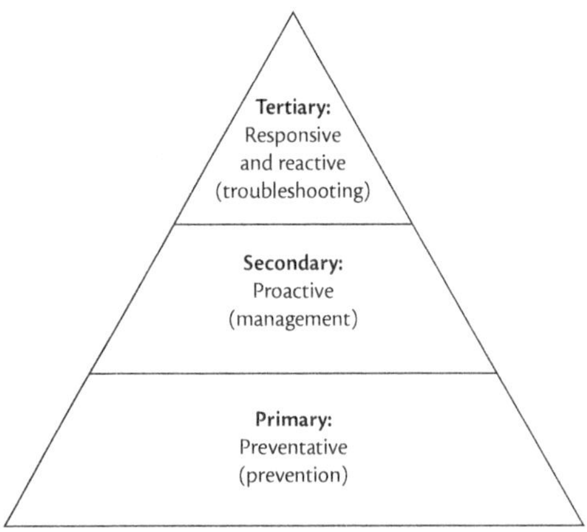

Figure 2.1 Management Strategy Hierarchy

> Primary strategies, for *Prevention*, are the foundation of fire safety: to prevent a fire from occurring in the first place. For example, the building is constructed appropriately; procedures, plans and training are in place to minimise fire risk.
>
> Secondary strategies, for *Management* of fire risk, could be in place for special cases – for example, cooking – where closer management and specific strategies, procedures and plans may be needed.
>
> But even with all this care, fire does occasionally happen. And that's when the tertiary strategies apply. Examples of tertiary strategies, for *Response and Reaction*, are fire extinguishers, fire alarms, evacuation procedures or calling the fire service.
>
> A positive model of managing fire is putting more time, attention and effort into the base strategies – *Prevention* – to make it less likely that *Response and Reaction* strategies will be needed.
>
> In a negative model the triangle would be upside down, with more time spent on putting out fires and relying on fire extinguishers than on putting measures in place to prevent fires.

Relating this metaphor to behaviours that challenge, the primary strategies are the everyday working practices, the environment and the behaviour of the caregivers within the setting.

Primary strategies include the culture, values and ethos of the setting as well as the physical environment. Also, education, attitudes, behavioural support strategies, positive relationships, person-centred practices, inclusion, reflection and support of the people working within the setting are vital at this stage.

The primary objective in any care situation is to improve the quality of life, to have happy people. Generally, happy and contented people are less likely to engage in maladaptive behaviours. So if an environment can be created where people's needs are being met, where they feel valued and where their self-esteem is growing, we should see an increase in positive, adaptive and social behaviours and therefore a reduction in behaviours that challenge. These principles should be applied to and by all individuals within the setting – staff, management and service users.

When we are working in a person-centred way, there will always need to be plans and strategies that are used to support and promote wellbeing on an individual level, which will allow the setting and caregivers to behave and adapt to an individual's specific challenges and deficits, to improve their personal outcomes.

Secondary strategies include individual behavioural support plans as well as response and de-escalation strategies for known maladaptive behaviours. This is where the 6STM becomes an active analytical process to create plans that support an individual day-to-day.

The important thing to recognise is that not everything goes to plan. The primary strategies aim to reduce behaviours that challenge through creating a positive environment. The secondary strategies allow caregivers to focus on an individual's strengths and positives as well as understanding any maladaptive behaviours, and to create plans to manage or adjust these – either through altering interactions, teaching new skills or adapting the environment.

However, change takes time, management plans may not work and need tweaking, information on individuals isn't always available and... people change. People can be unpredictable and can react very differently depending on numerous physical, environmental and psychological factors, and therefore there also need to be tertiary strategies. These tertiary strategies are for when the 'fire has already started' and when everything else has gone wrong.

Tertiary strategies include responding with de-escalation strategies to 'put the fire out' but may also include situations where caregivers have to react with personal safety strategies and restrictive and non-restrictive physical interventions (breakaway/disengagement techniques (self-defence)). Restrictive interventions may include physical, mechanical or chemical restraint, or seclusion.

One of the goals of the 6STM is to improve prevention, proactive management and responsive skills to reduce the need for reactions, particularly the need for any restrictive physical interventions within a setting.

THE UNFORTUNATE REALITY

Unfortunately, it is often the case in many care settings that the triangle of strategies described in the fire analogy is upside down. More time and effort are applied to the tertiary strategies than the primary and secondary strategies. The setting is forever 'fighting fires' – reacting to situations as they occur and increasing the risk to all, as well as impacting on the culture, available resources and quality of care.

Any environment that took the reactive strategy with fire – for example, 'We won't bother having regular checks on the electrical equipment – we'll just have lots of fire extinguishers' – would not last long.

There are a number of reasons why behaviour and fire are not managed in the same way. One is the perceived impact of the negative result. If a setting had regular fires:

- the problem would be obvious
- it would be considered unacceptable and unsafe
- the costs to rectify the damage would be prohibitive
- the time, effort and resources that would be applied to prevent further fires and prevent a major catastrophe would be significant
- there would be significant pressure from multiple parties to review all preventative and proactive measures to prevent a future occurrence.

Another reason is that maybe behaviour is seen more like a slowly leaking water pipe; the water damage may seem insignificant but it is building up over time, and the problem keeps getting patched up rather than improved. The problem is ignored but unfortunately it is slowly crumbling the foundations.

The effects of behaviour on caregivers or the setting can be significant but some are less obvious, such as:

- physical injuries
- low caregiver morale
- blocked care – where caregivers lose compassion due to feeling overwhelmed
- increased absenteeism
- high staff turnover
- recruitment costs and training
- lower quality of care
- reduced consistency and routines for individuals
- property damage.

It is also fair to mention that people are far more complex than fire; the three elements of the fire triangle – fuel, air and heat – are easily distinguished and can be planned around. But people are complex systems. The stressors, triggers and deficits of any individual may take time to learn and so fires may need to be handled while caregivers are learning about what causes them and how to improve understanding.

Knowledge and enforcement can also cause the triangle to be upside down; many people know far more about fire and fire reduction than behaviour management. Organisations invest in multiple fire prevention and management resources and plans because they are made to. There are mandatory guidelines that organisations must meet that include provisions, risk assessments, staff training, evacuation procedures, etc. This means there is a variety of resources, guidance and support to ensure an organisation knows how to meet standards. This does not exist around the subject of behaviour to the same extent. This book aims to provide a resource to help caregivers, managers, owners, parents and teachers to be better equipped to make their setting safe and positive, and to inform about actions, philosophies and principles to ensure the 'Management Strategy Hierarchy' triangle is the correct way up.

The next chapter looks at important actions that can be taken to prevent problems occurring.

CHAPTER 3

BUILDING A POSITIVE ENVIRONMENT

This chapter focuses on practical steps that can be taken to build the solid, primary strategies of the strategy triangle discussed in the previous chapter.

CREATE A WELCOMING ENVIRONMENT

CASE STUDY 3.1 THE SHOP

You walk into a shop. It's clean, tidy, well laid out. The person behind the counter gives a welcoming smile and offers to help if you have any queries. You feel positive about the shop.

But suppose the shop is a mess, the floor's dirty and the assistant doesn't acknowledge you and responds to a question with a huff and 'Just a minute...' You have a totally negative impression.

CASE STUDY 3.2 THE 'NOT A MORNING PERSON'

It's a bright morning in the family home. However, someone in the household gets out of bed on the wrong side and comes downstairs in a bad mood. Immediately, the atmosphere changes, the grump's attitude affects others' attitudes and vice versa. A negative spiral can develop, and the mood quickly deteriorates.

Commentary: In 'The Shop' case study, the first impression can have a huge impact on how we perceive the setting. What if we said that it was the same shop in both examples, just a different member of staff? That one person can matter to the atmosphere of the setting. Can these examples be mapped over to a care setting?

The key point therefore is the symbiotic relationship within any setting between every person and their neighbours. We are social animals that respond to each other. Caregivers have a responsibility to make sure: the environment has a foundation of positivity and kindness; people smile, take notice of others; the place is clean, tidy, welcoming.

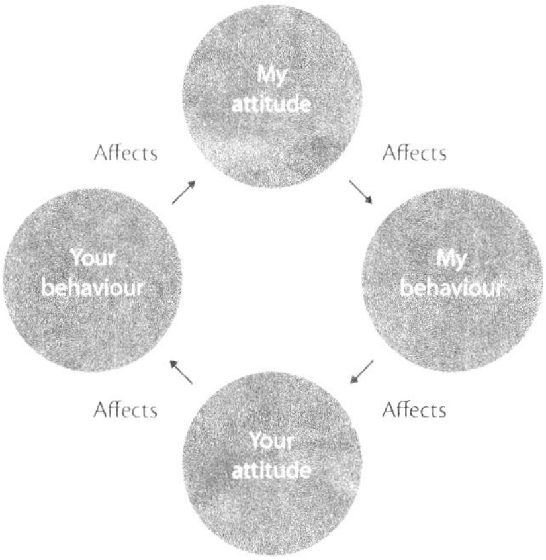

Figure 3.1 Betari's Box: The Attitude and Behaviour Cycle

The diagram above puts in a nutshell how interactions form a spiral. The spiral can twist in a negative or positive direction.

As caregivers, it is our responsibility to be aware of our own attitudes and to ensure the direction is positive.

The direction of the spiral works both at the specific, individual level and for the organisation as a whole. If the general pattern at the individual level is positive, this will permeate the organisation. The opposite is true as well.

CLEAR BEHAVIOURAL POLICIES + BOUNDARIES

Every environment needs rules to be able to function and for safety. There may be rules that are set by guidelines or even laws, but each setting will also have rules that they feel fall in line with their values. These values should be based on positive expectations that are not only for the individuals but also for the caregivers. Caregivers can be role models and should lead by example – for example, by showing punctuality and politeness, and being positive. Caregivers should always be showing their best version of themselves. If caregivers are criticising each other, undermining the organisation or not following the rules or maintaining boundaries, we are setting the system up to fail.

ETHOS

Individuals and caregivers should feel valued, safe, secure; they should feel that they are listened to and are part of a community. From a management point of view, caregivers should feel they are coming to work because they want to, not just because it's a job that pays the rent.

SUPPORT

This is primarily concerned with support for the *caregivers* – ensuring they have adequate training and have open channels of communication. Training improves confidence and competency, provides new ways of doing things, raises self-esteem, revitalises the mood and makes caregivers feel valued.

> **CASE STUDY 3.3** THE BROKEN HAMMER
>
> How does a workman feel if he has to cope with inadequate tools, such as a broken hammer where the head keeps flying off?
>
> Now imagine the reaction when a brand-new hammer is provided. An instant lift, plus better results.

CAREGIVER TRAINING

Caregivers should feel competent and confident in how to support and manage the individuals in their care. They should also have knowledge and understanding of potential conditions or challenges that a person may be living with.

When working with someone with autism or dementia or any other condition, staff should know about these conditions to help them understand the person and their behaviour.

Imagine the example given in Chapter 1 of swearing and Tourette's. If a caregiver didn't understand Tourette's, it would obviously affect how they would interpret any obscene language.

TRACKING AND ANALYSING BEHAVIOUR

When something goes wrong (as Murphy's law dictates, 'What *can* go wrong, *will* go wrong'), it should be taken as an opportunity to learn, not criticise. Questions asked should include: what happened, what worked, what didn't work, what can we do better next time?

Remember our fire analogy from Chapter 2... imagine we had a fire, and it was cleaned up and forgotten about. We shouldn't be surprised when that fire happens again.

Instead, after the first fire, we should be looking to find out what started the fire, how it could have been prevented or how we could improve what we did in response to the fire.

COMMUNITY BUILDING

Caregivers and individuals should be encouraged to build and feel a sense of community. There should be trust between all members of the community. There should be a support network for the caregivers and a promotion of positive relationships between different shifts, roles and responsibility levels. Staff that like and trust each other work better together.

REWARDS AND CELEBRATIONS

One of the aims of this book is to encourage whole organisations or settings to develop a culture and habit of targeting the positive. No setting is perfect, and perfection is always unreachable, but it's better to aim for the moon and fall short than aim for the ceiling and hit your head. It is so important to notice the positives and set the milestones of success. Improvements, no matter how slight, should be celebrated, appreciated and valued. How is everyone in the setting, including the caregivers, rewarded? Getting paid is rarely the best motivator to encourage people to care about their job, achieve their best outcomes and take pride in providing something special.

INVOLVEMENT OF FAMILY, FRIENDS AND PROFESSIONALS

There are cases where an individual is in care and living apart from the family, perhaps in a care facility or in their own accommodation. In other cases, the individual may be living within the immediate family; for example, a child with autism. In other cases, the individual may be living with just part of the family; for example, a child of estranged parents who lives with one parent.

Family do play a major role in many people's lives and should often be considered as part of care planning and support. Family can be a huge part of a person's identity (I am a brother, daughter, mother); these identities can matter a great deal to a person's wellbeing and sense of worth.

Family can often know the person in a different way to other people; they may have spent more time with that person than anyone else or cared for them at some point. Family input can be invaluable.

For other individuals, their friends may also play a huge role in their lives, and their friends may know more about their wishes and preferences than their family.

We ideally want a team around the person, with the individual at the centre helping the team to create plans and environments to maximise their wellbeing.

Sometimes, other people who want to have an input into an individual's life can seem to be challenging and part of the problem rather than part of the solution. Often, although the best interests of the individual are intended by everyone, the steps being taken to meet those best interests can be seen as wrong by some. Encouraging an inclusive role in the person's life, empathising with various views and promoting positive engagement can have a significant positive impact on an individual's support.

Communication is key.

Many of the principles in this book can help us to understand behaviours we find challenging from anyone we encounter in life, not only those we care for.

RESPONSIBILITIES, MEANINGFUL ACTIVITIES

We are often valued by what we bring to our own lives, to others' lives and to the environments we encounter.

Many of us take our independence for granted and may even complain about it from time to time; we all love a break from cooking, but how proud we feel that we can cook and feed ourselves and others. Our ability to help others, help ourselves and help our environment are a huge source of identity, self-esteem and sense of worth.

There are some individuals who have lost skills, struggle to learn new skills or have never seen the value in having such skills. For them, we need to provide opportunities to experience these feelings of pride and joy that come from helping themselves, helping others and feeling valued. It may be making someone else smile/laugh, making their own food, putting on their own socks, cleaning a communal space. Contributions and activities do not need to be big – just meaningful to the individual.

We want to encourage individuals to be active participants in their own lives rather than passive observers of it.

CASE STUDY 3.4 THE CRUISE SHIP FALLACY

People love a holiday – getting away from it all, no responsibilities, no alarm clock, all about the fun. For many people that is wonderful for a few weeks, but after a time many are feeling the itch to get back to some routine, meaning, worth and contribution.

Many care homes, particularly for the elderly, are set up like a cruise ship holiday... it's all about the fun.

'We have a singer on Monday, bingo on Tuesday, arts and crafts on Wednesday...' But these activities can be passive and, although enjoyable, potentially meaningless.

How much better would it be if the individuals could contribute – for example, by being asked nicely to distribute bingo cards and pencils and to tidy up afterwards – and be thanked for their help?

Chapters 4, 5 and 6 describe additional factors that contribute to a positive environment.

SUMMARY

The creation of a positive environment will bring the following outcomes.

- Happy caregivers make for happy individuals.
- Happy individuals make for happy caregivers.

CHAPTER 4

PERSON-CENTRED APPROACH

The basis of the person-centred approach is that an individual should be at the centre of their own care or support and be treated, first and foremost, as a person. The focus of the environment should be on the *individual* and on what they *can do*, not their condition, disability or challenges. Support should focus on the individual's aspirations, skills and abilities and be adapted to their unique needs and circumstances. Implementing a person-centred approach is vital to a positive environment.

Collaboration with the individual and maintaining their autonomy are key in supporting behavioural change. It should be standard practice to include the individual in this process.

However, age or incapacity may make it impossible or inappropriate to collaboratively work with the individual to have full control and autonomy over their own care and outcomes. In such cases we must justify that exceptional decision, seek consent and be as transparent as appropriate with individuals (or their advocates) about their care and behavioural support plans.

Many caregivers enter care with a concept of the 'caring hand'. This hand will support, care, promote wellbeing, independence and quality of life for the individuals they support... but then the caregiver tries to push that caring hand onto the individual, stating, 'Be cared for.' If someone tries to push something onto you, the instinct is to push back, not just accept it. This can soon become a pushing battle between the caregiver and the individual. It's easy to get caught in this trap, but we sometimes need to learn to relax the 'caring hand', stop pushing and focus on understanding the *person*. What seems right to the caregiver may not feel right for the individual.

We all have beliefs, values and attitudes that shape how we feel about what is right, wrong, good, bad and best. These views will be explored further in Chapter 5, page 34, but these views can sometimes cause us to focus on how the person needs looking after, protecting or changing – according to *our* beliefs rather than as an individual with their own values, beliefs and attitudes.

General values have changed over the years. For example, it was once believed that left-handed people had to be taught right-handedness, and so left-handed children were forced to write with their right hand and were punished if they didn't.

Nowadays this seems barbaric.

But it needed a big change of mindset to bring about a more understanding approach.

Could it be that in the present day there are built-in prejudices that affect the way we treat individuals?

If we were asked the following questions, how might we answer?

- How often should a person bath or shower?
- Should a person say please and thank you?
- Should we go to school as children?
- Should you look at someone when they are talking to you?
- Should you respect your elders?

The answers indicate our beliefs, values and opinions... not laws that everyone must follow.

Take bathing routines as an example. In general, most people will feel comfortable having at least one bath/shower each day, but this regime may not be desired by all. So, provided that irregular bathing doesn't cause societal issues such as body odour or skin integrity issues, why force an individual into daily bathing if it doesn't suit them?

Another example is eye contact. In the west, we are used to having eye contact with others as a sign of respect. But in some cultures, having eye contact with a superior, or any authority figure, would be considered insulting.

Changes in views over the last ten years have really moved the emphasis:

- away from other people deciding how an individual should be looked after
- to putting the person at the centre of their own care.

For example, encouraging children to have autonomy over their own lives or ensuring a person is consulted about their own care plan. It has been proven that these person-centred inclusions can reduce instances of aggression and behaviours that challenge by 60%.[2]

A person-centred approach isn't simply about giving choices – brown bread or white – because it may be that none of the choices are suitable for the individual; a person-centred approach is a holistic approach to find out how a person would like to live. This includes their physical, mental, emotional, spiritual and social wellbeing. For example, a person's ethnicity or religious background may need to be explored and understood when creating a person-centred environment. A Catholic individual in care may want to attend Mass on a Sunday, but if the option to do this is not facilitated, wellbeing may be affected; a non-religious person may find this difficult to understand.

'Maslow's Hierarchy of Needs'[3] and 'Kitwood's Flower'[4] state that a person's needs begin with the necessities for life – food, shelter and so on – but once these are in place, higher aspects need satisfying; for example, relationships and being meaningfully occupied. There is a danger that caregivers focus too much on the basic needs of the individual and accidently neglect the emotional and spiritual needs, which should be considered just as important to a good quality of life.

A person-centred approach promotes individuality. We express our individuality through our preferences, language, clothes and environment. For example, allowing an individual's bedroom to reflect their self-identity can be so important. We all tend to value individuality until it conflicts with our own values, so a child in care who has come from a neglectful upbringing may feel more comfortable in an untidy space but be perceived as lazy or dirty. Forcing the child to be tidy in the *one* place they can call their own can be detrimental to the child's feeling of acceptance and safety. Over time through role modelling and working to improve the child's self-esteem and confidence, tidiness may naturally result.

Maslow's Hierarchy of Needs is discussed in more depth later in Chapter 8, page 83.

To summarise, a person-centred approach will include:

- considering people's preferences and chosen needs
- ensuring people are physically comfortable and safe
- where possible, emotional support involving family and friends
- ensuring people have all the information necessary for them to contribute to decisions about their care and support.

CHAPTER 5

ENVIRONMENTAL CULTURE

Another element that affects the care environment is the culture within the setting. 'Culture' can be defined as: a set of shared values, ideas, beliefs and etiquette belonging to an institution or group.

Or, in simple terms, 'The way we do things around here.'

Most people are associated with more than one group, and the cultures of those groups can differ significantly in their behaviours.

'The way we do things around here' is a statement of fact; it's neither right nor wrong. However, just because a group has always done things in a certain way doesn't automatically make it right (tradition does not equal morality). And 'the way we do things around here' can change. For example, in the care industry, the concept of a person-centred approach has developed significantly. The Victorian approach to childcare (strict, almost barbaric discipline) differs massively from today's approach.

In the same way that technology progresses, so does our understanding of human behaviour and wellbeing. However, there is often a resistance to change. For example:

- 'I was raised like that and it didn't do me any harm.' How do we know... what's the comparable data? You might have ended up 'better off' if you'd been raised differently.
- 'I have 30 years' experience in the care industry.' Or is that one year's experience repeated 30 times?

HOW INDIVIDUALS AFFECT CULTURE

What we *see* in an individual is how they behave.

What we don't see are the *underlying reasons* for how they behave.

What we see is the tip of the iceberg. What's important for us to understand is the remaining 90%.

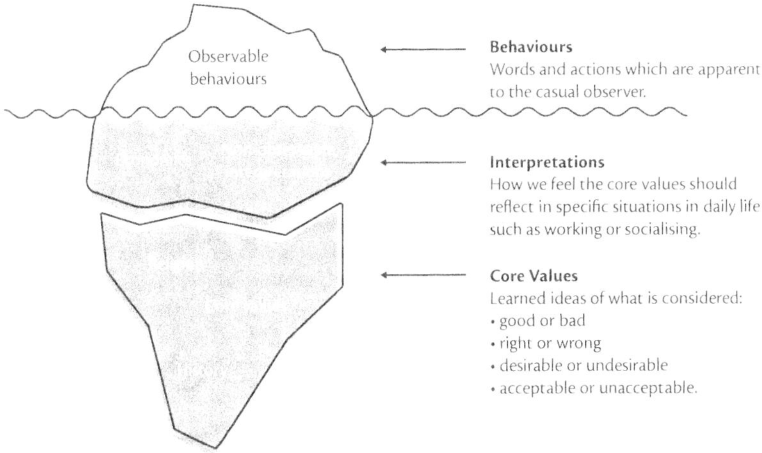

Figure 5.1 The 'Iceberg' Model of Organisational Culture

SOURCE: BASED ON A CONCEPTUALISATION BY SACKMANN (1991)[5]

Individual biases, values and attitudes influence the culture of an organisation; these factors affect how management and caregivers feel about how people should/shouldn't behave and the rules they follow. But the culture is also influenced by the individuals themselves.

One of the things this book tries to encourage is getting people to explore their own '90%' and how it affects their own views, attitudes and prejudices towards behaviour. For example, as mentioned earlier, is swearing necessarily a bad behaviour, or is our response based on our own '90%'?

Further, as will be explored later in the book, good people can do bad things and vice versa. So, although it's easy to judge a person based on their *behaviour*, that doesn't necessarily lead to a correct judgement about the *person*. Instead, a curiosity should develop about why the behaviour happens and what benefit it brings for the individual.

Rather than judging a single action or multiple actions of a person within one context or situation and feeling we can now define who that person is as a result, we aim to understand *why* a person may behave this way in this situation.

There is strong evidence that having judgemental attitudes and behaviours towards others has three undesirable effects:

- A negative impact on the person being judged by reinforcing their core beliefs about themselves or feeding into prejudices that others may have of them.
- A negative impact on the person making the judgement, as it increases the likelihood of self-criticism.
- When we focus on a person's flaws, we draw attention to them and

increase the likelihood of other people noticing them too. This can perpetuate the negative view of that person.

CASE STUDY 5.1 THE MEAL

A group of people go for a meal at a pub. The food and service are okay – not five-star but mediocre. Most of the group are fairly happy with the experience.

One of the group however isn't happy and starts to complain to the rest. The service was slow, they got your order wrong, my chicken was dry and the vegetables were soggy. On each complaint other members of the group are invited to criticise the meal and flaws are pointed out. By the end of this conversation, everyone in the group is now agreeing that the meal and service were terrible and they will never be going there again.

Commentary: It is easy to catch the negative and judge. One bad meal doesn't mean a restaurant is bad – it may mean they just had one bad night, but by focusing on the negative and directing judgement we may condemn and decide that they can never be better.

Whereas acting in an empathic and forgiving way towards others can promote their and our wellbeing. It can allow us to be self-forgiving and empathic towards ourselves when we make mistakes or behave in ways that feel wrong for our values.

Unfortunately, there are many examples in society where shame is used to reprimand behaviour and is considered appropriate. Examples include media reports and public attitudes towards crime, the labels about bad teenagers and knife crime, etc.

CASE STUDY 5.2 THE GOOD, THE BAD AND THE UGLY

Jessica (the good): Jessica is a well-liked girl who is doing well at school. She is often praised by her parents and teachers, directly and indirectly. Often this is done publicly, as the adults want to encourage other children to be more like Jessica.

'You look lovely today Jessica, you are a pretty little girl.' 'Well done Jessica, you are so smart.' 'Great work Jessica, you are such a good drawer.'

At first glance, these praises may seem like a good thing, but the issue is that Jessica is being praised for fixed ideas. Jessica is pretty, smart and talented. How might this feel to others?... 'I'm not pretty, smart or talented like Jessica as I don't get told I am, so I must be less.' Also, if Jessica *the person* is labelled 'smart' to explain why she does well... how will Jessica feel when she doesn't do well at something? Dumb, stupid? Failure is inevitable, but by praising Jessica herself rather than the process, a failure in outcomes can become a failure of self rather than indicating that more effort may have been required.

Praising Jessica for working hard, trying, making an effort – for the process rather than who she is or her outcomes – would promote growth ideas. 'If I work hard I can get praise like Jessica.' And if Jessica doesn't do well on something, she will know that maybe she didn't work hard enough on this occasion.

Billy (the bad): Billy is being described by a teacher: 'I am very concerned about Billy. He is disruptive in class, he doesn't listen or focus on his work. He is rude, he lies. I know he is smart as he can remember all sorts of information about Pokémon but try and get him to do any maths and he's just lazy.'

The teacher is hyperfocused on Billy's behaviour that challenges, and you can hear the undertone of 'always' in the description. For sure, this teacher is finding Billy's behaviour really challenging and that must be so hard to manage, but the labelling of Billy as a bad kid is not far away. And if Billy is just bad, how can anything he does ever be good?

Richard (the ugly): Richard was messing around with a ball in the house and lost control. It knocked an ornament which smashed on the floor. Richard heard the shout from the other room and the footsteps coming closer.

'What the hell was that?! That better not be you, Richie. I am fed up with this. You are a selfish little boy. I have told you a thousand times about a ball in the house. If you don't care about my stuff, then you shouldn't be allowed stuff of your own. There will be no more Xbox for you – if you can't stop being selfish, then no more nice things.'

The anger of the caregiver may be understandable, and the frustration of a repeated behaviour can get to us all. The narrative, however, is shame: you are not good enough, which is why you must be punished.

Later in the book, we will explore why shaming may be detrimental to improving outcomes and individuals' behaviour and how even the way we praise can impact on someone's self-identity and success (see 'Praise – a Secondary Reinforcer!', Chapter 25, page 233).

Mistakes are an important part of life; we can acknowledge them, learn from them and improve our skills and knowledge to avoid repetition. Such an approach should promote better outcomes than condemning a person or behaviour irreparably.

SHIFTING PERSPECTIVE

One way to increase our human connection and understanding is to shift to an opposite standpoint.

Often you may hear questions like – why are they so lazy? Why are they so violent? Why do people take drugs? Why are people greedy?

It can be interesting to take the opposite standpoint and ask the question in reverse.

Why are some people not lazy, as surely that would seem like the easier default position?

Humans are very good at finding the path of least resistance to meet a need. Many of us look forward to time off, we dream of holidays, we complain about work; so is laziness the reward? If we could always be lazy, would we take it? Or would we, if we'd had the chance to experience the joys of successes, achievements, independence, and even self-reliance, recognise that we prefer activity to laziness? But if we'd been role modelled laziness, only ever known it or didn't get pleasure from the opposites, why wouldn't we be lazy? Laziness is inevitable if we haven't discovered the right motivator.

Why are some people not violent? If we were bigger, stronger and more physically dominant than others, couldn't violence allow us to take more than our share? And be more advantageous to us? But most humans seem to have moved away from violence, as in most areas of society it doesn't earn the greatest rewards. But what if a person has been raised in environments or cultures where the 'survival of the fittest' is still rewarded?

Why isn't everyone addicted to drugs? See 'Case Study 5.3 The Rat Park Studies' below.

Humans are complicated animals. We have in most situations learned to manage our behaviours past our primal urges and innate responses to allow us to work together in society more harmoniously. Unfortunately, some people, due to circumstances, role models or cultural factors, may have the habits of what are perceived as negative behaviours; they may see them as the norm and as needed. This does not make such people bad, just different in their view and experience of the world. If certain behaviours are better for society or for their individual outcomes, we may need to educate and encourage a change in habits.

If we start from the position that the exceptions in society (the lazy, the aggressive, the drug addict, etc.) are the default positions that stem from innate, biological motivators, we can then explore the behaviour from an alternative perspective. We can ask why and how do most people go against their basic biology to engage in what society sees as positive rather than negative behaviour. We can then explore which of these reasons are things that the 'lazy/aggressive/drug addict' *do not* have or are unable to connect with... and then can we help.

CASE STUDY 5.3 THE RAT PARK STUDIES[6]

Original studies performed on rats found that, in tests to measure the nature of addiction, rats would choose stimulant drugs over food. This was used to demonstrate that drugs are incredibly powerful stimulants that can hijack even innate survival mechanisms. So why aren't we all addicted to drugs?

The original experiments were performed on rats who were kept in isolated, low-stimulus cages.

These experiments were later repeated but with rats kept in highly stimulating, enriched environments with other rats. The results showed that the environment significantly reduced the likelihood of the rats taking the drug over the food.

Commentary: A better environment for the rats decreased the maladaptive behaviour. The rats were getting their pleasure from the socially and environmentally stimulating setting rather than needing to gain the pleasure from a drug. So why aren't we all addicted to drugs? Because many of us find satisfaction, connection and pleasure from our surroundings, connections and achievements. But what would happen if we couldn't do this, due to circumstances, mental health or poor social support and dynamics?

> *It's easy to judge. It's more difficult to understand. Understanding requires compassion, patience, and a willingness to believe that good hearts sometimes choose poor methods. Through judging, we separate. Through understanding, we grow.*
>
> DOE ZANTAMATA

The views and attitudes of the caregivers will also be directly affected by the behaviour of the individuals and vice versa.

A staff team that is critical, aggressive and bullying will have a knock-on effect on the behaviour of the individuals.

CASE STUDY 5.4 KEV'S STORY

This is a paraphrasing of Kev's words from an interview about his childhood. Kev was raised in care.

I was in care from the mid 80s to the mid 90s, from about the age of 8 to 18. In that time I was in two different care homes and one boarding school. In all of those places I was restrained several times. Sometimes for fighting, but other times for almost nothing, like not doing what you were told. We'd all be restrained at some time or other.

It was restraint to intimidate, to control; to cause pain but without making it look like pain. You had no say.

Within a couple of days of entering the children's home I was restrained. I wasn't a violent person at that time, but by the time I'd left care I'd already been arrested for assault like three times. But before then, nothing.

I had been thrown into a situation where restraint and fighting were a way of life from day to day. I'd wake up thinking, 'Today, I'm either gonna have a fight with someone whether I want to or not, or I'm going to get restrained for not doing something that they want me to do.'

I reckon it influenced every kid there – to become more aggressive because

> of the aggressive nature of the life. There were kids that came in that were timid and soft. And by the time they left, they were more aggressive, more violent. Some went to prison. Some ended up dead. I wouldn't say it was all caused by the restraint. But being bullied by the staff – because you *were* bullied even if it didn't come across as bullying – also being bullied by the other children... that were also bullied by the staff. So it is a trickle-down system.

Commentary: This is only part of this case study. It will reappear as 'Case Study 34.6 Kev's Story – the Sequel', page 326.

It's often the case that individuals who get labelled as 'difficult' or 'challenging' create a culture around themselves, possibly of fear or intimidation. This can sometimes be intentional to assert control (not through any malignant motive but simply as a survival mechanism) or it can feed into the stigma around them, a self-fulfilling prophecy.

CASE STUDY 5.5 THE MISUNDERSTOOD

Adam had a distinct reputation of being 'extremely challenging' due to his physicality, demeanour and unpredictability. He created a culture around himself that was not in his best interests but may not have been understood by him in that way. Adam weighed 23 stone (150 kilograms) and had bipolar disorder, autism and other learning disabilities.

He would get very aggressive and, when distressed, would attack staff physically. Some of the staff found him extremely intimidating, to the point that some admitted hiding from him due to their fear.

If you saw people hiding from you, it may significantly impact your self-esteem negatively or it may reinforce the feelings of control despite the feelings of rejection.

This is a negative culture for both caregivers and Adam to be in. The setting was reaction-led by his behaviour.

When a new person enters a setting, they will have an influence on the culture through their behaviour and opinions. For example, one person who doesn't follow the rules, if not managed, will potentially influence others to break the same rules. However, in turn, their own views and behaviours will also be influenced by the existing culture. This is known as 'social conditioning'.

CASE STUDY 5.6 THE SOCIAL CONFORMITY WAITING ROOM*

An experiment was carried out where a waiting room was populated by actors and one member of the public (the subject) who didn't know the others were actors. From time to time a buzzer would sound, and each time the buzzer sounded all the actors stood up for a moment or two.

---

* Conducted by Brian Games on *National Geographic*.

After three times, the unsuspecting subject also stood when the buzzer next sounded, even though she had no idea of what was going on.

At intervals, an actor was withdrawn from the group, with the buzzer/standing activity continuing. Eventually only the subject remained – who continued to stand whenever the buzzer sounded.

Then, one by one, other members of the public were introduced into the room, and, without knowing why, they followed the lead of the first person and began to stand on hearing the buzzer.

The lesson: the power of peer pressure and social conditioning.

Social conditioning can be a power for good (discussed later as one of the most powerful and appropriate strategies for improved behavioural outcomes; see 'Teaching Technique: Role Modelling', Chapter 25, page 225). If all concerned have a positive outlook, are focusing on individuals' needs and so on, then the newcomer will adopt these habits. Yes, it is possible that one bad apple can spoil the barrel, but if the group is resilient that can be overcome.

REASONS WHY PEOPLE DON'T STOP NEGATIVE CULTURES DEVELOPING

Pluralistic Ignorance

Take a situation where a caregiver witnesses other staff behaving towards an individual in a way that feels inappropriate to some degree and is thinking, 'This doesn't feel right, but nobody else seems to be saying it's wrong, so maybe I'm wrong.' If other caregivers are thinking the same thing about this treatment but nothing is said, improvements are not made. This is known as 'pluralistic ignorance' and can act as a powerful barrier to progress.

Obedience to Authority

This is where individuals will continue to act against their better judgement if an authority figure says it's okay to do so.

CASE STUDY 5.7 THE MILGRAM EXPERIMENT[7]

This experiment began in 1961. An actor responded to fake electric shocks delivered by a volunteer who was told by an authority figure to progressively increase the level of shock. Most volunteers complied, even though it was clear that they were inflicting serious, perhaps fatal, harm to the 'victim', as long as an authority figure (a person in a white coat) told them they should.

Fixed Roles

People can fall into a pattern of conforming to a perceived role and learn to 'know their place' in the scheme of things. 'I am a manager', 'I am a subordinate'

– and behaviour mirrors that belief. In 'Case Study 5.5 The Misunderstood', had the bully/difficult person become a role for Adam to play?

CASE STUDY 5.8 THE STANFORD PRISON EXPERIMENT[8]

This experiment was carried out in 1971. Volunteer male students were assigned roles of prisoners and guards. Within a few days, the 'prisoners' were being severely abused by the 'guards'. After just 6 days of a planned 14, the experiment was abandoned.

Both the prisoners and the guards appeared to take on their respective roles and behaved as either dominant authorities that must be obeyed and would punish to dominate or subordinate/defiant prisoners who must create chaos and act to resist authority.

A Blame Culture

When things go wrong and caregivers lay blame on each other, criticising each other (potentially in public), it creates a culture of shame and a lack of solution focus. Blaming creates shame, and shame discourages reflection and limits the ability to understand why something went wrong. In turn, this blocks attempts to find a better way through solutions based on a positive approach.

If authority figures are doing this to caregivers, and caregivers are doing this to each other, then, based on the social conditioning principle, what will the result be for the individuals being supported?

CASE STUDY 5.9 IF...

If a person doesn't know how to read, we teach.

If a person doesn't know how to swim, we teach.

If a person doesn't know how to multiply, we teach.

If a person doesn't know how to drive, we teach.

If a person doesn't know how to behave, we... blame? Shame? Punish?

Why can't we finish the last sentence as automatically as the others?

Commentary: The answer is always to teach. With young children, this is often the natural philosophy. We don't punish a child for using their nappy, we teach them to use the toilet. It is only as we change our expectations – 'Well, you should know how to behave by now' – that we begin to feel that punishment is the right answer. The more we understand about the human condition, the more we understand that every person's ability to learn and their methods of learning, cognitive skills and emotional regulation are different. So we must adapt our teaching, improve our methods and person-focus our strategies to teach rather than punish.

HOW LANGUAGE CAN AFFECT CULTURE

The language used in any organisation can affect the culture in a big way.

Here are some examples:

Labelling a Person by Their Behaviour

For example, challenging, difficult, lazy, awkward, a nightmare. If a new caregiver is assigned to work with a particular individual, and a colleague says, 'Ha! Good luck! Right nightmare. Don't turn your back on him...', the new staff member could easily instantly adopt a negative attitude towards the individual and add to the negativity of the culture.

But suppose the new caregiver responds with 'Well, thanks for looking out for me... Now, can you tell me what he's good at, what he likes, what's his favourite subject?'

This response is based on the probability that the individual doesn't display behaviours that challenge for 100% of the time to 100% of people, but caregivers sometimes only see the negative. By asking about the person's skills and abilities, we can shift the focus and allow caregivers to reflect on the individual's positive attributes and that they are more than their labels.

CASE STUDY 5.10 THE OVERHEARD PHONE CALL

The following is an account from a mature adult, Tom, about an incident in his youth.

'I always remember, when I was 14/15 years old, overhearing my mum describing me as lazy when she was on the phone to someone. I felt that was a character assassination, I felt it was disregarding every bit of hard work I'd ever done – because she was just labelling me as lazy.

'I also had bad depression at the time, so if I didn't have a reason to get out of bed, I thought, "What's the point?"

'In hindsight, I get it. Because during the summer holidays, when I finally emerged from my pit about midday, I probably did very little, so I get her point of view.'

Commentary: By simply labelling Tom's behaviour as 'lazy', Tom's mum limited her understanding. There are things we know that she didn't. Often, during the summer, we find we're more energetic than in the depths of winter. That's because when it goes dark, our body releases a hormone called melatonin; it regulates our sleep cycle. But during adolescence that melatonin can be delayed in its release, by three to four hours. So if it doesn't get dark till 10 or 11pm, a teenager is not going to start feeling tired until 2 or 3am. But teenagers need more sleep – typically up to ten hours or more for full brain regeneration – than the seven to eight-and-a-half that most of us can cope with.

Unfortunately, by using the convenient label 'lazy teenager', Tom's mum was limiting her ability to understand Tom's behaviour, to relate to him and see how unhappy he was.

Derogatory Language

For example, 'He was kicking off earlier.' Immediately the assumption is that the individual was consciously choosing to behave that way. Instead of using the stigmatising 'kicking off', maybe 'he was in meltdown', 'he was overwhelmed', 'he couldn't cope', 'he was emotionally distressed' could be used – these terms recognise that the individual was struggling and that the behaviour wasn't just challenging for others, but also for the individual. Further, a nondescript 'kicking off' doesn't help to explain what was happening – maybe the individual was feeling crowded at the time, or not allowed to do something, or his favourite cereal had run out. Or did he run to his room, lock the door and put his music on at full volume? All much more descriptive than 'kicking off' and giving clues as to the cause and function of the behaviour.

'Attention-Seeking'

Well, what's wrong with someone who wants some attention? All human beings need 'attention' in the sense of attachment or connection. If someone is 'attention-seeking', the tendency is to ignore them rather than teaching them appropriate ways of gaining attention. If we understand human connection as being as vital as food, we can see that if someone were hungry, we wouldn't ever consider letting them starve.

The following case study is given here as food for thought.

CASE STUDY 5.11 NEGATIVE THOUGHTS AND LANGUAGE

Look at the following sums that 21-year-old Ben just attempted:

1. 1 + 1 = 2
2. 1 + 2 = 3
3. 1 + 3 = 5
4. 1 + 4 = 5
5. 1 + 5 = 6

What is your reaction?

Most people will state, 'Ben, number three is wrong.'

Few would say, 'Great, Ben! You got four out of five right!'

We are drawn towards the negative, instinctively.

If we see a bowl full of our favourite chocolates, but there's a cockroach sitting on top, the cockroach is definitely in the minority but puts us off the chocolates. The small negative overwhelms the much larger positive.

If we see a bowl full of cockroaches with one of our favourite chocolates on top – the chocolate is in the minority, but despite viewing it positively, the small positive isn't sufficient to overcome the negative.

Negative easily outdoes the positive.

We do this same thing with people all the time too. We notice their flaws, imperfections and deficits far more easily than their attributes and positives.

We want to catch people behaving well, not catch them behaving badly. Catching them behaving badly requires little effort and is easy.

If you have a manager, do you prefer one who recognises your good work with praise and thanks, or one who's quiet until you make a mistake, whereupon criticism is forthcoming?

Human nature dictates that we are drawn to the negative, we focus on it.

We are more likely to make the effort to give a bad review than a good one for a restaurant; we are also more likely to read the bad one.

It's easy to catch people behaving badly... it's a potentially lazy way to manage an environment. Catching people behaving badly gives them attention, and for them, *any* attention may be more rewarding than no attention and simply perpetuates the problem. We need to shift our attention to catching people being good! We need to become 'good managers' of the people we support and care for.

We want to create a culture where adaptive (good) behaviour is more rewarding than maladaptive (bad) behaviour.

This principle informs all stages of the strategy triangle, but working to change the everyday practice of caregivers to be positively focused gives a solid foundation to everything else we do. You will notice this positive theme repeated throughout the book.

Note: As an alternative, let's say we did the Ben case study again but with a difference.

CASE STUDY 5.12 BEN'S ARITHMETIC (PAGE 44) – REVISITED

Look at the following sums that Ben just attempted:

1. $465 \times 231 = 107{,}415$
2. $\sqrt{565} = 23.769728648$
3. $732 \times 3555 = 2{,}602{,}262$
4. $357 \div 45 = 7.93333333333$
5. $8999 \times 9888 = 88{,}982{,}112$

If Ben did these sums in his head and we were to check his work and notice that he only got number three wrong but it was only two away from the correct answer, would our instinct be different to when it was '1 +' sums? We would probably be far more likely to notice the positive and congratulate Ben. So what has changed?

It is our expectations that have now changed. We would expect a 21-year-old to be able to get 1 + 1 level questions right.

This is one thing that affects the attitude of a good and bad manager. A bad manager has expectations that you should get things right, just because it's your job. A good manager still recognises that being appreciated and valued for doing that job increases the likelihood of positive outcomes. A bad manager assumes that you will just know what to do and how to do it. A good manager recognises that we all have strengths and weaknesses and that we should build on the strengths and find ways to teach or adapt to any weaknesses.

CHAPTER 6

BEHAVIOUR MANAGEMENT OLD LOGIC: PUNISH/REWARD

Special terms used in this chapter:

'Operant conditioning': The simplified concept is that a behaviour that is linked to a pleasant consequence is likely to be repeated; a behaviour that is linked to an unpleasant consequence is less likely to be repeated.

'Reinforcer': This is described fully in 'Reinforcers', Chapter 25, page 228. In brief: a reinforcer is any stimulus (tangible or intangible) that whether provided or removed increases the likelihood of a behaviour occurring.

Function, purpose: These terms are used interchangeably to refer to conscious or unconscious aims of a behaviour.

Without specific training, most people's strategies for behaviour management come from learned parenting methods – how they were raised or how they raised their children.

Generally, many people tend to have been raised with what is called 'punishment/reward parenting': if the child does something good, there's some sort of reward; if the child does something bad, there's a consequence.

This strategy can work well to adjust behaviour and is used by many parents as their primary method of behaviour management.

It also mirrors how society tends to see appropriate behaviour management. Based on basic principles of behaviourism, rewarded behaviours will be repeated, while punished or non-reinforced behaviour will be extinguished. This is called the Law of Effect[9] that operant conditioning demonstrates. Animals tend to move towards pleasure and away from pain.

However, this strategy has its issues, as humans appear to be far more complex in our behaviour. Those who hold to the behaviourist theory recognise this complexity but often don't address it. Our concepts of self, our ability to analyse the past and look into the future, our emotional reactions and responses – these are affected by, and affect the way we respond to, environmental stimulus. We do respond to conditioning in a semi-typical fashion; however, our biology, psychology and previous experiences make reactions far less predictable.

In behaviourist experiments[10] where a pigeon was being rewarded or punished based on its actions, it is doubtful that a pigeon suffered an existential crisis about the meaning of its actions or reflected on whether the scientists watching liked or disliked him or whether the consequences occurring meant that he was a good or bad pigeon. But humans often do exactly these things. Behaviourist conditioning often doesn't consider an individual's psychological outcomes. Other animals don't appear to feel shame as humans do or reflect on consequences in the same way. So although the old logic can work to alter behaviour, it can actually neglect human emotional needs.

For example, if a child makes a mistake and receives a negative consequence, it may inhibit that behaviour being repeated but it might lead to feelings of lack of acceptance. 'If I'm not perfect I must be bad.' This kind of core belief can then be detrimental to mental wellbeing in later life.

Old-logic behaviour management of people actually varies in a number of ways from the operant-conditioning strategies used to train other animals such as dogs.

First, a reward is only a reward if it creates pleasure, and a punishment only works if it creates displeasure. Humans can have quite complex concepts of pleasure and pain; one person's pain is another person's pleasure. People can also be defiant, vengeful, spiteful and envious, emotions that are not typically seen in other animals but can hugely affect our acceptance of old-logic management. We have all heard the phrase 'cut my nose off to spite my face'.

Second, the way rewards/punishments are presented is often different. When training a dog, if we were to command 'sit' and then offer the dog a treat an hour later, we know this would prove ineffective in teaching this skill. If the dog chewed your furniture and you shut it outside to punish it, the dog is unlikely to be reflecting on the action that triggered this consequence after an hour outside.

Humans are often able to make connections from delayed rewards or punishment in a different way. We are often able to delay gratification or even experience pain to achieve a delayed pleasure. For example, no other animal would ever willingly get a tattoo – it's a painful process for an outcome that is less obvious in its reward.

For a reward or punishment to be effective, the individual concerned must be able to make a connection between the behaviour and the reward/punishment and then regulate their behaviour based on this connection and their desire to gain or avoid future experiences of that pleasure or pain. The ability to make connections between behaviour and consequences varies from person to person and can be affected by a person's cognitive abilities, memory and emotional/psychological state at the time of either the behaviour or the presentation of the consequence, as we will explore.

Third, there is a concept called learned helplessness. It appears that most animals and people, if they experience repeated situations where their actions seem to have no impact on their outcomes, develop an ingrained assumption that their actions are irrelevant. Author Geoff Thompson uses the analogy of an elephant and a twig.[11] In India, young elephants are trained by being tied to an immovable object like a tree. No matter how hard the baby elephant pulls, it cannot escape. Over time it accepts that it cannot escape, no matter what it does. These young elephants become fully grown adults weighing several tons; they can be tied to a twig and don't even try to escape. So a child who always seems to get things wrong or for whom life is always hard no matter what they do (due to their abilities or the behaviour of caregivers) may completely give up on ever trying to get it right. They may be happy because they develop the belief that their actions make no difference; this belief will often be pervasive throughout their life.

If an individual doesn't learn as we feel a typical person should – due to their experiences, developmental difficulties, insecure attachments or mental health disorders – then old-logic strategies can cause significant distress, reduction in self-esteem, reduced quality of life and relationship damage.

SO, WHY DOES THE TYPICAL 'PUNISH/ REWARD PARENTING' SOMETIMES WORK?

A newborn baby cries because it is hungry, in discomfort, is startled by a loud noise. The caregiver quickly attends, the baby's needs are met, distress is soothed and the baby feels good. The baby feels omnipotent, godlike, all powerful, and begins to develop a model of the world where they are really important in this world, they matter, they must be good and there are other beings that seem good too: 'I cry, someone comes, keeps me safe and meets my needs (maybe they are worth emotionally attaching to).'

Later in development, because of parental judgement or the practicalities of other children, changes in feeding methods, etc., the response of a caregiver is not as immediate but hopefully it is still consistent. The baby's needs are still met, but the lack of omnipotence is realised – maybe they are not a god. However, their model of the world, and their role within it, is still that they really matter in this world, they are good, they sometimes get attention and love even when they don't ask for it and so their sense of worth builds. This slight delay before their needs are met also helps them to realise that they don't die without having their needs met immediately. This helps them build resilience and be able to cope with emotions; and emotions are good because they draw people towards you. The initial model the baby formed – 'I cry, caregiver comes' – is modified. 'I'm not omnipotent but I still matter, I still have value, my emotions are still good and they draw these trustworthy beings towards me.'

This is what is usually classed as developing secure attachment.

At toddler stage, caregivers start to create boundaries and expectations of how the child should and shouldn't act. Sometimes the child will do something the caregiver disapproves of, and the caregiver communicates this through displeasure or punishment. As a result, the child experiences negative feelings, like guilt: 'I am good but I did something bad.' But despite these negative feelings, the previous experiences of love, unconditional acceptance, met needs and trust allow the child to overcome these negative experiences and typically aim to return to behaviours that stimulate positive reactions and results.

'Good' behaviour is being conditioned as the child moves towards the pleasure that good behaviour brings and moves away from displeasure that unwanted behaviour brings. So the law 'Rewarded behaviour will be repeated' is enacted for as long as there are still opportunities to receive the positive and reattach with trusted persons.

WHAT CAN GO WRONG?

Shame

Suppose the baby/child never consistently experienced the good feelings of having its needs met or unconditional love – perhaps due to neglect, abuse, the caregiver's incapacity, the child's hospitalisation and so on. The child develops a different world model: they don't feel worthwhile, they don't matter, they aren't loved. Maybe the child believes, 'I am bad, nobody cares, I'm of low worth, my emotions are bad.' Only negative.

Or maybe everything in the child's development started well. But then the child began having difficulties in maintaining expected good behaviour, perhaps because of increased caregiver expectations or a condition that affected their development resulting in lots of 'mistakes'. The negative reactions become the normal and the positive beliefs slowly disappear. Kierston Wareing, an actress with lived experience of physical abuse, said, 'If someone tells you often enough you're worthless, you start to believe it.'[12]

Unfortunately, this can mean that if, during their development, the individual does something 'wrong' and doesn't meet behavioural expectations and the caregiver shows disapproval – there may be no positivity in their background to be drawn to. There may be no sense that changing behaviour can lead to something positive, because they don't know what 'positive' is or what it feels like, or they don't believe that they deserve it or know how to get it. The resulting reaction is likely to be an internalised sensation of shame.

Brené Brown studies vulnerability, courage and shame and is a researcher-storyteller and author who described shame in this way in her TED Talk (Listening to Shame):

> Guilt is: 'I am good, but I did something bad.'
> Shame is: 'I am bad.'[13]

Shame doesn't allow for reflection or improvement. Self-esteem is needed to recognise that a mistake doesn't mean 'I am useless'. But shame is painful, shame emotionally hurts, and if something hurts and yet there is no resilience to cope with the shame – 'I know there is pleasure (attachments, etc.) to go to' – an individual must find other ways to protect themselves from the emotional pain of feeling useless, bad, worthless, etc. They become hypersensitive to this shame as well, so the smallest mistake can trigger a full reaction.

These defence mechanisms are referred to as 'shame shields',[14] and they often prevent learning from old-logic conditioning – punishment/reward strategies may have limited or no effect or can actually lead to worsening behaviours and negative outcomes for all.

This topic is reviewed in more detail in 'The Shame Shield', Chapter 15, page 140.

There are other factors that may affect the impact of old-logic behaviour management that may stem from these early life experiences.

Trust

Rewards that are offered by someone we do not trust may not have the desired effect of reinforcing the behaviour, as they may trigger anxiety rather than pleasure. Punishments given by someone we do not trust can trigger defiance, so the punishment could cause reinforcement rather than inhibition. What if compliance with any request by the caregiver is seen as a 'threat to survival' by the individual? No consequence will change the outcome.

Cause-and-Effect Thinking

CASE STUDY 6.1 THE MAN AND HIS MAGAZINE

Nathan has learning difficulties and had been agitated one Thursday morning; the outcome was that he had assaulted a caregiver.

It so happened that on Thursdays Nathan received his favourite magazine.

The question is... if Nathan is still allowed to have his magazine that day, would it be seen by him as a reward for his negative behaviour? And the opposite – would *not* receiving the magazine be seen by him as a punishment, which may stop him assaulting staff in the future? Let's compare that with a different scenario.

CASE STUDY 6.2 THE DOG WITH AN UPSET TUMMY

I go to work one day, leaving my beloved dog in the house as usual. Unfortunately, during the day, something upsets my pet's tummy, and he messes on the carpet.

I return home, see the mess, and go ballistic at the dog, who cowers in the corner.

Commentary: Most people with typical nervous systems who accidentally touch something that's very hot will immediately pull their hand away. This is an immediate response to a physical situation; there is no time between cause and effect.

But suppose that the cause and effect are not immediate, and a person doesn't have the normal capability of connecting the two. Without equating human beings with animals, in the above case of the dog messing the carpet, does the dog realise that the retribution received relates to the mess he made a few hours earlier? Probably not, a dog hasn't the necessary skills to make the connection between cause and effect. Will the retribution be effective in stopping the dog doing the same thing another time? Well, no – especially as the dog couldn't help his action in the first place; it wasn't done on purpose.

So the retribution serves no purpose; it's just the assertion of dominance over a vulnerable animal, and nothing positive has been achieved.

Relating this to Nathan and his magazine: if Nathan doesn't have the ability to connect cause and effect – for example, he may have problems with memory retention, concentration, the ability to make connections – it is unlikely that he would connect his behaviour with the loss of the magazine. Also, if Nathan has limited abilities to regulate his emotions or to communicate frustrations, or if that staff member pushed Nathan's tolerance past what he can manage, it doesn't make his behaviour okay but it does mean that punishing him will not give him these skills.

So withholding his magazine would serve no useful purpose; instead, it would lead to the outcomes described in the punishment cycle (see 'Punishment', Chapter 25, page 238).

Impulse Control

Humans have amazing brains that allow us to manage and control our basic impulses. We weigh up potential outcomes from our behaviours at lightning-fast speed to behave in ways that are socially acceptable. This is an ability that we tend to take for granted.

What if your brain doesn't act as quickly to control impulses? Even though logically you know an act is unacceptable, your impulse may act more quickly than your ability to stop yourself. Numerous neurodiverse conditions can, for many people, impair and impact on the natural development of impulse control. (This will be further explored in Chapter 10, page 93.)

CASE STUDY 6.3 DON'T SNATCH

As Amber brings the cakes to the table on a plate, before the plate makes it to the table, one of the children, Armie, snatches a cake from the plate. As Amber turns to tell Armie off for snatching, she sees a look of shame in his eyes. Armie has attention deficit hyperactivity disorder (ADHD) and he is learning to better control his impulses (he's currently doing training using a new computer game system), and although he is making improvements, he sometimes still struggles. Amber realises that telling Armie off will only impact his self-esteem and won't change the outcome now or in the future, and so instead she smiles and says in a joking tone, 'Wow Armie, that arm moved like a rattlesnake striking, give everyone a chance for cake.'

This allowed Amber to remind Armie that she still felt grabbing the food wasn't appropriate (which he already knew) but Amber's action didn't attack and shame him.

What if, due to emotional dysregulation, your emotions literally hijack your logical brain? Current understanding leads us to be aware that during emotional or stimulation overload the brain can enter a survival state, which overrules rational and logical impulse control. Most of our actions day-to-day are made up of a mix of rational and emotional processing. Logic without emotion is limiting. People who have had acquired brain injury to certain emotional processing parts of their brain struggle to make choices.[15] For example, why would we choose one dish on a menu rather than another based purely on logic? Part of the decision concerns what we feel like eating.

However, when you are feeling anxious when giving your first public speech, or you see a spider, or you are asking someone you like out on a date, you can't just convince yourself logically that there is no need to feel afraid. The higher stress of the situation makes it harder to think logically. Now, if a person experiences extreme stress, or their ability to manage/regulate that stress is impaired due to cognitive abilities, those emotions may bulldoze the rational brain. This can lead to behaviours and actions that may logically make no sense. It's not because the person is bad, but they keep getting into trouble because of their emotions, no matter how hard they try, because they haven't developed the right skills to better manage them.

Let's compare the level of control some people have over their impulses when they are in a heightened emotional state (survival brain) to a medical condition such as epilepsy. (This is not to belittle the plight of someone who lives with the awful condition of epilepsy but rather to underline the plight of someone who, due to cognitive decline, brain injury, neurodiversity, mental ill health or a traumatic past, experiences emotional dysregulation.)

When a person has seizures, we recognise that they don't *choose* to have seizures (although it was once thought they did, and individuals with epilepsy were once branded as witches and punished; thank science that we now know better!) and we know that they have no control of the seizure or their actions during it.

Therefore, we would:

- never punish a person when they have a seizure
- recognise that the seizures and condition negatively impact them more than us and therefore the plan must be centred on them
- understand as much about their condition as we could
- work with them to better recognise potential triggers and create plans of how these could be reduced or managed
- create a plan of what to do, and what we would need to know and do, if a seizure occurs
- ensure a person is safe during an episode
- comfort and empathise with them after it has happened
- explore if changes need to be made to the plan to improve prevention in the future.

You will notice that these principles will be common themes running throughout this book, but they will be applied to behaviour and emotional dysregulation.

Unintended Consequences of Punishment

Punishments include any stimulus presented or removed with the aim of reducing the likelihood of a behaviour occurring. More details about punishment can be found in 'Punishment', Chapter 25, page 238. Punishments may include acts of humiliation, criticism, removal of privileges or removal of attention/attachments. We have to realise that for those who already have negative core beliefs about themselves or others, punishment just reinforces those beliefs further. 'I am bad or others are bad.'

Even if those beliefs aren't there, the punishment itself has the effect of reducing a person's quality of life (missing out on privileges, enjoyment or connection, even if only temporarily).

The most likely effect of reducing quality of life is a reduction in self-esteem for the individual. Now, if the individual generally has positive core beliefs and self-esteem, they may well be able to overcome this one-off blip, especially if they get lots of positive regard and reinforcers in other areas of their life. If, however, they keep getting things 'wrong' and they are continually punished, thereby lowering their quality of life and reducing their self-esteem, the likelihood is extremely low that their overall behaviour will improve as a result.

Please don't misunderstand – punishment can be effective to reduce an undesirable behaviour. However, the cycle shows that relying on this model will inevitably lead to negative outcomes overall.

We also have to think about the effects of punishment on social learning: if we punish them... do they have a right and a responsibility to punish others? Are we creating a culture where these strategies are seen as appropriate?

CASE STUDY 6.4 THE NAUGHTY STEP

There was a popular parenting strategy called 'the naughty step'. It is often called something different now (e.g., 'safe space', 'time out'), but the model is similar regardless of the name.

When a child misbehaved, they would be put on the bottom step of the stairs for a set time. During that time the parent would not engage or communicate.

The aim was for the child to:

- calm
- experience the displeasure of connection being withdrawn
- recognise that their behaviour was wrong
- reflect and then make amends once their time was up.

It often worked. The child felt the immediate pain of disconnection, the shame of letting down the person they trust. The child had the resilience and core beliefs to know they were still loved despite the caregiver's dislike of the behaviour they just displayed. They could calm themselves, reflect, accept the guilt and make amends.

However, if the child is hypersensitive to shame, doesn't know how to calm, and/or doesn't trust the caregiver due to insecure attachments (fear of abandonment), this will only worsen all of these beliefs, and they will not be able to calm, reflect and make amends.

If the child has other difficulties of behaviour regulation, learning is unlikely as well.

But even if the child does learn and adapt future behaviours, they have been taught another lesson: 'If someone does not behave as I feel they should (as I believe), I should withdraw my affection from them until they behave as I want.'

When we see this sort of pattern of behaviour occur between two adults in a relationship, it is now societally classed as abuse and manipulation. But where was it learned?

Models of how to manage behaviour are often ingrained within our cultures, values and even laws, but, as mentioned, just because that's the way things have been done doesn't make them right – understanding moves us forwards.

We also need to be aware that when we are supporting individuals, we may not be 100% aware of how they have been cared for, treated and taught in the past. They may have insecure attachment models or be non-neurotypical. Their experiences or perceptions of behaviour management may have been detrimental.

If we take the extremes an individual may have experienced – neglect at one extreme (do what you want) and abuse at the other (do this or else) – we may find that even low-level versions of these behaviour management strategies can trigger shame shielding, anxiety, rage and defiance. We will explore this in more detail through the book, but to summarise: an individual who has experienced either physical or emotional abuse in childhood may perceive any shouting or raised voice as a return to that abuse, which may trigger survival tactics. If they have experienced abandonment or neglect, then a caregiver ignoring them may also create similar fearful reactions. Rather than learning from these consequences, they may just reinforce negative views of themselves or others.

See below for a fuller explanation.

OLD-LOGIC SPECTRUM

The diagram below shows the two extremes of a caregiver's potential responses to a child's behaviours during the child's developmental stages. The spectrum runs from severe abuse to total neglect.

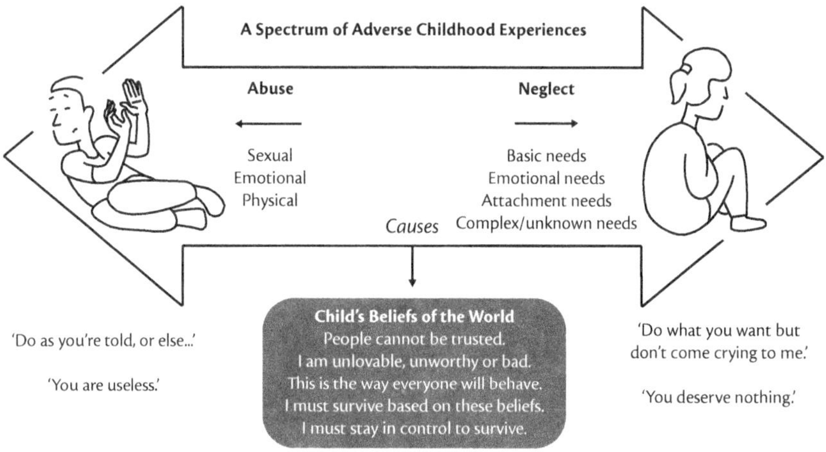

Figure 6.1 Old-Logic Spectrum

At one end we have abuse – physical, sexual or emotional.

'You do what you are told or else.'
'You are useless, stupid, a burden.'
'I will scare you or cause you pain because of your behaviour.'

At the other end we have neglect – emotional, basic attachment or unknown needs.

'Do what you like but good luck feeding yourself, comforting yourself, being on your own.'

These aren't necessarily purposeful abuse or neglect – some examples are given below.

- If a child has a developmental disorder, a caregiver may not know or be aware of how to meet the individual's needs; e.g., sensory processing issues – imagine that touch or eye contact is painful for the child. The caregiver comes to meet the child's needs and softly strokes the child and looks into the child's eyes, not realising this is adding to, not removing, the distress. The child cannot understand the caregiver's intent and instead interprets their treatment as punishment, not love. Or imagine being a caregiver supporting a child who doesn't seem to like your attention and recoils from it... it's hard to attach to a child who doesn't seem to like you, so the caregiver may withdraw.
- The caregiver may hold the child to behavioural expectations that they will always fall short of. This is not due to the child's purposeful misbehaviour but due to the child's delayed development or learning difficulties. These deficits may mean the child 'keeps getting things wrong' and is punished through an action somewhere on the old-logic spectrum. (Variations in the way the brain might function are further discussed in Chapter 13, page 120.)
- We also should be aware of mental health issues or learning disabilities in the caregivers themselves, or even illnesses in either the child or caregiver, that could all lead to non-ideal care for the child.

Whether intentional or not these experiences can leave the individual believing:

- 'People cannot be trusted'
- 'I am unlovable, unworthy or bad'
- 'This is the way everyone will behave'
- 'I must survive based on these assumptions'
- 'If I am controlled, it is dangerous'
- 'I must stay in control to survive'.

These beliefs can mean that even typical negative reactions to behaviour that society has thought appropriate for a long time can result in the individual's models of the world and their beliefs being reinforced. The version of Figure 6.2 shows the low-level reactions that might occur from shouting/criticising or walk away/take away strategies.

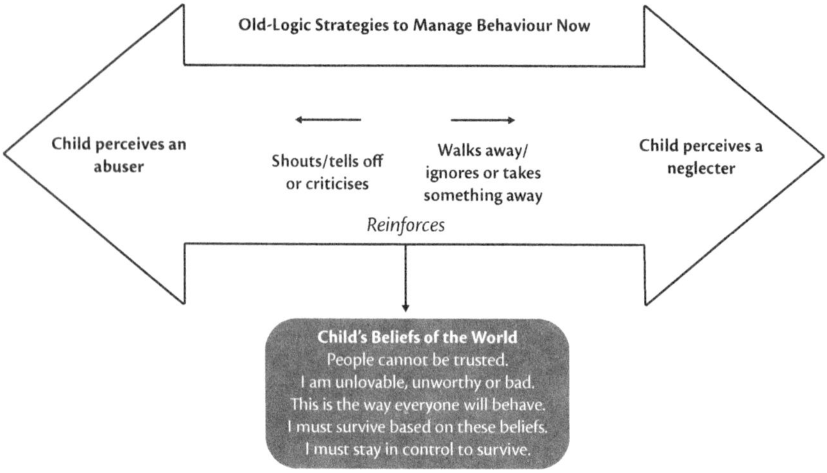

Figure 6.2 Old-Logic Spectrum – Low-Level Reactions

The old-logic spectrum is ingrained with the notion that bad behaviour should be punished by either presenting an unpleasant stimulus to stop the individual wanting to repeat the behaviour or removing a positive stimulus (e.g., a parent's/caregiver's attention or a preferred object) to create an unpleasant sensation that the individual wants to avoid in the future. This strategy can work to address some behaviours, but it often doesn't achieve the best overall outcomes. This is especially so for an individual who has experienced abuse (physical, sexual or emotional) or neglect.

Abuse may come in the form of the individual being judged as constantly 'getting things wrong'. 'Constantly getting things wrong' is the result of their caregivers' expectations. These expectations could be based on the caregivers' attitudes or beliefs associated with the individual's chronological age without understanding or adjusting to the individual's deficits and abilities.

Neglect may be the result of the individual having to be excessively self-reliant due to caregivers not being able to meet or not understanding the individual's needs or challenges (e.g., the child has sensory processing issues that make soft touch painful but a caregiver does not know this, which may mean they cause distress rather than relieve it) or the individual may have had to be a caregiver themselves to their parents or siblings.

CASE STUDY 6.5 'PLEASE SIR, I WANT ANOTHER BISCUIT'

A child asks if they can have another biscuit. The answer is 'no', and the child's response is to explode.

They go into a meltdown, full fight response.

You might think that the child has exploded because they can't have another biscuit. But actually it's the child's response to 'no' that's the cause.

'No' implies control. Based on the child's belief, the 'no' triggers their survival response. Control means danger.

Old-logic responses by the caregiver (based on the caregiver's assumption that this is just an overreaction to a biscuit) may include:

- **Telling off**: Raising the voice and stating, 'Don't talk like that to me, you won't get another biscuit behaving this way.' The caregiver has become the abuser in the child's eyes.

Or:

- **Walk-away, take-away strategies**: 'I'm walking away if you are going to behave like this and there will be no more biscuits for the rest of the week.' The caregiver inadvertently becomes the neglecter.

Referring to Figure 6.1, the shouting approach is at the abuse end; the walk-away approach is at the neglect end.

These actions reinforce the child's beliefs and assumptions about the world, and the pattern will continue.

We need to get off the old-logic spectrum and into new-logic approaches outlined in the next section (this case study will be referred to again with a new-logic approach in 'Case Study 34.23 "Please Sir, I Want Another Biscuit" – Revisited with New-Logic Eyes', page 344).

NEW-LOGIC APPROACHES

Throughout this book, we will be recommending a variety of strategies that fall under a new style of logic and thinking regarding behaviour management. The Target system includes a blend of different models and principles to provide the golden rules of understanding and managing behaviours that challenge.

The underlying principle of the system is to allow us to shift away from the old-logic principles and patterns like:

- judgement – they do/don't do it because they are bad, lazy, naughty
- individuals should do what they are told because caregivers know best
- caregivers should be in control as they know best
- caregivers don't make mistakes or do things wrong, so it must be the individual who is wrong
- bad actions should be punished – there must be consequences
- we should be respected as we are authority or here to help

to new-style thinking like:

- picking the right battles
- recognising skills and strengths
- unconditional positive regard of the individual
- curiosity about behaviours and the individual
- individuals should be at the centre of their own care
- empathy towards feelings
- collaborative support and teaching individuals about better strategies
- adjusting the environment or interactions to improve outcomes
- trust, connection building and earned respect
- self-awareness, self-reflection and self-management
- responding rather than reacting
- having a growth mindset through reflection and learning.

The following models or principles have been amalgamated into the Target system:

- Positive Behaviour Support (PBS) including Applied Behaviour Analysis but adapted to be person-centred
- Spell Framework from the National Autistic Society
- Trauma-informed principles and care
- Trauma-informed model – Therapeutic Parenting
- The PACE Model (Playfulness, Acceptance, Curiosity, Empathy) – by Dan Hughes[16]

There are also numerous psychotherapy models and concepts included.

These different models have all informed the principles and strategies within the Target system and the 6STM.

The strong focus on empathy and understanding repeated as a theme in the book encourages a person-centred, trauma-informed approach. The process applies these practices to numerous care settings with the aim of improving positive outcomes within the settings for all individuals and caregivers.

Although some of the models mentioned are aimed at specific settings or individual needs, there are many principles from these approaches that will benefit anyone.

One core principle of the 6STM:

> The behaviour management approach that a positive caregiver would typically offer a young child... applied to anyone.

CASE STUDY 6.6 THE CRYING BABY

When two-month-old Luna goes into an emotionally overwhelmed state, we do not say, 'If you don't shut up, I'll take your teddy away.'

No. We tend to try and calm her, let her know it's safe, let her know that everything's okay. We let her listen to our heartbeat and our breathing, where we're showing a lot of calm to let the child know, 'It's okay, you can be calm too.'

We also try to work out what's causing that distress and eliminate it; maybe she needs feeding or cleaning up. And during the process, we also develop our relationship with Luna.

If Luna never experienced this, she may not know how to emotionally regulate or may develop unusual ways to regulate or meet her emotional needs.

Using the positive approach of supporting someone in the way we would support a toddler is not aiming to infantilise anyone or treat anyone as a child. However, there are some underlying cultural norms of parenthood that are worth considering as we move into the Target system.

As new parents, we typically do the following things.

- We show unconditional regard towards the child – not only when they behave in a certain way, but just because they exist.
- We recognise that when they are emotional, they are telling us something and it is our responsibility to figure that out.
- We adjust the environment around them to ensure they are happy and safe and their needs are met until they are ready to manage these themselves. We focus on the behaviours we want and we develop strategies of how we will teach these.
- We accept mistakes as learning.
- We intuitively notice their strengths, their improvements and their abilities rather than their deficits.
- We allow the infant to dictate when they are ready to learn new skills and we patiently reinforce what they can do rather than criticise what they can't. (The child will talk when they're ready, but we praise every word or partial word rather than criticise mistakes; and if we correct, we do it gently with understanding rather than condemnation.)
- We recognise that we are learning about the child as much as the child is learning about the world.
- We focus on building connection and attachment at the same time as meeting their basic needs.

It is only social pressures or our own expectations that seem to alter these intuitive strategies. The 6STM aims to show how these same principles can and should be applied to everyone.

PART 2

THE 6-STAGE TARGET MODEL

CHAPTER 7

INTRODUCTION TO THE 6STM

CASE STUDY 7.1 THE CLENCHED FIST

Imagine you saw a person with their fist clenched and you were instructed by an authority figure that you needed to get the hand open. How would you approach this request?

Would you focus on the fist or the person?

Would you make assumptions about what that clenched fist was communicating – that they are angry, are scared, must be hiding something, have hurt themselves – and would these assumptions affect your approach?

Would the fact that an authority figure told you to do it affect your perspective?

As we examine this example, imagine the clenched fist represents any behaviour that we are finding challenging.

If we focus on the hand rather than the person in the example, we could try a multitude of strategies that may prove effective but may be considered inappropriate.

POTENTIALLY INAPPROPRIATE APPROACHES

Physically Trying to Prise the Fist Open

We would struggle to justify this as a reasonable use of force, i.e., it was necessary (last resort) and proportionate (the risk of prising the fist open was equal to or less than the risk of leaving the fist clenched), meaning it would be classed as assault, whether or not the action caused injury. It is also modelling the use of force to get an individual to comply with your demands, which is not a strategy we would want individuals to use against us or others.

Tickling

Depending on the relationship with the individual, this may also be perceived as assault, possibly even perceived as sexual in nature depending on the history of the individual or their perception.

Stroking the Hand and Trying to Comfort

This may not be inappropriate but may be perceived as patronising or may distress some people who don't like or want touch.

There are also incorrect verbal approaches:

Bribery

For example, 'Open your hand and I'll... give you a biscuit/a cup of tea/a cigarette/a quid.' So what's the problem with bribery?

- If the bribe isn't delivered, you damage trust; however...
- if the bribe works and is delivered, it potentially reinforces a negative behaviour, i.e., the way to get a biscuit is to clench my fist. It may be one biscuit the first time, but that price may go up. Many parents have made this mistake with their children.
- It's potentially manipulation (psychological abuse/emotional abuse) of the individual.
- What if the response to the bribe is 'No, but I'll have the cup of tea'? Can you stop them having the tea? No, because of the duty of care and human rights, you can't take away their rights. But some individuals with limited cognitive capacity may not know their rights; that is why we have safeguards in place to protect individuals from being manipulated.

Bribery = short-term solution, long-term problem.

Emotional Blackmail

For example, 'If you don't open your hands, we're not friends anymore; I thought you liked me.' As a type of emotional threat and manipulation, emotional blackmail may work, but that doesn't make it acceptable and it is often abusive and damaging to relationships and culture.

Threats

For example, 'If you don't open your hand, I'll have to tell the manager/you'll have to go to your room/you won't get any pudding.'

- If the threat isn't followed through, authority is undermined; however...
- it may cause a loss of trust between the individual and caregivers; we often don't trust people who threaten us to comply. 'It's easier to break trust than make trust.'
- It can cause escalation to aggression or feelings of defiance, retribution or fear (getting compliance because someone fears us is not an ideal outcome).

- If threats are the norm, what does that say about the setting's culture?... what kind of role modelling is being shown? Answer: threats can control my environment.
- Threats can lead to bullying or be classed as abuse.

Threats = short-term solution, long-term problem.

Note: There's a difference between a threat and a consequence. A threat tends to be 'me versus you', a power struggle; it's about who's in control. A consequence is more collaborative – for example, 'Look, you have a choice; make this choice and such-and-such will happen; make the other choice and so-and-so will happen. I think the best choice for you is (option), but it's up to you. The consequences are fixed, but the choice is yours' – with natural or balanced consequences being more appropriate. The use of punishment and consequences is covered extensively in Chapter 25, page 238.

Distraction/Redirection

This may be completely appropriate and one of the best approaches, but it all depends on why the fist is clenched. If the person needs help or to be understood, distraction may not meet the need. Where it is appropriate, ignoring the hand and just focusing on the person and redirecting their attention so they forget about the hand may allow us to de-escalate or prevent confrontation. If necessary, we could always go back later to exploring why their fist was clenched.

A BETTER APPROACH

Connection

The focus of the approach is on connecting with the individual and building rapport and trust rather than rushing into addressing the behaviour.

We could adapt the quote from the film *Patch Adams*,[17] changing it from 'You treat a disease, you win, you lose. You treat a person, I guarantee you, you'll win, no matter what the outcome,' to 'If we aim to change the behaviour, we win, we lose. If we aim for genuine human connection, we'll win no matter what the outcome.'

Curiosity

Try to find out *why* the fist is clenched or – more generally – *why* the individual is acting in this way. The object of the approach should *not* be to fix the behaviour as presented; it's to find out *why* the behaviour is happening. This may be done by asking directly or by indirectly exploring and being a detective.

Focus on the person

The two approaches shown above avoid the trap of focusing on the behaviour rather than the person, avoid falling into the trap of making assumptions about the behaviour and also allow the caregiver to assess whether the hand even needs to be opened. Even if an authority figure tells us to do something we should always avoid becoming task focused rather than person-centred and be able to act on our own cost-versus-benefit analysis of the behaviour.

> *The aim of the approach should not be to open the hand but to understand the person and understand: Why this? Why now?*

Unfortunately, many of the inappropriate tactics described above are quick and effective solutions despite their long-term negative outcomes, and they have been used in many settings, by many people, many times. These inappropriate tactics are often more intuitive than many of the more appropriate strategies depending on a caregiver's beliefs, experience, training and instruction, and the culture of the setting.

Caregivers often mistakenly invent a reason for the behaviour based on assumptions. These assumptions are commonly based on labels the individual has been given; for example, 'Oh, she's lazy/a liar/secretive/awkward/stubborn/manipulative/difficult/attention-seeking/a nasty piece of work.' These labels and assumptions cause caregivers to lose their curiosity about the behaviour.

Further, does it actually matter that the fist is closed or – more generally – is this behaviour actually a cause for concern? Does it affect the individual's or others' health, safety and welfare? Does it affect their level of care, their social inclusion? Or maybe it's the case that the caregiver (or authority figure) doesn't like or agree with the behaviour or even dislikes the individual. Which means it may be the *caregiver's* behaviour that's challenging, not the individual's.

Caregivers also often know exactly what they *don't* want a person doing but have no real idea of what they *do* want them doing.

This is why using a set system and models to give caregivers the skills and correct approaches to understanding and managing behaviour is so important. Common sense does not exist! A sense or understanding of the right way to do something can never be common to all people... unless it is created through teaching. This book aims to create a 'common sense' to managing behaviours that challenge that can be used as a full proactive management system that, over time, informs and creates a preventative culture. Or that can be used as a dynamic response system that aims to ensure the 'management strategy hierarchy' triangle is the correct way round and the overall aim of 'positive outcomes for all' can be achieved.

THE SIX STAGES OF THE TARGET MODEL (6STM)

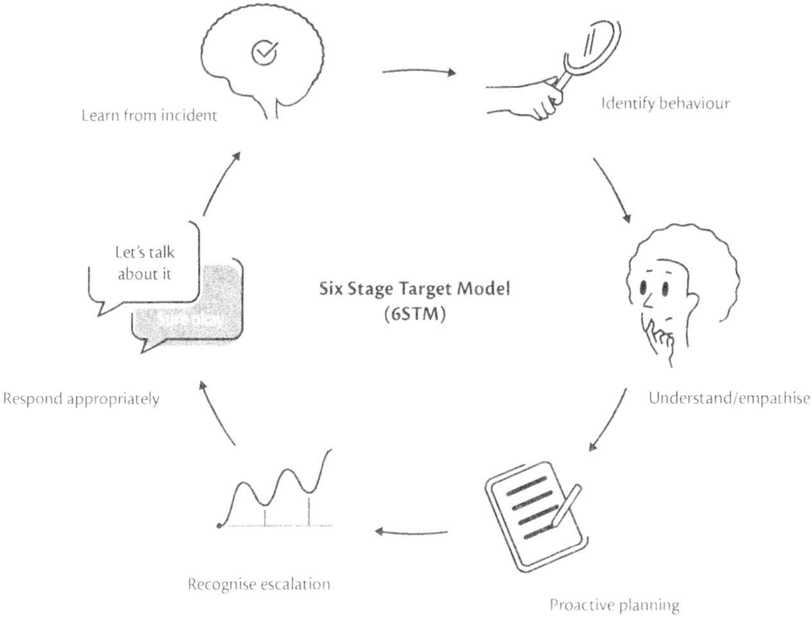

Figure 7.1 The 6STM

Introduction

The 6STM is a toolkit for organisations to ingrain into their systems, policies, training and day-to-day practice.

The toolkit has six stages that can be used as an ongoing proactive process, using stages (steps) as needed (in a semi-linear order) to move towards positive outcomes.

However, like a Monopoly board, we may not stop on every space, but we always go round in the same direction despite starting from different positions depending on the circumstances. Each stage will inform other stages as we progress and learn about the people we are supporting.

You will also find case studies scattered throughout the book that may jump around the stages and sections as demonstrations of how the process may develop.

This introduction to the model gives a summary of each component. Later in the book there are sections that describe each component in detail.

Summary of Each Component

1. Identify Behaviour

The identify behaviour process includes deciding if a behaviour is indeed one that presents challenges (for the individual and/or others), and if so, what are the costs/benefits to all concerned about tackling that behaviour. It's about identifying maladaptive behaviours and picking the right battles – those that we may need to manage or change.

We also need to identify adaptive behaviours and abilities – favourable behaviours that we can reinforce and build on.

2. Understand/Empathise

We cannot expect to tackle a maladaptive behaviour without understanding *why* the behaviour occurs. What benefit does the individual gain from this behaviour?

Most importantly, we should empathise with the individual to see the world from their perspective.

3. Proactive Planning

Proactive planning seeks solutions to the problem. For example, the individual may need to be taught new skills, or the environment may need adjustment (e.g., if something is stressful for an individual, can that something be removed?).

We also create plans for how to respond to ensure we reinforce desired behaviours but do not reinforce undesired behaviours.

(Note that we use the word 'respond' and not 'react'. 'Respond' implies 'rational', whereas 'react' implies 'emotional'.)

Stage 3: Proactive Planning includes a summary of the psychology behind resistance to change and practical techniques for implementing change.

4. Recognise Escalation

Behaviour doesn't occur in a vacuum, so learning to recognise pre-indicators or signs of escalation can allow us to respond in the right way at the right time.

We may need to recognise the warning signs and where on an escalation cycle the individual is. We can then choose the most appropriate response based on pre-planned strategies or ad hoc appropriate strategies.

5. Respond Appropriately

This describes how to respond to behaviours. The response may be based on proactive plans or may be dynamic based in the moment.

6. Learn from Incident and History; Monitoring

Once a plan for the individual has been implemented, its effects must be monitored.

If an incident occurs that isn't covered by the plan, or the outcome differs to what the plan expected, then the incident should be documented and a review undertaken to discover what went well, what didn't work and what could have been done differently to produce a better outcome.

Overall principle

Reviewing the six components, those numbered 1, 2, 3 and 6 (identify, understand, plan, learn) can be seen as behaving like a scientist or a detective, forming a hypothesis: 'I can see this happening, and I think this is the cause, and maybe we can do so-and-so to solve it.'

Components 4 and 5 (recognise escalation and respond appropriately) are 'in the moment', and our behaviour should be akin to a firefighter managing a blaze. This isn't the time to investigate what started it. Ideally we should be responding in planned ways to events as they unfold. This isn't the time to be looking for whys, should haves and prevention. The fire needs putting out for now.

CASE STUDY 7.2 THE FUTILE ARGUMENT

We may have come across (or even been involved in) an argument that begins in a rational way but after a while becomes detached from the subject and becomes an emotional slanging match. Rational analysis of the situation will not be possible until both people step back and take a deep breath. Only then can solutions be created and discussions be productive.

During the argument our rational brain is overwhelmed by our emotional brain; we enter the realms of black-and-white thinking and emotional reactions. The other person is wrong and seen as the opposition; everything they say is perceived as wrong or causes further emotion.

Supported individuals are no different. We shouldn't try to be proactive when we should be responding.

Note: When discussing the use of the 6STM, the 'Management Strategy Hierarchy' diagram as described in 'Case Study 2.1 Similarity to Fire', page 22, should be borne in mind. In brief: that diagram explains the three levels of management that apply to managing behaviours in a similar format to managing risks:

- **Primary/prevention**: The everyday practice of the workplace itself, policies, ethos, etc.
- **Secondary/proactive management**: The pre-planned interactions and procedures focusing on individuals' needs that are used to support the individual as needed.
- **Tertiary/responsive troubleshooting**: Responding to behaviours as they occur either based on planned responses or dynamic responses/reactions.

The Target system and the 6STM cover all three levels of the hierarchy.

- **Preventative**: All the tools, attitudes and understanding that are presented throughout the book can inform day-to-day practice. The more the Target system and the 6STM are studied and used, the more they will become ingrained in the culture of the setting, the greater the prevention and the better the outcomes. Strategies will become ingrained in the culture of the setting and the caregivers; thereby the strategies become part of the overall prevention strategy and improve quality of care, reduce occurrences of behaviours that challenge and produce positive outcomes for all.

- **Proactive management**: The 6STM is a process to develop behavioural plans that are individual specific. It allows caregivers to explore and learn about the individuals they support and to know how to interact, support and communicate with them in the best way to reduce distress. It also allows individuals and caregivers to create plans of how the environment can be adjusted and/or what beneficial skills, both for individuals and caregivers, can be developed.

- **Responsive trouble shooting**: In Stage 5: Respond Appropriately there are tools for planned situations where there is a planned response to incidents, but there are also multiple tools for managing unplanned situations. The Target system covers numerous de-escalation strategies (ways to put out fires). It also covers dynamic tools for recognising escalation in anyone and how these unexpected situations can be used to inform proactive management and ultimately improve day-to-day practice.

PART 3

THE 6-STAGE TARGET MODEL STAGE 1

Identify

CHAPTER 8

IDENTIFY MALADAPTIVE BEHAVIOURS

> *Treat a man as he is and he will remain as he is.*
> *Treat a man as he could be and he will become what he should be.*
>
> RALPH WALDO EMERSON

Stage 1 of the 6STM is where the behaviour of an individual is discussed from the point of view of caregivers:

- what behaviours caregivers assess as being maladaptive/adaptive
- what behaviour should be the priority for attention
- how that behaviour should be addressed.

We have written it this way to encourage caregivers to explore their conversations and decision making in an analytical and person-centred way.

If we want to improve an individual's quality of life, it is necessary to identify both the behaviours that *challenge* and the behaviours they exhibit that are *beneficial* to their outcomes.

As mentioned, many of the behaviours that challenge we might label as 'maladaptive' behaviours.

As discussed in previous chapters, when looking at what is a behaviour that challenges, many of the behaviours we label as challenging we class as *excess behaviours*. These excess behaviours impact the setting in some way, and many are considered hazardous, antisocial or detrimental to the individual's overall wellbeing, or may just be viewed as less appropriate than other behaviours (see 'Case Study 8.1 Class Clown').

Many of these excess behaviours are ways for a person to cope with their own behavioural *deficits*. A behavioural deficit shows a person's inability to meet their own needs or manage stress. The excess behaviours are behavioural adaptations the person has made, consciously or unconsciously, to cope, survive or meet needs.

Those excess behaviours that are self-destructive and that may actually fulfil a short-term need but create long-term detriment we call 'maladaptive' behaviours. For example, staying in bed for one day isn't necessarily self-destructive, but staying in bed every day probably is self-destructive.

These maladaptive behaviours are the ones that need to be identified and separated from those that are just disliked within the setting. This process will be explored in this chapter.

Once we identify which behaviours are truly maladaptive, we then need to understand their function or trigger or what behavioural deficit the cause may be.

CASE STUDY 8.1 CLASS CLOWN

Ian loves to be the centre of attention and make people laugh. He is a natural performer and can be very funny. Unfortunately, Ian can be disruptive in a class of other students as he can get silly and distract other students to make them laugh. The teacher has heard some of the other students in class getting irritated with Ian because he distracts them from their work. Ian sometimes struggles to engage with other students in more socially acceptable ways and so seems to use this silliness to connect, but actually this strategy is having an adverse effect on his engagement.

The teacher decides that Ian's behaviour needs to be managed due to its impact on others and on Ian's relationships with his fellow students. The teacher creates a strategy.

The teacher sets up a plan where if Ian gets his set classwork tasks done within the required time, he can earn a reward. Ian's reward is a five-minute slot at the end of the class to perform a short sketch or joke.

Over time this strategy seems to be making Ian more popular with his peers, and also both Ian and the other students are becoming more productive.

Commentary: In the example above, the 'maladaptive' behaviour is identified – connection-seeking behaviour. However, although the behaviour is *maladaptive* within the context (wrong time, wrong place), it is not *hazardous* and so needs only managing, not changing. In fact, in this example, by adjusting the perception of the behaviour, it was nurtured into an adaptive behaviour.

It is also essential to identify the individual's *positive* behaviours, skills and talents. These are 'adaptive' behaviours and can become the foundation for displacing the maladaptive behaviours and raising the person's self-esteem and wellbeing. This is the subject of the next chapter.

BE SPECIFIC

Behavioural assessment starts by *defining* an individual's behaviour.

This does not mean using general terms such as lazy, awkward, disruptive, defiant, selfish, attention-seeking and the like. As mentioned before, these are ill-defined; and worse, they are judgemental.

To make a useful definition of a behaviour, three elements should be recorded:

- **Appearance**: What the behaviour looks like; e.g., 'She put herself to the floor, lying on her front, and started pulling her hair and hitting her head hard on the floor while screaming.'
- **Frequency**: How often it occurs (e.g., 'daily', 'several times each day', 'at mealtimes').
- **Impact**: For maladaptive behaviours: how severe the outcome of the behaviour is for the individual and/or others – especially with regard to others' human rights and health and safety.

Details of how to record incidents are given in Stage 6: Learn from Incident.

PICK YOUR BATTLES

Having carefully identified an individual's maladaptive behaviour/s, the question must be asked: should we try to do anything about it? If we made a list of all the maladaptive behaviours that certain people exhibit and then tried to address all of them, we would create a very negative environment.

We should bear in mind that there's a risk of reinforcing a behaviour by paying more attention to it.

So we need to look down the list and decide: 'That one cannot be ignored.'

We also need to use this principle dynamically, in the moment. We may have a list of behaviours in advance that are being proactively assessed. However, new behaviours – and as a result, new habits, prejudices and strategies – develop all the time. Any change or transition may result in a new behaviour arising. If, as mentioned, we are not selective in reacting to these, we carry the risk of reinforcing or falling into the trap of negative focus.

Note: When we refer to 'ignoring', this does not mean we ignore the person or use ignoring to eliminate the behaviour. Ignoring means we don't directly confront the behaviour in the moment with the aim to stop it. We ignore the behaviour... not the person.

Being Honest with Ourselves

Is this a case of me simply disagreeing with it because it goes against my own values and beliefs, rather than it being potentially maladaptive?

Context

Is this behaviour a one-off? Did the individual kick the door in an isolated fit of temper? Drawing attention to it may accentuate the negative – negative self-esteem, for example. Do we need to spend/waste time on what is probably a one-off?

Again, consider context. If the individual has dementia and is trying to break through a door because they want to go 'home', they may be disorientated. We cannot change this behaviour and so we may need to ignore the behaviour. Instead, we can focus on the *person* rather than the behaviour, and perhaps try to redirect or distract or adjust the environment to reduce disorientation and distress.

We should always consider an individual's *developmental* age rather than their physical age. Neurodiversity, developmental conditions, cognitive impairments or mental health concerns can lead to individual discrepancies in an individual's functional abilities; this topic will be explored in more detail in Stage 2: Understand/Empathise.

CASE STUDY 8.2 PICK YOUR BATTLES

Take a look at the following graphic.

A study of an 18-year-old youth with FASD revealed that they were functioning at the following developmental age levels:

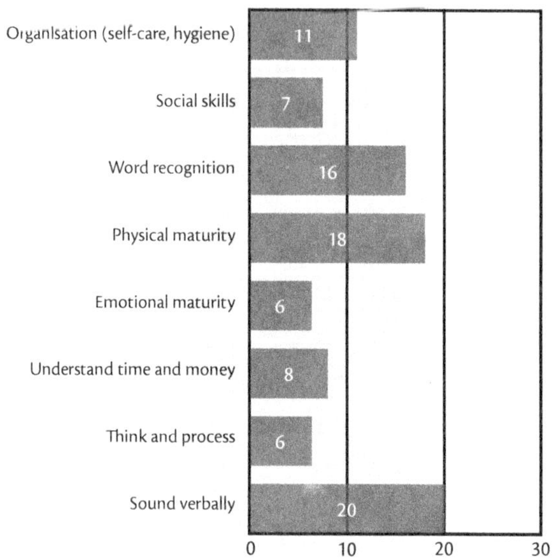

Base your expectations realistically.

Figure 8.1 Developmental Timelines

These are real results taken about an 18-year-old with FASD (foetal alcohol spectrum disorder).[18] But similar results could be found in individuals with autism, ADHD, dementia, etc.

The point is that many individuals in care have cognitive imbalances (split skills). A child may have high intelligence for certain faculties and do well at school, and yet *not be able* to organise their books or timetable. Just because the child is clever at one thing doesn't mean they'll be at the same level for all things, because there are different forms of intelligence.

We must work hard to avoid the mistake of assuming that just because an individual is 18, they should react in all circumstances as a typical 18-year-old.

If that incorrect assumption is made, individuals may not meet our expectations, and as a result this could reinforce the individual's belief that they're not good enough.

Many caregivers find it hard to allow a child or adult to behave in line with their emotional age, often due to external pressures and the judgement of ignorant people. But setting a standard too high, so a person will always fall short, is to set up failure; but not *the person's* failure – it's a failure of those supporting them.

Commitment: Change takes time, and some behaviours are heavily ingrained in habit; we need to consider the level of commitment and consistency that might be required for change. If we're only going to see the individual for two weeks on respite, or maybe for one hour per week, is it worth spending all of that time on a behavioural issue? This could put stress on the individual when realistically, given the time available, nothing can change. Now, if it's part of an individual's overall care plan within a variety of settings, then of course, for consistency's sake, it may be worthwhile.

Human Rights

We need to be mindful that when changing a person's support/care strategies without their consent, we may be impacting on their autonomy and choices. Under the European Convention on Human Rights, all human beings have the right to express their thoughts, make choices about their life and have freedom of movement. We must make sure that if we are restricting any of these, we must have legal justification (e.g., a person lacks the capacity to make a particular decision – Mental Capacity Act 2005). Also, under the Equality Act 2010, we must ensure that a person is not being discriminated against and treated differently to anyone else purely based on their age, disability or any other protected characteristic. For example, we cannot assume that, because an individual with a cognitive disability makes an unwise choice (in our opinion), they don't have the mental capacity to make choices themselves (Mental Capacity Act 2005). We must always ensure any infringement of a person's freedom or choices is in the person's best interests and only applied in the least restrictive manner.

CASE STUDY 8.3 DIABETES

Elwood has diabetes and is also living with dementia. He likes sticky toffee pudding but some caregivers think he shouldn't be allowed it due to the risks with his diabetes. In the following discussion, 'A' = giving him sticky toffee pudding, 'B' = not giving it. Let's explore using a cost-versus-benefit analysis.

- **Cost of A**: Physical risk to health due to blood sugar management. Increasing the risk of numerous medical issues.
- **Benefit of A**: Emotional – Elwood really enjoys sticky toffee pudding; it makes him happy. Physical – the custard he has with it is fortified with additional vitamins. Mental – he has made the choice and feels empowered.
- **Cost of B**: Emotional – lower mood from seeing others get the pudding he is not allowed. Mental – Elwood has had his choices restricted so feels bullied. Social – reduces positive relationship with staff. Behavioural – has become aggressive when told 'no'.
- **Benefit of B**: Physical – easier to manage blood sugar, healthier.

The staff may be able to argue that Elwood doesn't have the capacity to know what's best for him regarding his diabetes, and so they should make the choice for him if they are focused only on his physical wellbeing rather than the holistic benefits (see 'Cost Versus Benefits' below). However...

Could the setting offer a low-sugar version? Can his sugar intake be reduced elsewhere to compensate for the pudding? Can his insulin be adjusted to compensate – how are his sugar levels usually?

These options may or may not be necessary depending on the risk, but they are examples of less restrictive options to manage the concern.

CASE STUDY 8.4 BIZARRE CLOTHING

A young man, who is autistic, with learning disabilities, in a supported living environment, enjoys going into a town. The young man requires support and supervision to be safe and so he is always accompanied by a caregiver.

One morning, prior to a trip into town, the young man dressed himself in a mishmash of clothes, an ensemble of colours and patterns that would not generally be described as socially typical.

The caregiver who was meant to be supporting the lad with going into town felt unhappy with the lad's clothing choice and tried to persuade him to change into something more suitable, but the lad resisted. Eventually the caregiver set an ultimatum: change or no trip to town. The lad reluctantly complied.

Commentary: In a review of the incident the caregiver was asked why she acted in that way. She said that she didn't want to see him laughed at or bullied when in town.

Well, didn't the caregiver bully the lad to make him change? Was her bullying any better than anyone else's? She had taken away his human rights of autonomy and free choice. Did the lad care what other people thought of him? Probably not. Did *she* care what people thought of him or even how they may judge her? Probably more so. The individual probably felt proud that he'd dressed himself and liked to express himself. In this example, the behaviour that challenged was not the lad's behaviour, it was the caregiver's.

Cost Versus Benefits

We all behave as we do because our behaviour brings us benefits. If a behaviour does not bring benefits, we won't repeat it.

There are various types of benefits of behaviour:

- **Emotional**: Emotional pain relief or giving positive feelings.
- **Spiritual**: Giving feelings of validation, meaning, importance.
- **Social**: Feelings of attachment, belonging or concepts of self-identity ('I am funny,' 'I am a father,' 'I am kind,' etc.).
- **Physical**: Relief from pain or discomfort.
- **Mental**: Learning, problem solving, confidence in choice making, having our thoughts about the world or ourselves validated (even if those beliefs are negative; e.g., 'See I knew I'd get it wrong,' or 'Told you I was right.'). This is the opposite of cognitive dissonance.

But when we observe behaviours that challenge, it's not always obvious to us what benefits there are for the individual. A thought worth remembering is that all of us at some point have acted or behaved in a way, or made a choice, that maybe even we can see, in hindsight, was a bad idea or had a cost. However, in that moment, when we took that action or made that choice, we felt it was right. No one behaves in a way that they know is a bad idea; they must have thought it was a good idea at the time. So there must be a perceived or subconscious benefit to every behaviour.

- In 'Case Study 1.3 Behaviour That Challenges... Maladaptive or Not?' we read about the boy who relieved his tensions by jumping on his bed. That behaviour is certainly one that challenged his caregivers, but by jumping, the child obtained relief from sensory overload – a benefit.
- Take another example: smoking. Smoking is known to be physically and physiologically bad for a person. So, perhaps a person smokes to cope with emotional pain or to relieve stress – benefits.
- But what about self-harm, cutting for example? Again, the individual may be gaining relief from emotional pain – benefit.
- The person who repeats a bad behaviour. Maybe they feel shame, and cover it up or take control of it by revelling in their bad reputation – a benefit.

The question is: does the benefit from the behaviour outweigh the cost to the person or the setting? If the answer is no, then clearly some action needs to be taken. We must find a way to retain the benefits but perhaps by using a more appropriate behaviour.

TRIAGE

If we are supporting a person with several behaviours that challenge, it is important that we not only assess which of the behaviours are maladaptive rather than just disliked, but also decide a plan of which behaviours need managing as a priority. If we try and address all behaviours immediately, it can be overwhelming for both the individual and the caregivers. It may also be that we need to ensure we address certain behaviours at a certain time in a person's care journey.

To start this process, we can use a cost versus benefit assessment.

If we list any behaviours that challenge in a risk matrix (below) we can use this matrix to explore the costs to both the individual themselves and to others (including the staff). This process is subjective, and so including the opinions of others can increase the chances of reaching a balanced assessment. The exact scores do not matter too much as long as the same measurement process is used for all behaviours.

Frequency / Impact	1. Rarely	2. Occasionally	3. Regularly	4. Daily	5. Multiple times per day
1. Insignificant impact	2	3	4	5	6
2. Potential over long term	3	4	5	6	7
3. Affects wellbeing and outcomes	4	5	6	7	8
4. Life-altering effects	5	6	7	8	9
5. Immediate risk to life	6	7	8	9	10

Figure 8.2 Cost Versus Benefit (1) – Risk Matrix

Table 8.1 Cost Versus Benefit (2) – Frequency

Behaviours that challenge	Frequency	Impact	Cost
	Add together for cost		
Hitting staff when angry	5	3	8
Refusing showers	3	3	6
Sleeping in till 11am	2	2	4
Refusing to eat vegetables	4	1	5
Stealing property of others	4	3	7
Cutting their arm when upset	2	5	7

We now need to assess the benefits as perceived by *the individual* who is showing these behaviours.

If we take the following five areas and allocate a score system of 1 for potential benefit and 0 for no benefit perceived, we may have a maximum total of 5 points: emotional, spiritual, social, physical, mental.

So in the example chart (Table 8.1), we could say that hitting has emotional and spiritual benefits. It's an emotional release, and depending on the reaction of staff, this may make the individual feel validated in the moment.

Refusing showers could have emotional, spiritual and mental benefits, as they have control and choice over their own hygiene.

Part of this process is to ensure caregivers are recognising that all behaviour has benefits, even if we struggle to understand them. Just having control over a choice or situation can be a good thing.

Table 8.2 Cost Versus Benefit (3) – Benefit to Individual

Behaviours that challenge	Frequency	Impact	Cost	Benefit to individual =	Total
	Add together for cost			Minus for total	
Hitting staff when angry	5	3	8	2	6
Refusing showers	3	3	6	3	3
Sleeping in till 11am	2	2	4	3	1
Refusing to eat vegetables	4	1	5	4	1
Stealing property of others	4	3	7	2	5
Cutting their arm when upset	2	5	7	1	6

In the example above, it may seem obvious that 'hitting staff' and 'self-harm' are a greater priority than 'sleeping in', but it does allow us to see in black and white which behaviours need examining and managing first. It doesn't mean we ignore the other behaviours forever, but we are picking our battles and not becoming the 'critical parent' who keeps reminding the individual about all their negatives. We may find disagreements in the figures given by different caregivers and other people involved; this is good to explore as these people may have different backgrounds and values or be experiencing the behaviour differently.

The other factor we need to consider when evaluating whether a behaviour is priority or when it should be addressed is Maslow's Hierarchy of Needs and an individual's previous experiences in relation to it.

MASLOW'S HIERARCHY OF NEEDS

American psychologist Abraham Maslow created the well-known 'Hierarchy of Needs', as shown in Figure 8.3.

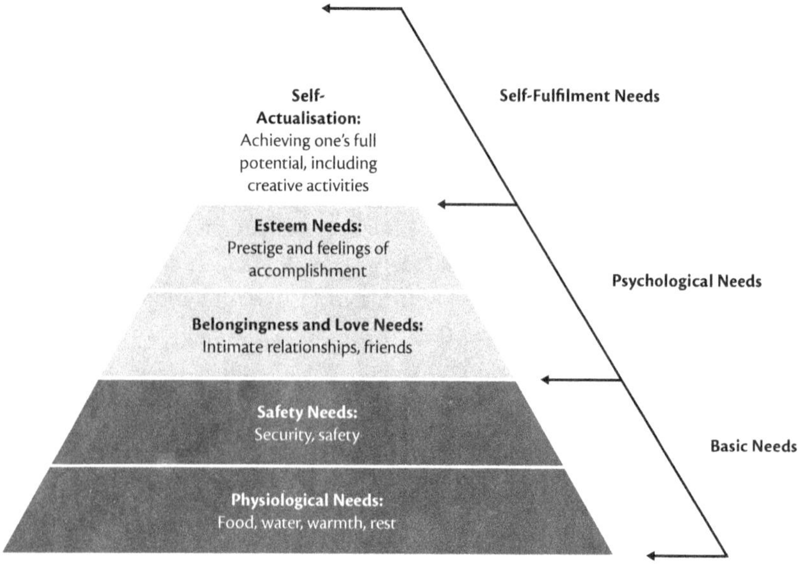

Figure 8.3 Maslow's Hierarchy of Needs

Maslow's Hierarchy of Needs is a motivational theory comprising a five-tier model of human needs.

From the bottom of the hierarchy upwards, the needs are:

1. physiological (food and clothing)
2. safety
3. love and belonging need
4. esteem
5. self-actualisation.

This five-stage model can also be divided into:

- deficiency needs (which includes the basic needs)
- psychological needs
- growth needs (the self-actualisation area).

Deficiency needs arise due to deprivation and are said to motivate people when they are unmet. Also, the motivation to fulfil such needs will become stronger the longer they are denied. For example, the longer a person goes without food (as measured in hours/days), the hungrier they will become; and the longer they have experienced a shortage of food (measured in weeks or longer), the more they will believe that hunger is their normal.

As we will explore more in Stage 2: Understand/Empathise, some individuals may have historically lacked access to the basic needs. (Think about what a typical primary caregiver provides an infant: first, food, warmth and comfort;

then safety; then attachment.) Some individuals may need to be built or rebuilt from the bottom up; for example, we can't expect someone to immediately develop trusting relationships with a caregiver if they don't even trust whether they're going to get a meal today.

Ideally, individuals must have lower-level deficit needs met before progressing to meeting higher-level growth needs. However, needs don't have to be satisfied 100% before the next need emerges.

It is important to note that this model is not rigid; individuals can move up and down through the hierarchy due to changes in circumstances and transitions. For example, let's say an important relationship breaks down in a person's life; as a result, the individual may lose self-esteem.

When we are prioritising behaviours that need to be managed, it is worth using the hierarchy as additional input to the process: the lower on the hierarchy, the higher the priority. Table 8.3 gives an example.

Table 8.3 Cost Versus Benefit (4) – Relevance to Needs

Behaviours that challenge	Frequency	Intensity	Cost	Benefit to individual =	Total	Hierarchy
	Add together for cost			Minus for total		
Stealing and hoarding food	5	3	8	2	6	1
Refusing to talk to staff	5	2	7	1	6	3

In this example, we may decide that the priorities of both behaviours are similar but using the hierarchy we can see that food hoarding is potentially meeting a basic need, whereas social engagement is a psychological need. And therefore we may initially focus on the food-hoarding problem.

As a rule, any transition can cause us to feel unsettled until we recognise that in this new setting our needs will be met. How long this will take is going to be affected by a person's models of the world, previous experiences and habits.

TRAUMA-INFORMED CARE

Severe adverse life events, either as a singular incident or as an ongoing state of being, will impact on how individuals see the levels of the hierarchy within their models of the world. Trauma can trap people in a past state due to the way the emotions and memories invade the present. Our brains are environment expectant and environment dependent. If the neurons in our brain have been laid down in a world of neglect, abuse and chaos, then that is how we will expect the world to be.

To fully satisfy a level of the hierarchy, two elements are needed:

1. The actual need must be met. (Here, in this place, you are fed. Here you are safe. Here you can build connections. Here you are valued and can build self-esteem. Finally, here you can grow and meet your potential.)
2. The individual must *believe* that the need will continue to be met.

Initially it may only be possible to satisfy point 1 – meeting the actual need at each level.

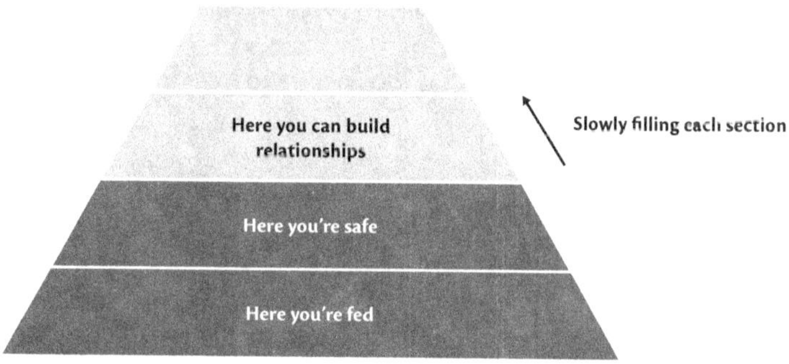

Figure 8.4 Maslow's Hierarchy – Belief

We may then have to help the individual realise that their present is different, that this is the new norm. We can help them to rewire their brain to this new model of understanding. This process takes time.

We may be building a column of trust and habits at each level. This column may be fragile to start with and easily broken.

This development of trust is part of the stabilisation process in the trauma recovery model and needs to be considered in Stage 1: Identify as it may dictate whether addressing certain behaviours should be postponed until the person believes that their basic needs are met and that there is hope and potential for their psychological needs to be met.

There is more information on the trauma recovery model in Chapter 21, page 187.

CHAPTER 9

IDENTIFY POSITIVE BEHAVIOURS

The previous chapter discussed how to identify maladaptive behaviours. This chapter describes the benefits of identifying positive behaviours.

In 'Case Study 5.11 Negative Thoughts and Language' about Ben's arithmetic, we saw that we have a bias towards identifying the negative.

The human brain also has a built-in cognitive bias.

CASE STUDY 9.1 COGNITIVE BIAS – THE NEW CAR

Isn't it the case that when we've just bought a new car, we begin to notice more of the same make and model as our car on the road than before?

It's not that there *are* more of our car type; it's just that we are noticing them more.

And, just as in the case study about the new car, if negative behaviour is identified, suddenly caregivers will start to identify it more often.

The same is true if *positive* behaviours are identified, and so it is essential to identify the individual's positive behaviours, skills and talents. These are 'adaptive' behaviours and can become the foundation for displacing the maladaptive behaviours and raising the person's self-esteem and wellbeing.

There are three parts to identifying positive behaviours.

1. DEFINE AND LIST

Identify what the setting, culture or society views as positive behaviour. What types of behaviours are advantageous to a person's quality of life and overall wellbeing? In Stage 3: Proactive Planning we will look at how to do this on an individual level but here is a general list of a few behaviours we may consider positive.

- Being kind to others.
- Being kind to oneself.
- Treating people with respect.
- Respecting property.

These are very general headings and would need to be more detailed and specific to the setting, but creating a values list of positive behaviours can help an environment to set up strategies to make these behaviours rewarding and valuable and be recognised by the caregivers and the setting as a whole.

For example, can we make 'being kind to others' a valuable behaviour in the setting?

An initial list of behaviours that can be admired, encouraged, rewarded and supported can be the trigger for positive cognitive bias; more and more such behaviours will be observed. Such incidents can be recorded, just as negative behaviours are recorded.

For example:

- 'I was doing the washing up and she came and stood next to me and dried a few of the pots, without saying a word, and then she left the room.'
- 'While I was engaging with him, I noticed he smiled when I talked about my horses. So I showed him a photo and he looked at the pictures with me for approximately six minutes before he disengaged.'
- 'I noticed he was getting agitated, but he went to his room for half an hour and when he came back he seemed in a better mood.'

Part of this recording may include how caregivers reacted or responded to this positive behaviour – was it acknowledged or rewarded in any way?

These observations can help us to develop a better understanding of the individual and their likes and dislikes. This is an important starting point for developing a plan of what reinforcers (see Stage 3: Proactive Planning) seem to work for them and what current abilities we can develop and work with.

2. INDIVIDUAL PREFERENCES

The second step in identifying positives is noting and observing an individual's preferences that seem to stimulate positive behaviours or have a negative or no real impact.

This preference list may be created separately for each setting where the individual spends time; for example, home, school, place of occupation, residential facility, even transport, etc. Where possible, the individual themselves should be involved in its creation, along with a number of key caregivers, depending on the setting.

The following observations can be noted.

- **Preferred activities**: These are activities where there is a consensus that the individual finds them enjoyable or at least not aversive.

- **Disliked activities**: These are activities that the individual seems to get no pleasure from and needs only do insofar as they may be absolutely necessary.

- **Preferred and disliked conversation topics**: Are there topics that seem to increase engagement or any that seem to bore or upset?

- **Preferred people**: These are people with whom the individual clearly enjoys spending time. The more sophisticated the observations done here, the better; e.g.:
  - 'He likes spending time with Anne at home but hates it if Anne visits the school.'
  - 'She likes spending time with Alan, and she likes spending time with Ben, but she doesn't like spending time with them both together.'
  - 'He likes spending time with just one person at a time, and he certainly doesn't like it if he is in a group of more than three people.'

- **Non-preferred people**: Although nobody likes to be a non-preferred person, it is important that we are clear here. Equally, we hope that those named don't take it personally!

- **Interactions between activities and people**: It is important to note any relevant observations; e.g.:
  - 'She likes going to football with John but likes watching films with Ian.'
  - 'She likes watching films with John but televised football with Amy.'

- **Preferred foods, disliked foods or foods that are neither liked nor disliked**: Again, the observations may be quite detailed; e.g.:
  - 'He loves a boiled egg at breakfast time but gets really agitated if you offer him one at teatime.'

- **Finally**: Any observations about any behaviour or activities that can help the individual live according to their preferences and choices.

Such observations can be highly relevant and acted on as far as is practicable.

3. IDENTIFY AN INDIVIDUAL'S ABILITIES AND SKILLS

Make a note of any abilities an individual may have, and encourage staff to spot additional skills.

Examples may include: imagination, assertion, organising, caring, dependability, honesty, curiosity, focus, attention to detail, knowledge, determination, hard work, introspection.

These attributes are skills an individual may already have that we can nurture and direct positively to improve self-esteem and improve outcomes. There are many maladaptive behaviours that, if reframed, we could fit into those skill categories. For example:

- lying requires imagination
- defiance requires assertion
- being nosy requires curiosity.

By focusing on the positive and identifying both the behaviours we desire and the strengths and preferences of the individual, we are already working towards shifting the culture of the environment. And as we will explore in the other sections/stages of the 6STM, this is a vital step.

PART 4

THE 6-STAGE TARGET MODEL STAGE 2

Understand/Empathise

CHAPTER 10

REFLEX

Causes of Behaviours that Challenge

Special terms used in this chapter:

Reason, trigger, cause: These terms are used interchangeably to refer to factors that increase the likelihood of a behaviour occurring.

Function, purpose: These terms are used interchangeably to refer to conscious or unconscious aims of a behaviour.

Benefit, cost, consequence: These terms are used to refer to the outcome of the behaviour whether that was the consciously or unconsciously desired outcome or not.

The causes of behaviours that challenge are many and complex. Over the following chapters we will be exploring the causes, functions and benefits of behaviours and why some people may behave in ways that may seem strange, inappropriate or hazardous to us but are based on their environment, biology and history.

Initially we will break the cause of behaviour into three categories:

- **Reflex**: The person may struggle to control behaviour due to their neurological, cognitive or emotional abilities.
- **Reactive**: The behaviour is triggered by stressors, events or occurrences.
- **Intentional**: A learned response.

Each of these is discussed in its own chapter. This chapter deals with 'reflex'. A reflex is an involuntary or automatic action that your body does in response to something – without you even having to think about it. If your knee-jerk reflex is tested (by tapping just below the knee) you don't decide to kick your leg, it just kicks.

Most people will have experienced a situation where they acted in a way they regretted almost immediately afterwards; for example, saying something nasty when cross, or making an inappropriate statement in a situation by accident, or maybe even breaking something in a fit of rage. These things may not happen constantly, but they do happen. In these examples there was a reflex action that occurred without planning or rational thought.

We often act before thinking, and yet we also so often manage to control, regulate and inhibit these very same reflexes. For instance, let's imagine a situation where someone has wronged you in some way or is irritating you to the point where you feel so angry you feel like hitting them... However, you don't.

But why? Why don't we hit people as our reflexes may want to?

Answer: inhibitors.

Inhibitors override the natural urge to react impulsively; they make us stop and think.

Let's explore a variety of potential inhibitors in the context of hitting someone.

INHIBITOR 1: CONSEQUENCES – I.E., PLANNING

'If I do "X"... result "Y" may happen.'

The first reason we don't hit the person could be the recognition of potential or actual consequences that we perceive as a 'cost' to ourselves.

There could be *legal* consequences from our action, and in turn these could lead to a loss of employment, and restrictions on movements and whom we're allowed to see.

There could be *social* consequences, such as loss of standing in the community or damage to a relationship.

There's the risk of *retaliation*; maybe the other person is stronger or has the ability to make life difficult.

There's the risk of *harming* oneself or the other person in any sort of violence – breaking a hand or accidentally killing someone, for example.

There's the *emotional* risk that feelings of shame and guilt could be induced after carrying out the action.

There could be *financial* consequences, such as having to pay for compensation or repairs, a fine or higher insurance premiums.

Consequences are dependent on our values as we will explore in inhibitor 2; as an example, though, let's take social consequences. If a person belongs to a social group that sees violence and losing one's temper as a weakness, then that person will view the consequences of hitting as negative. However, if they belong to a group where the culture is 'you hit first' and 'don't back down ever', then that person may view not hitting as the weaker action.

Therefore, consequences and values are connected.

INHIBITOR 2: VALUES

Is a violent act wrong?

On the face of it, the answer is 'yes'.

But suppose it was in self-defence? Or you were in a boxing match? Or in a military battle?

So violence may be appropriate, given the appropriate setting, although a pacifist who renounces violence may stand by a fixed view that all violence is wrong, with no exceptions.

What about lying? We tell children off for that behaviour, and when our politicians do it we condemn them, but think about occasions when we teach people to lie.

Perhaps a child receives a Christmas gift from Granny, but the gift isn't liked. Nonetheless, the parents might ask the child to write to Granny saying it was a lovely gift, because telling the truth could be hurtful. This is the 'white lie'.

Or stealing. Should someone steal medication to save their sick mother's life if they have no way to afford it? Should someone be punished for taking, without asking, that stationery from work for a home project as it's only small?

The above examples show that our *values* about any topic aren't fixed, aren't absolute. They dynamically adapt according to the context, our perception and our justifications.

So, how do we acquire our values? This is an age-old philosophical and psychological question that may always be asked, but here are a few simple factors:

- **Primary caregiver experiences at an early age**: The household might have a value of 'Never raise a hand in anger'. Another household might habitually smack.
- **During child development**: Our values can be acquired from such sources as peer pressure, role models (such as teachers, gang leaders, group leaders) or even celebrities.
- **Society**: The values exhibited by the society, as seen through media and social interaction.
- **Cultural values**: A set of ideas, beliefs, attitudes, etiquette and rules that belong to a certain group or institution. Most people belong to more than one group, and each may have slightly different cultures, and so our behaviour may vary depending on the group we are with.

So, to repeat: our values are not quite as fixed as we might imagine, and everyone's values will vary and change over time due to experiences, environment and circumstances.

INHIBITOR 3: TRAINING AND PREVIOUS EXPERIENCE

Many people at some stage in their lives have exhibited aggressive behaviour and other behaviours that challenge. That stage has become known as 'the terrible twos'. Most children learn and/or are taught that life is easier if such behaviours are dropped – it's not the best way of engaging with other people, or meeting our needs, or coping with our emotions. Unfortunately, that isn't the case for everyone, and sometimes even the well-adapted can regress. This will also be looked at in significantly more detail in Chapter 15, page 135, where intentional behaviours that challenge are discussed.

The three inhibitors just covered are the reasons why we don't hit. The next inhibitor covers our ability to recognise our emotions and the alternative strategies we may choose. What did we do rather than hit them? We... walked away... took deep breaths... kept it verbal... planned our revenge.

INHIBITOR 4: SELF-CONTROL

There are three factors related to self-control.

1. Learned Behaviour, Either Positive or Not So Positive

CASE STUDY 10.1 THE HOLE IN THE WALL

Ned was Jack's father. Ned had a quick temper, and he knew it. When he was angry, he had a habit of throwing his fists towards inanimate objects like boxes, doors and sometimes even walls, which had twice resulted in him breaking his hand in the process. Jack had witnessed this act on multiple occasions during his childhood.

Years later, when Jack was an adult, his parents came to decorate his bedroom; they found a hole in a partition wall that, in a temper, Jack had punched through. The hole had been concealed with a poster. The parents called Jack to criticise him for the damage they had found.

Did Jack's parents have a right to be annoyed at Jack, or should it have been annoyance at their role modelling? Because as much as parents say 'It's do as I say, not do as I do!', children learn what they see, as we will explore in 'Teaching Technique: Role Modelling', Chapter 25, page 225.

Jack had learned this method to release his anger. Some may argue that it's better to hit some-*thing* rather than some-*one*.

Nonetheless, it's important to note that although damage to another person may have been avoided, there is potential damage to Jack's hand and property (hitting objects is a form of self-harm). And what happens if there is no object to hit – only a person – and we have no other way to manage our feelings?

Violence can be an effective release of tension and feel cathartic; there is often some immediate lowering of stress levels. However, that doesn't mean the person is calm after hitting... they're just not as aroused as they were before they hit. There are other methods that will be explored through this book that look at coping strategies that allow a person to actually feel calm in stressful situations.

2. Self-Control Based on Emotional Intelligence

We all have different types of intelligence; for example, artistic, engineering, social (someone with high social intelligence tends to be great with people, for example).

We also have emotional intelligence, which includes the ability to recognise our own emotional stress and manage it. If the emotion is anger, our emotional intelligence will warn us that corrective action needs to be taken.

All types of intelligence have a spectrum... some people have high artistic intelligence, some low and so on.

There is a condition called alexithymia where an individual does not recognise internal signs of emotions, know how to label them or react to them. They are almost emotionally blind. This condition can be caused by numerous factors but can be found in those on the autistic spectrum and those who have experienced trauma. It is harder to control your anger if you didn't realise you were getting angry in the first place.

3. The Window of Tolerance

We will explore the window of tolerance within polyvagal theory in more detail at the end of Chapter 12, but within the context of inhibitors it is worth looking at the following analogy. The window of tolerance concept was coined by Dan Siegel in his 1999 book *The Developing Mind*.

CASE STUDY 10.2 THE WINDOW OF TOLERANCE

Imagine every person is born with a different size container: some people carry a thimble, some carry an egg cup, others a mug, a jug or even a barrel.

This container represents their window of tolerance.

Imagine I take two people and give them identical experiences where bad events kept happening – little things like a broken clock, bad traffic, a small fall, a little argument. Every bad thing is represented by a marble. Each marble is placed into each person's container. After five marbles, the containers of some people are full and overflowing. Others can fit lots of marbles in their container with room to spare.

We often look around and assume that everyone has the same size container. 'I can cope, their sibling can cope, that other person can cope, so why can't they?' Maybe their container is smaller or their container already had marbles in it before you started counting.

Another case study explores a similar phenomenon about how angry different people get when faced with the same triggers (see 'Case Study 14.2 How Angry Do You Get?', page 127).

Commentary: In this case study, the containers represent our emotional resilience, which is made up of both biological and psychological factors. These will be explored more in the further chapters on understanding and empathising throughout Part 4.

WHERE DO INHIBITORS COME FROM?

The inhibitors above all involve the use of a particular region of the brain called the frontal lobes. The brain is the most complex structure in the known universe, so the following is a fairly simplistic breakdown of neurological processes to allow a layperson some basic understanding.

The Frontal Lobes

> The frontal lobes of the brain are located directly behind the forehead. They are the largest section of the human brain, and they are also the region that is most commonly affected by traumatic brain injury. The frontal lobes are important for voluntary movement, expressive language and managing higher-level executive functions.
>
> Executive functions are a collection of cognitive skills that include the capacity to plan, organise, initiate, self-monitor and control one's responses to achieve a goal. The frontal lobes are considered our behaviour and emotional control centre and home to our personality.[19]

'The executive functions' role is similar to a conductor's role within an orchestra. The conductor manages, directs, organises and integrates each member of the orchestra. They cue each musician so they know when to begin to play and how fast or slow, loud or soft to play and when to stop playing.'[20] This is how your frontal lobes manage the rest of your brain functions.

It's this part of your brain that allows you to plan: 'If I do this, this could happen next.' It allows you to see consequences. It allows you to predict other people's reactions – 'If I do this, this could cause them to do that' – and to empathise, to understand how another person might be feeling.

Empathy and experiencing how actions affect others are factors that also affect our values and how we want to make the other person feel.

This is also the part of the brain that allows us to have a theory of mind: 'Well, I think this but maybe they think that, and maybe they think that I think this. There are different ways of looking at this. So maybe I'm not right.'

This 'conductor' checks all other factors like environmental risks or social implications of actions to decide at lightning speed on the right action in the moment. It does a split-second risk assessment for reflexes. Think about how the same person may have different reflexes to the same emotion depending on if they know they are on CCTV or they're in a car, on the internet, in the privacy of their own home, in public or in front of their children.

So, this part of the brain acts like a filter; it makes us stop and think. It inhibits our impulses.

The Limbic System and the Amygdala

But behind the frontal lobe, our filter, there is an area of the brain called the limbic system – your 'thrive to survive' area of the brain. This area of the brain processes emotions and memory; it's our reward centre and where we form habits, as well as where we manage our basic survival requirements of hunger, thirst, temperature regulation and pain regulation among others. Within this part of the brain is the amygdala. Simply stated, the amygdala is primarily associated with emotional processes and is the trigger for our fight-or-flight response.[21]

CASE STUDY 10.3 TABLE MANNERS

You see some food on a table, you're really hungry, you haven't eaten all day. Your limbic brain says, 'Let's eat.'

Problem is... you're in a restaurant and the food is in front of someone else. You don't just take it – your frontal lobe activates your inhibitors.

For example, you realise that a consequence of taking the food could be that you get thrown out of the restaurant or the person may hit you if you take their chips. Your values may say that stealing is wrong; you also recognise that although you are hungry, you can wait a little longer, you can delay gratification.

Your learned experience also informs you that if you sit down and order some food and have money to pay for it, you'll be able to meet your needs in a more socially acceptable way.

Whereas an animal would have no such inhibitions and would be eating that food if its flight response wasn't triggered instead.

The frontal lobe is more developed in humans than any other animal.

We also use the frontal lobe for certain social interactions.

CASE STUDY 10.4 WEIRD HAIR

You meet a person with a slightly unusual hairstyle. Your impulse might be to laugh or tell them that they look strange. But you don't just come out and say that, because maybe they'll be upset by the criticism. Maybe they won't like you if you say that.

So again, you look at the consequences and your values, and you inhibit that behaviour and ignore the impulse.

But what would a young child say on meeting a person with an unusual hairstyle? They're likely to just come out and say something. Now that may be down to some social learning and experience, but it is also because the frontal lobe is the last part of the brain to fully mature.

The frontal lobe is the most human part of our brain, and it takes time to develop. On average, full brain maturity is attained around the age of 26; generally, maturity comes slightly later for males. The range of ages for brain maturity is quite wide: for females, it can start in the early 20s; for males it can even reach the early 30s.

CASE STUDY 10.5 THE STROOP EFFECT

(Note: There is a wealth of information available online about this effect that is named after its main proponent, psychologist John Ridley Stroop.)

Experiments show that impulsive reactions occur much more quickly than rational reactions. The basic test is to measure the difference in time it takes for volunteers to name the font colour of a list of words that are also colours. When the words don't match the colour of the font (e.g., the word is 'red' but it's in green ink), it takes significantly longer to name the font colour than when the font colour and word correspond. There are many variations of the basic test.

Try it yourself at: https://faculty.washington.edu/chudler/java/ready.html.

There are numerous complex processes occurring in the Stroop test but put simply: your impulse is to read the word, as that is an automatic habit. Your executive function must inhibit that impulse and allow the actual target behaviour to occur. In the list where the colour and word match, there is no conflict between the impulse and the required action. In the non-matching list, the conflict of the two causes a slight delay and feels harder. The Stroop test shows our ability to control behaviour. If asked to state the colour of the font rather than the word, we must overcome the initial and stronger stimuli to read the word.

Commentary: Research shows that the time it takes to read the non-matching list decreases with age from early childhood through early adulthood. This reinforces the idea that executive function and speed of processing improves with development of the frontal lobes.[22]

CHILD DEVELOPMENT

Children and adolescents have an underdeveloped pre-frontal cortex. Adolescents undergo a significant rewiring and reorganising of the brain that impacts on the functioning of the frontal lobes and adolescent behaviour. The adolescent period typically begins at about the age of 11 and ends around the age of 30. During this time, the limbic system (the 'thrive to survive' area) develops faster[23] and is relied on more as 'unused connections in the thinking and processing part of our child brain (called the grey matter) are "pruned" away.'[24] The front part of the brain is remodelled last.

It's like a defragging computer. While the system is clearing unused files and reorganising to make the computer more efficient, it must rely on its more basic programs to keep functioning.

Additional Information

There is also a change in brain chemicals during adolescence: the levels of the neurotransmitters dopamine and serotonin in the limbic system change. Neurotransmitters are chemicals that allow information to be transmitted around the brain. These two chemicals can make adolescents 'more emotional and more responsive to rewards and stress.'[25] Dopamine is a neurotransmitter in the brain associated with pleasure and attuning to the environment during decision making. During adolescence, dopamine levels increase. The increased dopamine activity in adolescence increases risk-taking behaviour, novelty- and pleasure-seeking behaviour and vulnerability to boredom and social pressures. 'Serotonin is involved in the regulation of mood and behaviour.'[26] It is known as the 'calming chemical'. Serotonin eases tension and stress and can inhibit the excitement and sometimes recklessness that dopamine can produce. If there is a defect in the serotonin processing in the brain, impulsive or hazardous behaviour can result.

Lumen Learning explains that: 'When stress, arousal or sensations become extreme, the adolescent brain is flooded with impulses that overwhelm the rational brain and can result in risk-taking behaviours, emotional outbursts and reduced inhibitions because of the chemical imbalance and the frontal lobes still developing.'[27]

Should we be surprised when teenagers act selfishly or impulsively or about why they struggle to see how their behaviour impacts on other people? The explanation often given by observers is: 'Oh, it's their hormones kicking in.' A better explanation would be: 'Oh, their frontal lobe is underdeveloped and their neurotransmitters are all over the place.'

Other than basic child development, there are many factors that affect the way the brain works and can impact on reflex.

In the next chapter we'll explore more about how our brain and nervous system work to manage and regulate our behaviour, and examine numerous conditions, illnesses and factors that may impact on this.

CHAPTER 11

THE HUMAN NERVOUS SYSTEM

Causes of Behaviours that Challenge

Let's look at the human nervous system.

Extract from *An Introduction To The Sympathetic and Parasympathetic Nervous System* by Roxanna Salim

The nervous system is split up into the central nervous system and the peripheral nervous system. The central nervous system refers to the brain and spinal cord, while the peripheral nervous system is split up into the somatic and autonomic nervous systems.

The somatic nervous system is involved in the movement of our skeletal muscles. The autonomic nervous system – which as the name suggests is involved in a number of typically automatic, regulatory functions – is then further split into the sympathetic nervous system (SNS) and the parasympathetic nervous system (PNS).

These two systems are activated in times of arousal or recovery. Put simply, SNS activation triggers a 'fight-or-flight' response, and PNS activation leads to a 'rest-and-digest' response; or in extreme situations of danger the PNS may trigger 'freeze or fawn/submit' responses.

The fight-or-flight response is a mobilisation/hyperarousal state and involves the SNS changing bodily processes to mobilise for action and help prepare for a perceived threat. Changes include inhibition of the digestive and immune systems, increases in pupil size and heart rate, expansion of the lungs and the release of adrenaline/noradrenaline. These processes are meant to optimise functions in the body when it's under attack – you won't benefit from digesting food, but you're likely to need more oxygen from the lungs.

To facilitate the rest-and-digest response, the PNS alters several functions in the body to help it recover. These functions are largely mirror opposites of SNS activation, and include stimulation of the digestive and immune systems, decreases in pupil size and heart rate, and contraction of the lungs. These processes optimize functions in the body at rest and allow it to focus on maintenance.[28]

This rest state also allows facilitation of social engagement and connection.

However, in extreme circumstances of danger, it's possible that fight-or-flight responses are either perceived as unavailable or appear to have failed. The only other survival responses available involve immobilisation/hypoarousal. This is where the PNS jumps in and slams a brake on the SNS to increase survival chances. These responses may include 'play dead', 'don't move and maybe I can survive this' (freeze) or 'I'll do whatever you want, just don't hurt me' (submit/fawn). In this survival mode, once the danger is over, the body is in a charged state of fight/flight that has been paused by the freeze response and so reactivation of the SNS tends to happen immediately following the immobilisation state.

CASE STUDY 11.1 THE GAZELLE

A young gazelle is with its mother. The mother spots a leopard; initially the mother becomes alert but stays still, watching. The young gazelle senses the mother's stress and so stays close, hiding behind her (social engagement to feel safer).

The leopard starts to move closer; the mother moves into flight response and the young gazelle does the same.

The leopard catches the young gazelle; the young gazelle struggles to escape for a moment, with no success. The young gazelle goes limp (freeze).

The mother tries to fight and tries to ram the leopard. The leopard responds back with fight and runs at the mum to back her away, but to do this it releases the young gazelle.

The young gazelle suddenly bursts into life (flight) and runs back to its mum. The leopard, now tired, has missed its kill.

Humans react in many of the same ways as the young gazelle; the difference is that it's often not a leopard that triggers these survival responses. The triggers range from genuine threats like a confrontation with a person (although this person could be a family member, who may or may not be an actual threat) to a job interview, an exam or anything our brains perceive as a threat, whether rational or, like a phobia, irrational. The reaction we exhibit may also be different. *Fight* may be displayed as controlling or confrontational behaviour; *flight* as anxiety; *freeze* as silence and withdrawal; *submit* as people pleasing and avoiding confrontation.

It is also understood that we learn from these experiences and begin to adapt our responses based on the strategies that we perceive as successful.

So a gazelle may instinctively run from a leopard, whereas a rabbit may freeze when faced with a fox; a rat may attack a cat when it's cornered, and a dog may drop its head in submission to another dog. We often learn to be the gazelle, rat, rabbit or fox from early life experiences and may continue to use that strategy in other similar events, whether or not it is needed.

CASE STUDY 11.2 THE SPIDER AND THE CHILD

A spider lands on a young child; the child immediately freezes in fear. The spider moves on. The child's brain makes a connection. Because you froze, you survived. Now the child is an adult, but whenever a spider is spotted the adult is frozen to the spot.

CASE STUDY 11.3 THE SHOUTER

A dad gets very angry with his son Jim... 'Look at me when I'm talking to you, and don't you move.' Jim stays still (freeze) to not cause further anger. Although Jim wasn't in true danger, the brain has made a connection.

As an adult, a colleague shouts at Jim for something that wasn't his fault. Rather than defend himself, Jim says nothing; he just stands and takes it. Afterwards, Jim sits at his desk. A colleague comes to ask Jim a question. Jim loses his temper and shouts at the colleague to leave him alone. (The fight response has now been activated.)

In the gazelle example, you can follow the activation of the SNS, then the PNS and then back to the SNS again. Within minutes of escape, that young gazelle will be back to a full PNS response and be nibbling on grass.

In Case Study 11.3, you can see a similar activation of the SNS to the PNS and back to SNS again. However, due to the developed human brain, the neocortex gets involved in recovery and prevents the natural emotional brain from acting out its response and releasing the charge (the built-up adrenaline/noradrenaline). It holds on to the charge and then potentially releases the brakes at inappropriate times (e.g., when the environmental or social inhibitors are reduced, allowing the individual's primitive brain to recognise the reduced risk of SNS activation*) or in maladaptive ways. If the charge can't release, it can build and build until a trigger causes full mobilisation and the SNS overreacts to events that really don't deserve that reaction.

---

* When we feel stressed, having an attachment figure to whom we can turn to re-regulate is the fastest and most effective way to de-escalate. If we don't have a secure attachment figure available, our SNS can get charged up with fight-or-flight potential. However, if environmental or social inhibitors prevent release of that charge, our PNS kicks in and puts the SNS on pause; we may just go quiet and hold it all in. Unfortunately, when inhibitors change, that charge may then be released and the SNS reactivated. This may be displayed as directed aggression towards someone we are actually attached to, who was unconnected to the original cause. This description can help us to understand why a child may behave at school but then pick an argument with mum as soon as they are picked up. Or why a person who is stressed at work keeps snapping at their partner at home.

The next section explores the process of amygdala hijacking to further explain these responses.

AMYGDALA HIJACKING

CASE STUDY 11.4 'OH! IT'S YOU!'

Your friend sneaks up behind you, and yells, '*Boo!*' It triggers a flinch response (you jump). But you don't end up punching them or running out of the house, because almost immediately you realise, 'Oh, it's them, they aren't a danger.'

So what has happened here? Psychologist Daniel Goleman coined the term 'amygdala hijack'.[29]

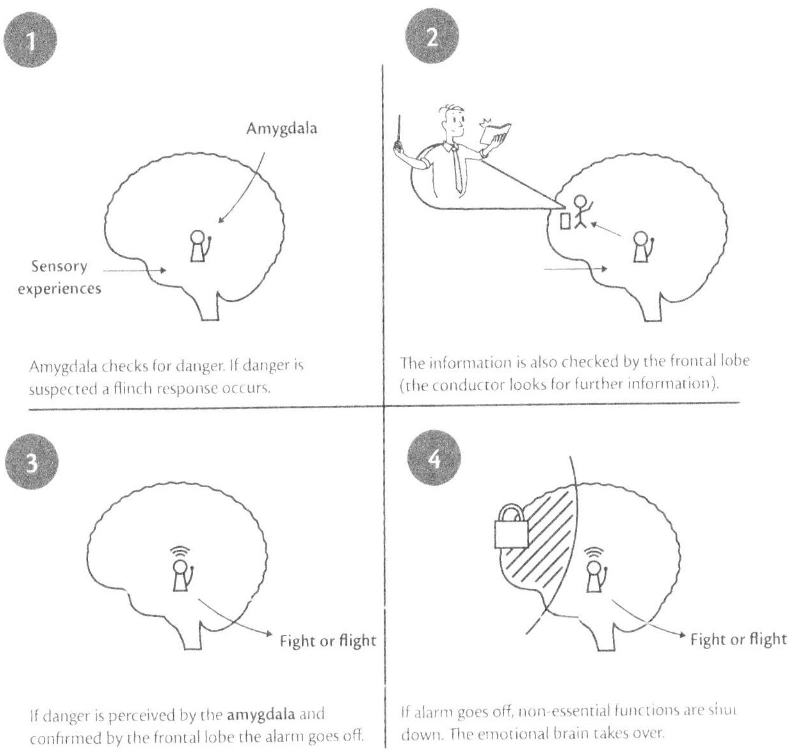

Figure 11.1 Amygdala Hijacking

Information enters our brain through our senses. If something alarming occurs, we may instinctively flinch, preparing for survival (fight/flight/freeze/submit).

So everything we see, smell, feel, hear and taste enters the brain to be processed. The information goes through the thalamus, which is like a gateway. The thalamus then splits the information to two areas, one of which is the primitive amygdala. The amygdala, which is in the limbic area of the brain (or emotional area of the brain), acts like a smoke alarm that fires when it perceives danger, triggering our primitive survival behaviours.

The sensory information is also passed to the rational part of the brain, the neocortex (the frontal lobe (the conductor) and temporal lobe). This happens milliseconds after the amygdala's reaction.

The mechanics are complex and made up of multiple variables, but in some instances of alarm, the amygdala's fight/flight/freeze/submit response is calmed by the neocortex that assesses the situation, recognises our friend and decides 'no danger', and so we don't hit our friend who yells 'Boo'.

But in other instances, the amygdala's fight/flight/freeze/submit response takes control before any calming process can occur. In some cases, this might be appropriate action – I see a hungry lion coming towards me. However, in other cases, I may indeed lash out at my friend if he ambushes me in a dark alleyway. Only after I've hit him does the rational brain realise the error.

When the amygdala takes control, it is known as 'adrenal hijacking' or 'amygdala hijacking', and the rational brain is shut down. Emotional management is all about controlling and inhibiting this amygdala takeover and acting logically instead.

CASE STUDY 11.5 SURVIVAL

I'm walking across the savanna when I see a lion approaching. I don't have time to wonder if, perhaps, the lion is friendly, is vegetarian or has already eaten today – do I run or fight (black-and-white thinking)?

I also don't need to talk to the lion, sleep or digest food. All these are a waste of valuable energy, so these functions are deactivated to allow energy to be used for running or fighting.

CASE STUDY 11.6 TONGUE-TIED

I'm in a job interview. I'm nervous. Suddenly my vocabulary seems to have disappeared – I can't find the words and I'm stumbling over my words.

Two guys are squaring up to each other outside the pub. Their argument has deteriorated to swearing and monosyllabic communication: 'Yeah... so!'

CASE STUDY 11.7 THE ROW WITH YOUR PARTNER

We're arguing. It's become heated. The original point of the argument has been lost, it's become just emotional content and nasty comments we don't even mean (nasty comments and swear words aren't stored in the same area of the brain as regular language, which is why swearing is more likely when we are angry, have hurt ourselves or have a condition like dementia that can impact on Broca's area of the brain where expressive communication originates). Everything they're saying is wrong (black-and-white thinking – I'm right, so they must be wrong). The anger grows further. We walk away before we act in a way we would regret.

Humans have ingrained survival mechanisms where the rational brain can become overwhelmed by the primitive – amygdala hijacking. The more the alarm (amygdala) goes off, the harder we find it to engage our logical brain and inhibit our survival responses.

There are many factors that can affect this ability. Some people's alarm bells can become hypersensitive, making it hard to regulate and unpredictable; a major cause of this is trauma, which we'll look at in the next chapter.

CHAPTER 12

TRAUMA

Causes of Behaviours that Challenge

We can summarise trauma with the following definition:

> Trauma is the response to a deeply distressing or disturbing event that overwhelms an individual's ability to cope, causes feelings of helplessness, diminishes their sense of self and their ability to feel the full range of emotions and experiences.[30]

The important aspect of this definition is that there is not an external threshold for what counts as trauma. It's the internal experience that makes it traumatic.

Suppose something bad happens to you in a 'green room'. Not a catastrophe, but something unpleasant. Next day, you happen to walk into another 'green room'. You may be reminded of yesterday's incident and may feel a slight emotional response but be able to shrug it off.

A similar example might be... while waiting at a red light in our car, we might get bumped from behind. Next time we get into the car we may feel apprehensive. But the memory of the bump has been stored as an emotional and a rational memory, and the rational brain will decide, 'Different day, different situation,' and maintain control over the emotional response.

Now suppose that what happened in the 'green room' was something we perceived as life threatening to us or someone else and we felt helpless to escape or avoid it. In such a circumstance, walking into another 'green room' the next day could, by association, trigger another alarm. Although it wasn't the colour green that was the danger, the information coming through your senses triggers the amygdala hijack.

Returning to the car accident example... suppose the accident was really bad. It could be the case that the emotional alarm is retriggered by getting into a car, so much so that as we go to get into a car again we are overwhelmed by an urge to avoid and take flight.

The immediate alarm response and the effect it may have for a few hours to a few days is known as Peri trauma. If this same emotional response effect lasts up to a month, it could be classed as acute stress disorder. If it lasts longer than a month, it could be classified as post-traumatic stress disorder (PTSD). The trauma effect may not occur immediately following the event; it may develop over a period of time after the event.

The following diagram indicates the normal process flow of an emotional incident.

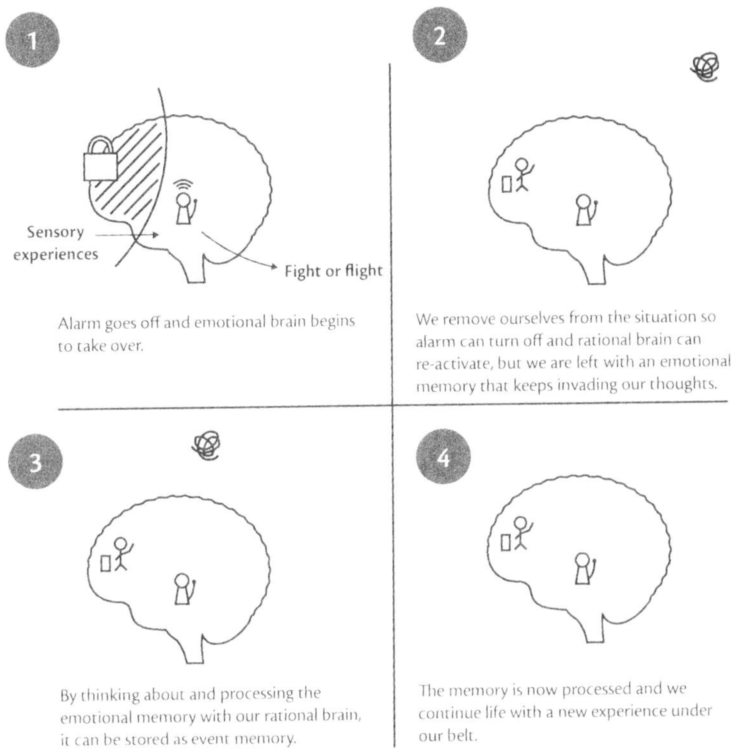

Figure 12.1 Normal Emotional Processing

The incident occurs, the alarm goes off and an emotional memory is created. When the amygdala determines that there is no longer danger, the alarm bell subsides and the rational brain reactivates and allows us to process the fragmented emotional memory over into an event memory.

CASE STUDY 12.1 THE ROW WITH YOUR PARTNER (PAGE 106) – REVISITED

We're arguing. It's become heated. The original point of the argument has been lost. The alarm bell has gone off.

But inhibitors such as my emotional intelligence kick in. They tell me that if I don't move away, I might do or say something I'll later regret.

So I move away, calm down, and let the rational brain process what happened.

As I'm calming, though, I may keep replaying the argument in my head: 'I should have said that,' or 'Them saying that hurt.' Emotional memories are disjointed though. You don't replay the argument from start to finish, you remember random parts of it, often out of order (therefore even when calm, you and your partner may have very different recollections of what happened as you will lay down the memories differently based on your experience, perspective and emotions).

Being able to turn off the alarm and be safe and calm allows us to engage our rational brain – to process the event from emotional memory to event memory, where we can revisit the event but not be emotionally triggered by it. Once we have processed the memory in this way, we are able to reorganise our understanding of the person we argued with, reintegrate with the person and then adapt our relationship based on this experience that no longer triggers emotional feelings.

However, suppose that the event is not just emotional and unpleasant but also overwhelming. The diagram changes, as follows:

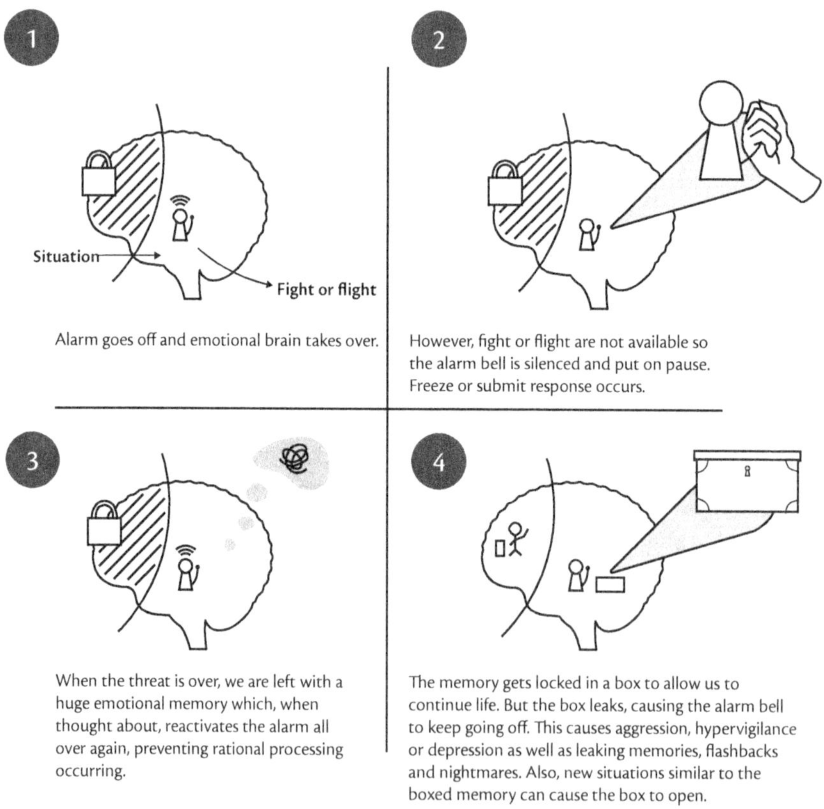

Figure 12.2 Trauma-Related Stress Disorders

In this case, amygdala hijacking has occurred. The alarm is triggered, and the emotional memory is created. However, the difference now is that neither safety nor, therefore, calm can be reached or, due to the individual's severe response to the event, the emotional memory is so big, strong and terrifying that even thinking about the event causes it to replay and retrigger the alarm. The rational brain keeps being deactivated and doesn't have the opportunity to process the information and turn what happened into event memory.

So the person is stuck with this emotional memory that keeps invading their thoughts – just like after the argument – but it is debilitating, as it keeps triggering survival responses. The person has to adapt because they have to get on with their life and continue to function; so their brain protects itself by saying, 'I just won't think about it anymore.'

Imagine the memory is locked inside a box in the non-conscious. The only problem is that the box tends to leak, and when it leaks it retriggers the alarm. And the person can, for example, show fight/flight through behaviours such as hypervigilance, anxiety or aggression, or show the freeze response through numbness, withdrawal or depression. Flashbacks and nightmares can also be triggered as the box leaks those disjointed emotional memories. The sufferer will also try to avoid situations that might reopen the box, and, using the earlier example, will avoid all 'green rooms'.

All the above effects are symptoms of PTSD.

The diagnostic criteria of simple PTSD include:

- exposure to death, threatened death, actual or threatened serious injury, or actual or threatened sexual violence
- the traumatic event being persistently re-experienced – flashbacks, nightmares
- the individual avoiding trauma-related stimuli after the trauma – avoiding 'green rooms'
- negative thoughts or feelings that begin or worsen after the trauma
- trauma-related arousal and reactivity that begins or worsens after the trauma fight-or-flight responses
- symptoms lasting for more than one month
- symptoms creating distress or functional impairment (e.g., social, occupational).

SIMPLE PTSD AND COMPLEX PTSD

In the previous chapter, we reviewed innocuous events, such as preparing for a job interview, that nonetheless can cause anxiety, sleepless nights and so on, temporarily affecting a person's life.

Earlier in this chapter we also reviewed a singular traumatic event – a serious car accident – that caused PTSD. This is termed 'Simple PTSD'.

There is also a condition known as 'Complex PTSD'. This is characterised by an individual experiencing any of the following:

- Childhood abuse, neglect or abandonment.
- Trauma that lasted a long time.
- Situations where escape or rescue from a traumatic situation were unlikely or impossible; e.g., being tortured, being kidnapped and being a prisoner of war.
- Multiple traumas.
- Being harmed by someone close (e.g., a relative).
- Ongoing domestic violence or abuse.
- Repeatedly witnessing violence or abuse.
- Being forced to become a sex worker.[31]

The effects of these events on an individual can be especially noticeable if they happen in early life when the young brain doesn't have the ability to rationalise the experiences.

An example might be a child who has experienced domestic abuse every weekend for the past five years. How many 'green rooms' or 'leaking boxes' might they have? And as the years go by, if the individual hasn't managed to safely process these events, their general mental health can be significantly affected.

It is worth exploring the study of adverse childhood experiences and how they have long-term impact on physiology, psychology and even neural development. See Appendix 2, 'The Adverse Childhood Experiences (ACE) Study'.

It is fair to say that most people have experienced some traumas in their lives whether they were extreme or low level. These experiences can shape how we see the world, how we expect things to happen and how we react to it. At any time we can get stuck in past events and re-experience thoughts, feelings and reactions of our past selves. It is one of the reasons we can all overreact to situations in the present.

CASE STUDY 12.2 CHEATED IN LOVE

The love of your life cheated on you when you were 18 years old. You were devastated and spent the next month wallowing in a self-induced pity party. You kept imagining the event, and when you did, you re-experienced the pain, anxiety and anger. You grieved the relationship and slowly recovered.

You are now 32 and despite numerous failed attempts have just met the partner of your dreams and you are starting to fall for them.

One evening, on a night out with your partner, you nip to the toilet and on your return you see them talking to an attractive member of the opposite sex. Your chest suddenly feels tight, you feel sick, all your muscles feel tense and your heart is racing. You keep your composure, and as you reach your partner, the stranger has already moved away. You ask their identity and are told they are 'just a friend'.

You struggle for the rest of the night; you become quiet and it's impossible to let loose, relax and have fun. When you both get home at the end of the night, you end up in a blazing row with your partner because they said they weren't hungry but are now stealing the chips you bought for yourself. You realise the chip argument is petty and stupid and you don't really understand why this little thing has triggered your anger.[32]

Commentary: So, what has happened here? The following diagram explains it:

Event severity 1–10	Baggage	Reaction severity 1–10
→	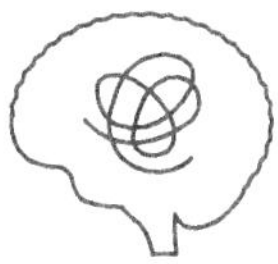	→
Event severity 1		Reaction severity 8
Partner talking to an old friend, no matter who they are, should not really be a bad thing.	Hits emotional baggage from past experiences of being cheated on. The event is accelerated to an 8, triggering feelings of loss, fear, anger.	Fight or flight is being activated, but because of inhibitors, the argument cannot happen there and then. We may also be wrestling with our rational brain ('it's fine, don't react...') but the event keeps emotionally invading. Unfortunately, when home is reached, the environmental inhibitors are no longer there, and the freeze response now becomes fight.

Figure 12.3 Emotional Baggage

Trauma, adverse childhood experiences and our early experiences of care and attachment figures (or lack of them) will stay with us throughout our lives and guide our models of who we are, how others will treat us and whether other people can be trusted. In turn, this can affect our behaviour and reactions to situations. It is worth understanding more about attachment theory as all of us are affected by our early-life attachments.

THE ATTACHMENT PROCESS

When born, human babies are more like baby birds than babies of other mammal species. Most mammals, within a few minutes of being born, are capable of moving independently, of finding the source of their mother's milk and so on. Whereas human babies are like nestlings – totally dependent on a caregiver.

In fact, human babies are effectively born prematurely. This is because the human brain is large in comparison with other mammals, and if birth were delayed until brain maturity, the size of the baby's head would make passage through the birth canal impossible.

Human babies are born with the brainstem (the alarm bell system) more developed than other functions. They lie down and cry for assistance: 'I'm hungry,' 'I'm uncomfortable,' and so on. Therefore, attachment to a caregiver is massively important.

The attachment is like a piece of string with the baby at one end and the caregiver at the other. Both can pull on the string at times. The baby can cry for attention, the caregiver attends. Or the caregiver can pull the string to get nearer to the baby to show love, to smile, to engage, to be there.

Later, the baby's limbic system within the brain grows, and the baby starts to develop a core belief that it matters in the world: 'If I need attention because I'm hungry, or in pain, or scared because I've heard a loud bang and I don't know what it means – I get the attention. And I learn that other people are good and kind – they come and make me comfortable again.'

The baby is incapable of calming itself; it needs the caregiver to turn off the alarm bells that the baby is experiencing.

The baby and caregiver share eye contact, the baby follows the gaze of the caregiver and the two look at things together. The baby smiles; the caregiver smiles.

The baby is developing a cognitive understanding of the world.

This is known as the Arousal Relaxation Cycle, as shown here:

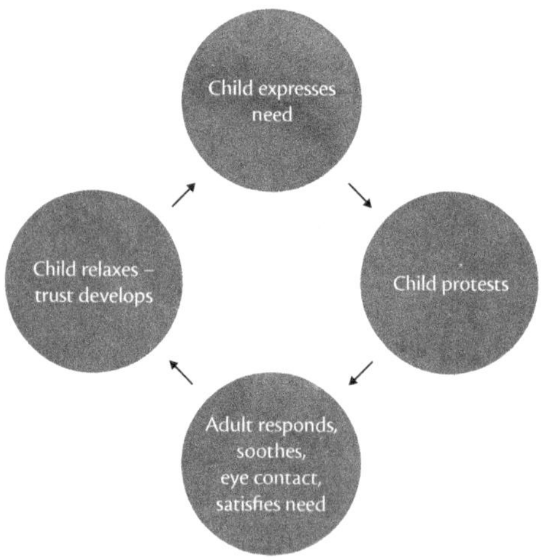

Figure 12.4 The Arousal Relaxation Cycle[33]

In this process, the primary caregiver consistently provides basic necessities (food, shelter and warmth) as well as emotional essentials (touch, movement, eye contact and smiles).[34] This process is repeated and repeated, and a *secure attachment* is built between the child and caregiver or caregivers.

But what happens when attachments do not develop securely?

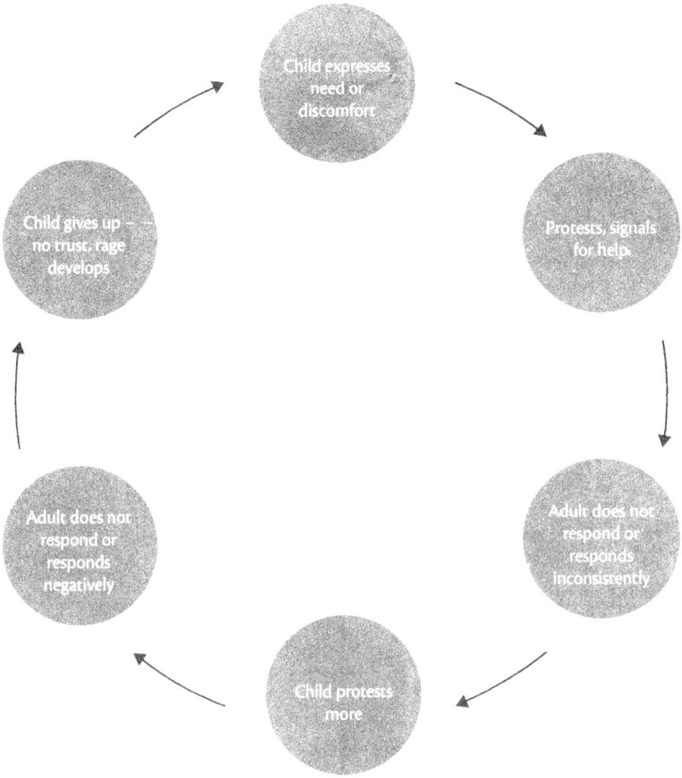

Figure 12.5 Disturbed Attachment Cycle

The child experiences the same need or discomfort and therefore protests. But the caregiver responds inconsistently or not at all.

If the caregiver responds inconsistently, the child is left with uncertainty: 'I don't know whether they're going to come or not.'

And if the child doesn't know whether something's going to happen or not, that can increase the likelihood for anxiety: 'I don't know what's happening, I don't know what works, I don't know what doesn't work.' The increased uncertainty about whether the need will be met or not makes it even harder for the child to soothe itself.

When eventually a caregiver arrives, this can cause the child to experience frustration with the caregiver, leading to further negative responses such as anger towards the caregiver and lack of trust. As a result of the lack of trust, the child may be unable to allow the caregiver to soothe the anxiety.

This is known as 'insecure ambivalent attachment'.

If, however, the caregiver doesn't respond at all, except perhaps at set times – 'I feed you at this time, I toilet you at this time, but otherwise you cry' – it's as if the caregiver has dropped the string.

This then tends to cause the child to see the world as hostile: 'Nobody's going to meet my needs, I need to do it myself.' So the child may learn to turn their alarm bell off through strategies they develop, but the child is learning that the world is untrustworthy, and they can't rely on anybody else.

This condition is known as 'insecure avoidant attachment'.

Perhaps the child protests more. The response from the caregiver is negative: shouting, hitting, crying. The child comes to believe that the world is bad, that they are bad. The child creates a very complex understanding of the world. So the child gives up, no trust develops and they don't develop attachments.

This condition is known as 'insecure disorganised attachment'.

Relating these unsuitable attachment models[35] to trauma, we can see that alarm bells are being triggered but not calmed down. This restricts activity in the parts of the brain that can rationalise alarms; those parts of the brain may therefore not develop in a typical way.

The following summarises the four attachment models and how they affect the way individuals behave:*

- **Secure**: I am loveable, worthy, effective. Others are available, loving, interested and responsive.
- **Insecure ambivalent**: I don't know whether I can trust people or not. You may leave me; you may not meet my needs. No matter how much love you show me, I never believe that that love is enough. Therefore, I may take action to protect myself from being hurt; e.g., I cheat to stop you cheating on me first.
- **Insecure avoidant**: Nobody's there for me so I have to look after myself. I can't trust others; people are merely functional. So I might engage with you if I feel I need something from you. But otherwise, I don't see a benefit of connecting with you.
- **Insecure disorganised**: I am bad, and other people are bad, and the world is a bad place. Therefore I may not have any empathy towards other animals or human beings. I feel I need to stay in control because other people controlling me have meant bad things; if I hadn't kept that control myself, I wouldn't have survived.

* These were developed by Mary Ainsworth and Mary Main from John Bowlby's theory of attachment.

One final point is that, depending on the child's circumstances, it is quite possible for the child to develop multiple attachment models. Therefore, the attachment model being displayed by an individual can change depending on the environment. Perhaps a child will display 'avoidant' at school but 'ambivalent' at home. These attachment styles will continue to affect relationships, future attachments and reactions to perceived attachment figures throughout the person's life from childhood to old age.

How might an elderly person with dementia, who has an avoidant attachment style, react to being in care? They may be very rejecting of any care or help.

THE WINDOW OF TOLERANCE AND POLYVAGAL THEORY

On page 97, the concept of a window of tolerance was introduced as a container that we all have that allows us to manage stress and emotional regulation.

This section will further explore how polyvagal theory and the window of tolerance model help our understanding and planning for certain aspects of behaviours that challenge.

This concept is shown in the following diagram.

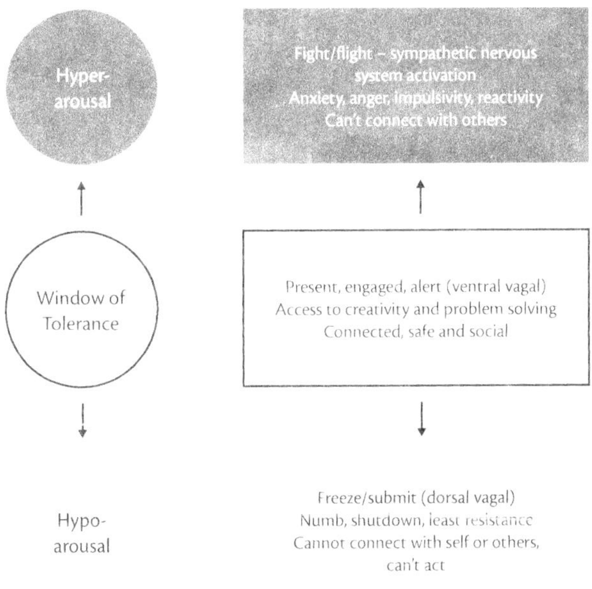

Figure 12.6 Window of Tolerance

The central area is the 'window of tolerance', where homeostasis – emotional balance – is king. This area is where an individual's SNS and PNS, explored in Chapter 11, are in balance with each other. This area is where an individual can engage in rational processing, focus and attention, and also social engagement and connection.

When a person has a healthy window of tolerance and they experience stress, they are often able to maintain emotional regulation, manage their feelings and engage in social connection when feeling stressed. This is a typical healthy emotional management process.

In polyvagal theory[36] this window of tolerance uses the brain's ventral vagal system to regulate emotions by using 'most aspects of social contact and pleasure. It guides eye contact, hearing, eating, speech, singing, nursing, kissing, smiling and, some would say, direct heart-to-heart contact'.[37] Polyvagal theory refers to the development of the ventral vagal system through early-life secure attachments and attunement (the process of communication that occurs in early life where a primary caregiver uses eye contact and facial expressions, skin-to-skin contact and their heartbeat to settle and engage with an infant). A good example of this is how a child goes to Mum when upset or how adults who have experienced a crime often want to call a parent or partner before calling the police (remember the actions of the young gazelle in 'Case Study 11.1 The Gazelle', page 103).

This window of tolerance can be shrunk by multiple biopsychosocial factors as discussed in this book through the information on trauma, adverse childhood experiences, numerous developmental conditions and mental ill health conditions.

When stress situations become too great, or for stress that pushes a person out of their window, the two outcomes are either hyperarousal or hypoarousal.

Hyperarousal is the SNS reaction (fight/flight). This state allows a person to regain regulation through mobilising the body into action. However, this process takes much longer than connection (typically 15–20 minutes) to re-regulate, and many of the actions associated with this state are considered antisocial and challenging for others.

Hypoarousal is where the PNS applies the brakes on the system to allow re-regulation through immobilisation (freeze/submit). This is where the dorsal vagal system activates and pulls us away from connection, out of awareness and into a state of self-protection. The benefits from this state of re-regulation apply when it exists for very short periods. However, if this state continues, it impacts on a person's engagement with the world, meaning they forfeit relationships, as well as reducing their opportunities for experience and growth. They are also left with a reserve of built-up charge, as explored in several parts of this chapter and Chapter 11.

We have seen that emotional dysregulation can be a contributing factor in causing individuals to display behaviours we find challenging. It's important to be aware that an individual's window of tolerance is not fixed.

As we move into proactive planning, we will explore ways to help individuals expand their window.

SUMMARY

So far, Part 4 has discussed one cause of behaviours that challenge: inappropriate *reflexive* responses. We have also seen that many of the reasons for such behaviour involve early life experiences and trauma. Our brains are environment dependent and environment expectant. When the events we experience in early life are not positive they can lead to trauma.

Such trauma-related behaviours include:

- intense and ongoing emotional upset
- depression and anxiety
- anger, irritability and mood dysregulation
- negative core beliefs about self and others
- difficulty with peers and forming relationships
- attention and academic difficulties
- hypersensitive fight, flight, freeze responses (combative, running, spacing out/numbing)
- physical complaints, aches and pains
- difficulty eating/sleeping (nightmares).

In Chapter 1 of this book, there is a non-exhaustive list of behaviours that challenge. We can expand on that list and roughly categorise the behaviours according to emotional reactions, as described in Pete Walker's *The 4Fs: A Trauma Typology in Complex PTSD*:[38]

Table 12.1 Behaviours Related to Emotional State

Freeze	Fight	Flight	Submit/Fawn
Disassociation	Rage	Anxiety	Trauma bonding
Withdrawing	Aggression	Hyperactivity	Passivity
Daydreaming	Shouting	Hypervigilance	Aiming to please
Hiding	Destruction	Fidgeting	Never drawing unnecessary attention
Self-harm	Confrontation	Inattention	Unquestioning
Avoidant	Demanding	Absconding	Inappropriate strategies to appease
'Masking'	Lying	Disruption, being loud	
	Blaming		

In the last chapter of this section on reflex, we will explore and introduce a number of different labels, conditions and illnesses to expand our understanding about the individuals we may support and how these factors affect their reflexes.

CHAPTER 13

FACTORS THAT AFFECT BRAIN FUNCTIONING

Causes of Behaviours that Challenge

So far, we have looked at how normal brain functioning and automatic nervous system responses work. We then explored a number of different *experiences* that affect and impair a person's ability to manage and inhibit their reflexes.

But there are many *conditions* that affect the way the brain works and which have a direct impact on a person's psychology and behaviour.

These variants in brain functioning may impact on the inhibitor function of the brain and therefore directly affect the ability to weigh up consequences, to assess values, to recognise emotions, to exercise self-control and to develop learning through experience. Some conditions affect the way an individual interacts with the world. Some of these conditions are pervasive, and some fluctuate depending on multiple factors, but understanding a condition can help us to understand the individual in many ways.

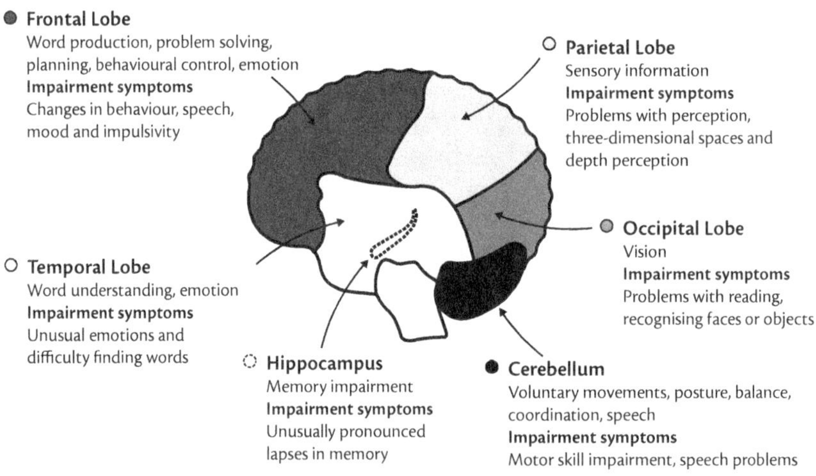

Figure 13.1 Areas of the Brain

Many of the conditions, labels and disorders mentioned below can affect a person's psychology and behaviour. This can make the individual seem different to someone whose brain works in a typical way. There are three main areas that can be affected.

The first is emotional dysregulation – this is either the brain's inability to control or regulate emotions due to impairments in the neocortex, or is due to hyperarousal/sensitivity in the limbic system/emotional brain. We have already introduced this effect in child development, trauma and attachment issues.

The second is a significant increase in the stressors experienced by a person because of communication challenges, sensory difficulties, memory problems, physical abilities, inflexibility, distortions in thinking and even hallucinations. As we will explore later, when stress goes up, our ability to inhibit goes down.

The third is the way a person interacts with the world or other people. It may be considered societally inappropriate, but because of the way the person thinks, they cannot see the issue or understand how their behaviour is in any way maladaptive.

Any combination of these three effects can be present.

One way we may be able to relate to these effects is by using the example of alcohol. Many people have directly or indirectly experienced the effects of this substance on the brain.

Alcohol directly affects numerous areas of the brain and the way they function. We can see how that effect manifests itself in the way a person responds to events/stimuli, how it affects their judgement and impairs their ability to foresee consequences and how it amplifies their emotions, but alcohol also inhibits their ability to imagine other people's perspectives and to empathise with others.

Many of the areas of the brain that alcohol impairs are also affected by the conditions listed below. Many people claim that they have acted differently when drunk to how they would act when sober. If we follow this analogy through but realise that the condition a person experiences is not one that they can just 'sober up' from, we can potentially empathise with how the individual's ability to act 'acceptably' or 'normally' in the world may be a real challenge for them; they should not be judged, but instead be understood and supported.

> Understood – to increase acceptance and reduce shame.
>
> Supported – to develop better strategies and skills where possible or by adapting their environment to work around their deficits and play to their strengths.

It should be noted that if an individual is diagnosed with any of these conditions, it does not mean that the person will engage in any specific behaviour, nor is the condition always the cause of the observed behaviour. Every person, regardless of diagnosis, must be treated as an individual. However, ensuring we understand the condition to its fullest can allow us to better understand an individual's experience of the world and how we may need to adapt our strategies or the environment to support them in the best way we can. If we are working with someone affected by dementia, we should do all we can to understand dementia through training and research.

Conditions of note that should be explored include:

- autism spectrum condition (disorder)
- sensory processing disorder
- pathological demand avoidance
- oppositional defiance disorder (ODD) and conduct disorder (CD)
- ADHD
- attachment and trauma
- foetal alcohol spectrum disorders
- learning disabilities and chromosomal disorders
- mood and anxiety disorders
- schizophrenia
- personality disorders
- cerebral palsy or acquired brain injury
- dementias
- drugs
- alcohol
- psychosis
- delirium.

CHAPTER 14

REACTIVE

Causes of Behaviours that Challenge

Special terms used in this chapter:

Core beliefs: A term used to describe the conscious or non-conscious way we see ourselves, the world, other people and events. Core beliefs affect our thinking, and significantly shape our reality, behaviours and perceptions of the world.

Scripts: Ways we feel we should behave or who we should be, whether positive or negative. Scripts are created by influences in our life but mainly by early-life caregivers and include examples such as: 'You must be perfect to be successful.' More information about these and their relevance appears later in the book – see 'Teaching Technique: Role Modelling', Chapter 25, page 225.

THE SYMPTOMS

CASE STUDY 14.1 THE COKE BOTTLE

There is a bottle of Coke on the countertop in the kitchen. What you don't realise is that the bottle has been on quite a journey to get there. It has been shaken and dropped on multiple occasions. It looks like any other bottle of Coke but you open the cap and... POW! The internal pressure is released, and you get covered in Coke.

Imagine that every person you interact with is like a bottle of Coke. You may not know that the bottle has been shaken; you are just the unfortunate one who walks into the room and inadvertently takes the lid off, which results in you being covered in Coke. Is it personal? No, but can it feel personal? Absolutely – if the person is directing their frustration, stress or anger towards you, of course it can feel personal.

It is worth remembering that we are like bottles of Coke too, and if we feel attacked, we get shaken and feel defensive. We may end up retaliating and snap, 'I'm only trying to help you!'

The result of our reaction can be like adding Mentos to the Coke bottle, causing a full-on explosion.

However, if that person sees us as being in a position of dominance over them, they may suppress their reaction (freeze/submit), but the pressure is still there and will emerge sooner or later in some way. This can affect that individual's self-esteem, along with our long-term therapeutic relationship with them.

If we know a bottle of Coke has been shaken, or we are aware of certain activities or situations that can shake up this particular bottle of Coke, and we go in and shake it some more... who is to blame when it explodes? Especially if we know that this person's ability to keep their lid on (reflex control) is not great.

So, if we know a bottle has been shaken, what should we do?

- **Option 1**: Leave it to settle. (If we know that works for the individual.)
- **Option 2**: Use any tricks we know to prevent the bottle from exploding, like turning it upside down and tapping the lid three times. (This is not a valid scientific solution and definitely shouldn't be applied literally to a person! However, if we are aware of an effective calming technique, then we could try that before attempting to open the bottle. Or even use that technique to settle the bottle before exposing it to an event that we know is likely to get it shaken.)
- **Option 3**: If we *have* to open the bottle, then doing it slowly and gently, maybe holding it at arm's length, or even outside in the garden, might prevent us from being covered... which still works as an analogy.
- **Option 4**: Give it to someone else to open. But at least warn them first. If the other person is either calmer themselves or better able to open this bottle without getting covered, it's not a weakness to pass it over; it may be an act of kindness and the most appropriate course of action.
- **Option 5**: Being very aware of our own bottle of Coke and how that could be affecting our behaviour and approach.

We may not always know when a bottle of Coke has been shaken; however, learning more about the individuals we support, using the 6STM to build a prediction and recognition tool, allows us to be better prepared. If we are not sure... we should always assume the bottles have been shaken.

If they have been shaken and we are gentle and careful, we avoid getting covered.

If they have not been shaken and we are gentle and careful, we still avoid getting covered.

But if we are not careful and gentle, we may be washing the Coke from our hair later.

Note: Many caregivers describe the individuals they support as unpredictable. But this makes them predictable: they are predictably... unpredictable! It's the one predictable thing about all of us really.

THE CAUSES

Let's look at what can cause this build-up of internal pressure. We can identify four categories of potential stressors, as shown here:

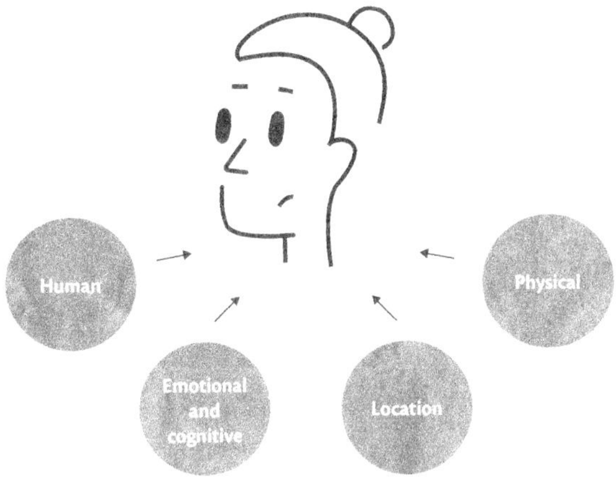

Figure 14.1 HELP Stressors

The acronym 'HELP' can be useful in remembering these:

H – Human
E – Emotional and cognitive
L – Location
P – Physical

It's often not one thing that triggers escalation but an accumulation.

HUMAN STRESSORS

The individual needs a person for:

- help
- connection

- attention
- validation, acceptance or recognition.

Or the behaviour of other people is making the individual feel (this is a non-exhaustive list):

- threatened
- insulted
- ignored
- made to do something
- bullied
- patronised
- criticised
- teased
- shouted at
- coerced into doing something
- like their choice is restricted
- controlled
- disrespected.

These interpersonal stressors can affect the individual's self-esteem, their rights, their feelings of freedom, and their choices. In turn, the result is a deterioration in the individual's overall wellbeing.

It's important to note that the stressors shown are as *perceived by the individual*, not by the perpetrator. For example, an individual may feel bullied even though the 'bully' was only joking or doing it for the individual's best interests. Other caregivers in the setting may not perceive the behaviour as bullying – depending on its regularity and what their threshold and values might dictate. (A good example of this stressor was explored in 'Case Study 8.4 Bizarre Clothing', page 80, when the staff member made the lad change his clothes.)

Even how we address individuals is important. Use people's preferred names rather than a diminutive (Michael prefers to be called Michael, not Mike); avoid the terms 'poppet', 'darling', 'mate' and suchlike. Some people may not mind being addressed in this way but some may dislike it and not be assertive enough to say so.

EMOTIONAL AND COGNITIVE STRESSORS – THE WAY THEY ARE FEELING OR THINKING

Here is a non-exhaustive list of emotional and cognitive stressors:

- Hallucinations and delusions

- Memories
- Mood and mood disorders
- Anxiety and fear
- Feelings and emotions
- Unstructured time (lack of predictability or routine)
- Disorientation, memory loss, disassociation
- Grief and loss
- Control
- Core beliefs and scripts
- Automatic negative thoughts (see some examples in Stage 6: Learn from Incident).

CASE STUDY 14.2 HOW ANGRY DO YOU GET?

Appendix 1 of this book is a self-test; you may like to try it. The test presents 20 potentially annoying scenarios and asks you to rate each as A (untroubled), B (annoyed) or C (angry).

This self-test is often used in training courses covering conflict management or de-escalation training.

Students are asked to complete the questions based on a general day and then asked to reveal their ratings for each item.

The scores and answers vary wildly from person to person; for example, one person giving an 'A' to a scenario that others in the room have labelled as 'C'.

So, what conclusions can we draw from the results of this test?

Every person's reaction to the scenarios differs from the next person's. There is no absolute rule about what should or shouldn't make people angry.

It is also worth considering the following points:

- This test is taken at a certain time, with individuals who have different life experiences and on that particular day have certain things happening in their lives, either positive or negative. So you might find the same person would give different results on different days.
- Some individuals may have very fixed expectations about how people (or objects) are supposed to behave, and outliers make them angry. So a person's beliefs, attitudes, experiences and values can all affect the given ratings.
- Is it also highly likely that in real life an accumulation of several 'A' incidents in the same day might lead to the next 'A' being classed as 'B'? Or that several 'B's might lead to a 'C'? That the individual's normal ability to rationalise mistakes or negative events may get worn down? That the Coke bottle is gradually getting shaken? For example, when one traffic light turns red just as you get to it, no big deal, but if five

green lights turn red on you in a row, it's harder to not take it personally (despite logically knowing the universe is unlikely to be interested and intervening in your journey to the shops).

CASE STUDY 14.3 BAD DRIVER

You were cut off in traffic, and you reacted negatively by waving a fist or giving the finger.

Why were you angry? Was it a near-miss that triggered feelings of fear; e.g., 'I was put at risk' or 'My car could have been damaged'?

Or a feeling that people just shouldn't drive like that?

Or a prejudice against certain types of vehicles; e.g., taxis, white van drivers?

Either way, our thoughts affected our feelings, and our feelings affected our behaviour.

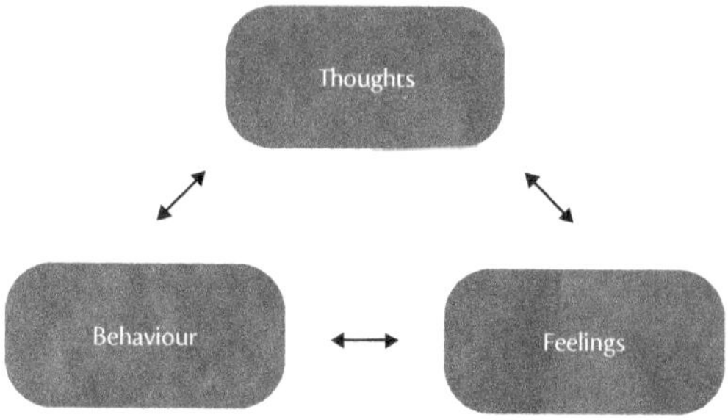

Figure 14.2 Thoughts–Behaviour–Feelings Cycle

Commentary:

1. Whose day was ruined? Not that of the bad driver. It's the person who was cut off who gets angry, while the other driver may not even realise what he's done.
2. Why did anger result? Nobody can make you angry without your permission. As we explored in the section on amygdala hijacking in Chapter 11, emotional reactions and triggers are complex and not necessarily under our conscious control. Anger/aggression is part of our fight response to a threat that may be triggered by either the near miss or the negative thoughts. There is a useful metaphor for this principle in the box below.

The Inner Chimp

In his books *My Hidden Chimp* and *The Chimp Paradox*,[39] Steve Peters refers to our emotional brain as our inner chimp brain and gives a great simile to better understand and relate to our emotional self. The inner chimp is our primitive brain that is there to keep us safe, to fight or flight ourselves to safety. The chimp gets triggered into action by all kinds of stimuli. Some triggers may be genuine dangers or threats, where the chimp is useful. The chimp is why we have survived as a species. Some triggers may only be perceived threats, or sometimes they may not be threats to our safety but threats to our values or core identity/self-concept; for example, fear of rejection, failure, humiliation, challenges to our beliefs, damage to pride.

The chimp can be strong and very dominating. However, it is only a part of us. The chimp is our pet that is useful for survival but can cause maladaptive responses to situations if it's not kept in check.

We have the responsibility to manage our chimp, to pull it to heel or put it back in its cage when not needed. This isn't always easy, and as we can deduce from Chapter 12 about trauma, some people's chimps are really big and strong because they had to be in their past, and other people have limited resources or strategies to keep the chimp under control. But the statement 'Nobody can make you angry without your permission' refers to the fact that we should not blame an inability to manage our emotions on other people. It has to be an individual's responsibility to manage their own chimp. No one can do that for them. However, some people may need help to recognise their chimp and see how its behaviour impacts negatively and unnecessarily and may need support and help with knowing how to control and manage it. This is where empathy comes in (recognising the chimp in someone else and why it may have been triggered, relating our feelings to theirs and adapting our behaviour to accommodate and help the chimp to feel safe before we offer ways that the chimp could be managed better).

3. Maybe the bad driver was oblivious to what had happened because he was rushing to hospital because of the unexpected premature birth of his child. Or perhaps the driver had just been fired from his job. Or had just been diagnosed with terminal cancer. None of which makes the bad driving acceptable, but there is a reason behind that behaviour.

Let's explore how the need to be in control seems to drive many reactions to stress.

CASE STUDY 14.4 FEAR OF THE FALL

Christine is terrified of heights; one of her biggest phobias is being in the car when it is on a road with a steep drop on one side.

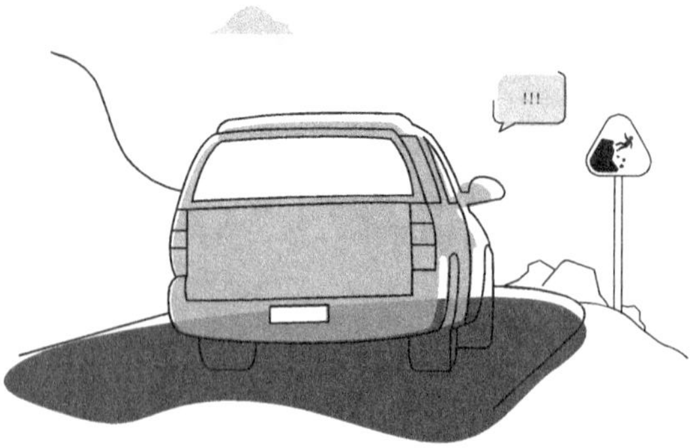

Figure 14.3 Driving at the Edge

She describes the feeling: 'I feel sick, my vision goes blurry, every part of me wants to leap from the car away from the drop, it's overwhelming. I can cope with it if I'm driving, but if someone else is driving, I close my eyes, hold my breath and pray for it to be over.'

Commentary: Most people in Christine's situation would not be so seriously affected. But while the car is on the mountain, Christine can barely function. Why? She needs to be in control ('I can cope with it if I'm driving'). We all feel safer when we are in control. This case study is revisited later in the book in the context of things being different if Christine has trust in the driver (page 257).

A need for control in all areas of their life may be stronger in individuals who have experienced harmful people or inconsistent or neglectful caregivers in their life.

This is why 'no' is such an emotive word. 'No' demonstrates that someone else is in control. For example:

- a salesperson who finds 'no' hard, as it feels like personal rejection
- a toddler who is told 'no' and it triggers a meltdown
- a teenager who can't cope with a 'no' because that word's representation of control has become like the 'green room' we mentioned in Chapter 12 on trauma, and it triggers a survival response.

CASE STUDY 14.5 WAITING, WAITING...

You are told, 'The engineer will be along sometime between 9 and 5.' So you take time off work, and you wait. And wait. As the day progresses and there's no sign of an engineer, you become increasingly anxious and annoyed.

Commentary: Many people feel more comfortable if there is structure and predictability; humans generally like patterns, and so patterns feel safer. The situation in this case study may create heightened anxiety because it is something we have limited control over. This 'stressful day' may increase the likelihood of you snapping at your kids or partner for traipsing mud into your kitchen. You may react to this trigger, passionately. And potentially in a way that surprises not only your kids/partner, but even yourself.

CASE STUDY 14.6 ARE MY KIDS OKAY?

Margaret is elderly and living with dementia. She is found trying to open a locked door. A caregiver asks, 'What are you doing, Margaret?' Margaret replies, 'I want to go home.'

The caregiver tells Margaret that this is her home and she needs to calm down.

Margaret shouts at the caregiver, tries to hit out at her and says, 'Get away from me!' Margaret then walks down the corridor and tries another door.

CASE STUDY 14.7 HERE TO HELP

Later that evening, Margaret is calm in her room. A caregiver comes in to help her undress for bed. Margaret seems cooperative but quiet. However, when the caregiver starts removing Margaret's underwear, Margaret screams, 'Get off me,' and slaps the caregiver in the face.

Commentary: Margaret's reactions may be due to disorientation and memory loss associated with dementia. The Alzheimer's Society uses a metaphor of two bookcases to explain the impact of dementia on memory which is a useful way of understanding what may be happening to Margaret.[40] Watch the video at https://youtu.be/aVXTVMoMQ50 to understand what is happening for Margaret.

LOCATION STRESSORS

Here is a non-exhaustive list of location stressors that can contribute to internal pressure:

- Poor ventilation
- Privacy
- Overcrowding
- Offensive smells
- Under-stimulation
- Temperature
- Noise
- Lighting
- Overstimulation
- Linked associations (trauma or disorientation)

On the face of it, location stressors such as temperature, noise and lighting should be easy to modify. However, in a communal setting, it's likely that there will be differences among individuals about what level of these factors is acceptable – one person thinks it's too hot, another feels it's too cold. Depending on the facilities available, it would be ideal to provide a quiet area, sound-proofed rooms with individual temperature control and so on, but clearly, this is often not possible.

Person-centred care will try to ensure that an individual has their preferred level of privacy and dignity. Lack of these becomes a stressor.

The stressor 'linked associations' refers to the memories triggered when the senses detect a similarity to an environment where something bad happened – the 'green room', as discussed in Chapter 12.

PHYSICAL STRESSORS

Here is a non-exhaustive list of physical stressors that can contribute to internal pressure:

- Physical discomfort
- Physical disabilities and disorders
- Sensory disabilities
- Sensory processing issues
- Hunger
- Tiredness
- Hormonal, e.g., menstruation, puberty
- Medication

It's fairly obvious why these problems will cause stress; if an individual isn't feeling well, they may have less patience with others. Similarly, an individual who is on a drug or alcohol withdrawal programme will be more susceptible to stress. Or perhaps they are taking medication to reduce hyperactivity, but this makes them feel lethargic and that they 'can't be bothered'; in turn, this can lead to apathy, which may be interpreted as laziness, which is often seen as a behaviour that challenges.

SENSORY PROCESSING

'Sensory processing' was touched on in 'Amygdala Hijacking', Chapter 11, page 105, and in Chapter 13, but needs a little more explanation here.

There are the five senses that we are all familiar with – sight, hearing, touch, taste and smell.

But there are other complementary senses:

- Temperature recognition
- Balance
- Hunger, thirst
- Pain
- Emotions
- Proprioception (the awareness of the position and movement of the body; e.g., we can walk without looking at our feet, or we can touch our nose with our eyes closed)

If an individual has sensory processing difficulties – either being oversensitive or undersensitive, or struggling with discriminating the information coming in – the information to process can become overwhelming or be ignored. Difficulty with sensory processing might result in an individual with dementia not being aware that they have broken a hip; they just become more irritable and aggressive. Or an autistic person becoming overwhelmed in a noisy place.

SUMMARY

This chapter has discussed one reason for behaviours that challenge: inappropriate *reactive* responses caused by HELP stressors:

H – Human
E – Emotional and cognitive
L – Location
P – Physical

CASE STUDY 14.8 I'M HUNGRY AND ON A DIET

I haven't eaten all day. But I'm meant to be on a diet and not eating any rubbish food. I slept through my alarm and had no time for breakfast. I've been really busy, but it's now 2pm and I still haven't eaten, and I reach the point where I must eat *now*.

I go to the fridge to meet my need, and I find ingredients that, given 20 minutes, I could cook to create a nourishing meal.

But there's a bag of crisps on the counter. Now, even though I'm on a diet, it's quite likely that I'll grab the crisps. The stress of my hunger has reached a point where the inhibitors no longer matter.

Now consider what happens if I have no food in the house, and I have no money. Will the stress of my hunger cause me to go against my values and steal some food?

Commentary: When stress goes up... inhibitors go down. As my limbic system is activated by stress, my frontal lobe becomes deactivated.

The higher the stress, the less our inhibitors are available. So where possible we want to eliminate as many stressors within an environment as we can if we want the best chances of improving outcomes, teaching new skills and reducing behaviours that challenge. We can't eliminate all of them, and so, as we will explore, we want to also build individual resilience to keep the Coke bottle lid on and also help the individual to learn how to release the pressure in a safe way.

CASE STUDY 14.9 I'M HUNGRY AND ON A DIET (PAGE 133) – REVISITED

I go to the cupboard and it's bare – there's no food in the house. I am hungry but I realise that I'll have to go shopping... but it's raining, I know the car's low on petrol... In this case, I might decide that the level of pain to assuage my hunger isn't greater than the pain of the hunger and so wait and end up giving up the diet and ordering a takeaway delivery later.

But...

Consider what may happen if I was on that diet and when I went to the fridge the food available was pre-prepared, healthy food choices and there were no crisps in the house. I would be able to better stick to my diet because I had created proactive strategies rather than reacting to the hunger.

Commentary: Human beings usually move towards pleasure and away from pain, and we often have non-conscious strategies for achieving those outcomes based on conditioned responses from our past. Let's explore these intentional strategies next.

CHAPTER 15

INTENTIONAL

Causes of Behaviours that Challenge

Behaviour is a form of communication.
All behaviour has a function.
This function will have benefits. Although the behaviour may be challenging.
Bad behaviour doesn't make a person bad.

CASE STUDY 15.1 ATTENTION-NEEDING

No one is interacting with Janet. Feeling invisible, she bangs her head on the table hard and repeatedly. She uses this to cope with anxiety, but she also finds she feels better because the staff attend and comfort her.

Graham lives in a care facility and commonly follows the staff around the home, standing near them, always close. The staff often get annoyed and walk him back to the lounge, where no one talks to him. He gets bored and lonely so goes looking for someone to be with.

Amir is non-verbal; when he is overwhelmed, he makes himself sick by sticking his fingers down his throat. This upsets the staff a lot, as it is very distressing. Sometimes, though, the boy approaches the staff and makes sick noises and pretends to vomit and only stops when the staff attend to him and hold him tight. This is his way of asking for a hug.

When Joey lived at home, his mum was very busy. She had lots of 'friends' coming round. His mum and her 'friends' would often go to his mum's room and would not come out for ages. Sometimes Joey would get so hungry because his mum was too busy with her 'friends' to feed him. Joey found the best way to get food was to be really loud – to shout and bang and stand at the bedroom door asking lots of questions. Mum would often shout at Joey but she usually got him some biscuits to eat to shut him up.

Commentary: In all of these cases, the individual's behaviour is being reinforced with some form of attention. The individuals have consciously or unconsciously made a connection that their behaviour receives that benefit.

For Joey and Graham, even bad attention is better than no attention.

In all cases, the caregivers are actively trying to stop the behaviour they are finding challenging but are unwittingly encouraging the behaviour they want to discourage.

In Janet's case, she is causing herself harm to gain this benefit. The benefit must outweigh the cost for her, and she doesn't know what else to do.

Amir's need and behaviour is similar, but he has adapted his self-harming behaviour to a mimicry of the actions to reduce the cost but still gain the benefit.

In all cases, the individuals have learnt that the behaviour works and therefore repeat it as required. The behaviour has become intentional in so much as it has a predictable function.

This does not mean that they are aware or even in control of this intention. It can be as automatic as folding our arms.

CASE STUDY 15.2 EXERCISE: ARM FOLDING

Note: The following exercise involves both arms, so if you are reading this as a book, please read the instructions before starting – you will have to put the book down!

1. Fold your arms however you normally do this (see diagram).

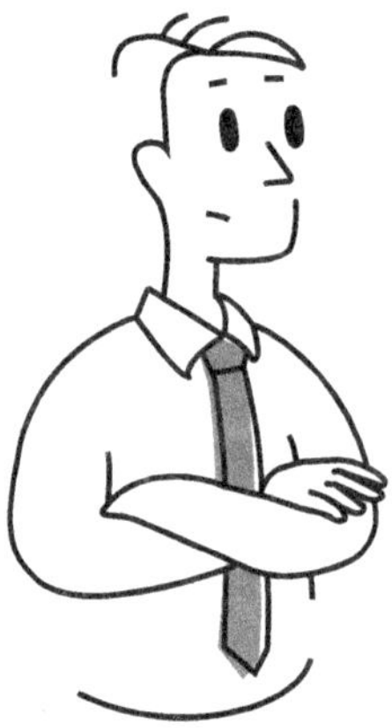

Figure 15.1 Folded-Arm Activity

2. Note which arm is on top – the right or left (the left arm is on top in the diagram).
3. In one quick movement, open your arms, tap your thighs with both hands and then refold your arms with the other arm on top.

4. Repeat a couple of times – thigh tap and refold, alternating which arm is on top.
5. End of exercise – you can relax and pick up the book now!

How easy was it to change arms? Many people find it quite difficult, some almost impossible. It normally requires some concentration. (It's worth noting that there is no correlation between left-/right-handedness and which arm naturally goes on top.)

Generally, people feel a little less comfortable doing it the 'other way'. Even if they manage to change, it feels odd.

Is there a right and wrong way to fold your arms? Clearly, no.

If someone asked you 'Why do you fold your arms that way?' you would probably answer, 'I don't know.'

If you have children, would you accept 'I don't know' in answer to the question 'Why did you do so-and-so?' (e.g., hit your brother or lie). You probably wouldn't.

We often expect people to know why they do what they do.

People do things the way they do because it's comfortable, it's automatic, it feels safe, it's kept them alive. Doing it any other way is less comfortable, more challenging, makes them feel vulnerable and takes more effort, but they may not be aware of either set of reasons.

Commentary: In the arm-folding exercise above, the way we fold our arms is just a habit; habits feel comfortable. Changing habits can be hard and uncomfortable.

Think of all the habits you may do in a day without thinking.

Do you always snooze your alarm once in the morning, do you always put your slippers on before going to the bathroom, do you always wash your hair before you wash your body in the shower, do you wash your body in a set order? Do you know the reason for all those habits?

There may be some habits that you are aware of and have a rationale for. There may be some that are completely non-conscious; you weren't even aware of that habit, but if it became conscious, you could create a rationale for it (whether true or not). Other habits, well, you don't really know why you do them; they are completely automatic.

In total, 95% of our behaviour is non-conscious; we really don't know why we do what we do – we often act on impulse, automatically, reactively (as shown in the Stroop test in Chapter 10 – you don't know why your brain tries to read the word first, it just tries to do it; you must consciously stop it from its automatic action to name the ink colour).

Figure 15.2 shows that much of our non-conscious is made up of ingrained programmes and learned concepts/abilities – learned ways of thinking, feeling and behaving in response to stimulus. You won't necessarily remember learning many of them, but you have been developing them throughout your life. You can test your own non-conscious biases at https://implicit.harvard.edu/implicit/takeatest.html.

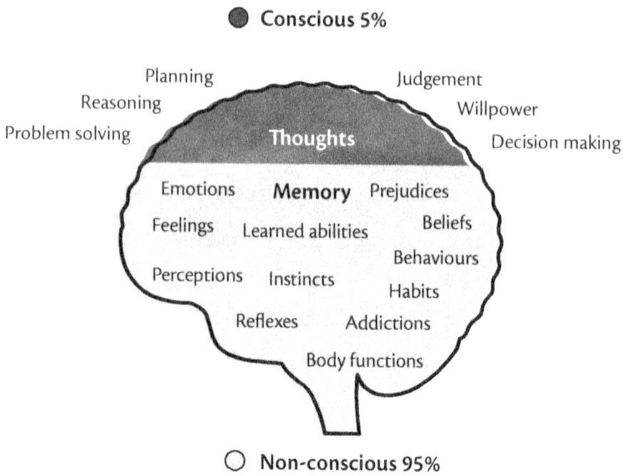

Figure 15.2 Conscious/Non-Conscious Thinking

THE ACTOR-OBSERVER BIAS[41]

When it comes to explaining *our own* behaviour, we are very likely to overly attribute why we behave in a particular way to the external forces of other people, the environment, the situation... whereas the Fundamental Attribution Error (FAE) (correspondence bias) is our tendency to underemphasise situational and environmental explanations for the behaviour *of others* while overemphasising personality-based explanations. This effect could be described as the assumption that a person's behaviour reflects their personality.

For example, 'I was going over the speed limit because I was really late for a meeting, but I didn't realise how fast I was going.' 'They were speeding because they're impatient or just want to show off their fast car.'

In the Stroop test, described on page 100, we are usually able to take conscious control of the automatic behaviour, like we could in the arm-folding exercise, but it wasn't necessarily easy and was even a little uncomfortable.

What if you were told that folding your arms the opposite way to your normal way was better for you? That it would be a better behaviour for you, socially or physically, and it could even improve your mental wellbeing?

Would you change the way you fold your arms?

It's extremely unlikely.

If you didn't trust the source of the information, change would not even be considered. A trustworthy source may be considered but still may not be motivation to change.

Would Janet stop banging her head just because someone told her to?

Would Graham stop following staff just because someone told him to?

Would any of us change any habit, just on the request of someone else, even if they presented good rational reasons?

That's not to say habits cannot be changed; we constantly adjust our habits (you can train yourself to fold your arms either way).

But there must be a motivation to change – a net benefit in making the change.

Atomic Habits[42] describes four principles that increase the likelihood of a person changing a habit. The alternative must be:

- obvious – I can see the alternative
- easy – I feel I can do the alternative (the easier the alternative the better)
- attractive – I can see the benefits of the alternative
- rewarding – I experience a benefit from the alternative.[43]

(These principles in reverse can also help to extinguish an unwanted habit – e.g., if it becomes harder to do the current habit than the alternative, it becomes less attractive than the alternative or there is no longer a reward or benefit from the current habit.)

The principles above mean that most people wouldn't bother to learn how to fold their arms differently (unless they like a challenge).

In the case study below, look for the different functions of the behaviour and then make a note of the different alternatives John creates and how he sets up rewards.

CASE STUDY 15.3 THE SMOKER

John has smoked for years, and lots of people have told him to stop. Even people he cares about. John has always been adamant that he will quit when he feels ready.

John visits the doctor, as he keeps getting chest infections. John is told that he has a lung condition that means if he doesn't stop smoking, his health will get worse very quickly. John decides it is time; he can now see the cost to his behaviour and the benefit of stopping, and he knows what he must do.

John feels he will struggle to just stop smoking – there seems to be no short-term reward to that. John decides to use nicotine gum as an easy initial alternative.

John also wants to make it harder to get cigarettes, so he gives his remaining packet to a friend.

John makes a plan. When he gets the craving for a smoke, he will chew his gum. He also thinks he uses smoking when he's bored, not just from a craving. So he also downloads a game on his phone, so if he gets bored and craves a cigarette, he also has an easy alternative there to occupy his mind.

John also sets himself a reward. He puts the money he usually spends on cigarettes into a jar and at the end of the week he is going to treat himself and his partner with the money he saves.

Commentary: In this example, there are a couple of benefits mentioned that John gets from smoking:

- Nicotine
- Relieves boredom

There will be lots of other benefits that John or others may gain from smoking, such as stress relief and sensory or social associations. Some may be conscious, others subconscious.

John creates a number of new habits, with each one being obvious, easy, attractive and rewarding:

- **Nicotine gum**: This meets his nicotine need.
- **Game**: This keeps his hands busy, distracts him from cravings and reduces boredom.
- **Not buying cigarettes**: This inhibits his current habit and saves money.
- **Money in jar**: This provides a visual representation of his progress for a short-term reward and a weekly treat for a mid-term reward.

The long-term reward is hopefully a healthier longer life.

John's strategies would not suit everyone, nor would John's motivation be a motivator for everyone, but this is an example of someone having intentional behaviours. The example acts as an introduction to strategies that can be used to manage or change behaviours in ourselves or in others.

THE SHAME SHIELD

The shame shield is an intentional strategy with a specific purpose. Like the attention-needing examples earlier, it is a conditioned response, but rather than being used to gain a benefit, it is a way to avoid a cost or pain.

Shame shield strategies are very common in children who've experienced early-life trauma, abuse and neglect, but the behaviours can occur everywhere.

There are many different definitions of shame; Arlin Cuncic defines shame as 'a feeling of embarrassment or humiliation that arises from the perception of having done something dishonourable, immoral or improper.'[44]

Shame differs from guilt or regret, though, as shame is not the result of doing something wrong (although this can trigger it). It is about a feeling we have when we perceive that we are not good enough in some way. Shame refers to something about our character or who we are as a person that we believe is unacceptable.

Shame can be problematic when it becomes internalised and results in an overly harsh evaluation of oneself as a whole person. This internal critic might tell us that we are a bad person, that we are worthless or that we have no value.

If a shaming narrative is repeated – someone being told they are not good enough or that they keep 'getting it wrong' as they don't behave or manage their emotions 'properly' (remember, this inability to manage their emotions or behaviour 'properly' may be a behavioural deficit due to various factors discussed in Stage 2: Understand/Empathise or preconceived prejudicial expectations around developmental milestones) – this can result in these internalised core beliefs being adopted. Their behaviour and their self-concept become inseparable.

'I'm told I do bad... I must be bad.'

'They tell me I am stupid... I must be stupid.'

Shame differs from guilt in that guilt is the negative feeling we get when we act in a way that is counter to our values. Guilt can be a positive emotion in that it allows us to experience pain when we don't meet our own expectations about ourselves. This pain teaches us not to repeat what caused it.

> Guilt is: 'I am good, but I did something bad.'
> Shame is: 'I am bad.'[45]

As discussed in 'How Language Can Affect Culture', Chapter 5, page 43, we often hear examples of shaming in our culture. Whether it's from the media (particularly social media), managers or teachers – we hear judgements of a person based on their appearance, personality traits or behaviours that don't just label the trait or behaviour but also label the person themselves. This shaming narrative can easily become part of the shamer's daily habit.

It is important to understand that shame is emotional pain, and if you don't believe you can escape that pain by being able to change who you are, for example:

> 'I am bad, I can never be good.'
> 'I am stupid, I will always get it wrong.'

then you will develop strategies to cope with and defend yourself from those feelings. A hypersensitivity to shame will develop, and shame will be avoided in a similar way to other emotional pains like failure or rejection.

> 'If I don't try, I can't fail.'
> 'If I never ask someone out, I can never be rejected.'

'If I don't try to be good, I will never feel the shame of being bad.'

The shame shield uses this strategy and comes with multiple tools that all work to deflect the painful sensation of shame.

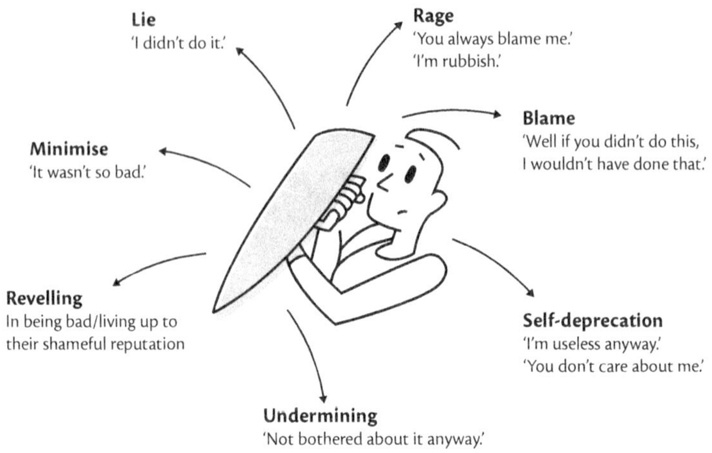

Figure 15.3 The Shame Shield[46]

So...

I lie: 'It wasn't me.'

I minimise what happened: 'Does it really matter in the grand scheme of things?'

I revel in my badness and revel in my shameful reputation: 'See, I've done it again, because that's what I do, because that's who I am. I'm not bothered about it or the consequences anyway.'

I find an excuse and turn attention elsewhere: 'It's his fault.'

I rage: 'You're always blaming me, it's always my fault. Everybody's always picking on me.'

I self-deprecate: 'I'm useless anyway, you don't care about me, you hate me anyway.'

By using the shame shield, the individual is taking control of the shame, defending themselves from feeling shame and often turning it back on the person that they feel is trying to shame them.

Ultimately, the individual can't learn, reflect and improve on their actions, because they can't accept that they can be any different; their core beliefs define their identity.

In restorative practice,[47] which is a therapeutic process used in numerous environments like youth justice, individuals are encouraged to explore their shame while allowing them to move past their shame-shielding behaviours. The aim is to nurture acceptance of their deficits and the deficits of others, but also, through the process of empathy, to help them realise that deficits don't define a person's identity and are not fixed.

This book will also explore overcoming these shame shields. Shame shields are maladaptive, as the cost to the individual is a limitation of their own outcomes due to a fixed model of who they are and their potential – their shield prevents the opportunity for growth and restoration.

Brené Brown says: 'Ultimately, shame resilience is about moving from shame to empathy – the real antidote to shame.'[48]

As we explore the use of empathy in the 6STM, we will see how using empathy and promoting the development of empathy in others is a huge step to allowing a person to overcome and process their shame and the shield that may hold them back.

SUMMARY

This chapter has discussed how behaviours can be learned, become intentional and become automatic. This is because the individual has learnt that the behaviour produces some benefit.

CHAPTER 16

THE BIOPSYCHOSOCIAL MODEL

Causes of Behaviours that Challenge

So far in describing Stage 2: Understand/Empathise we have explained how causes of behaviour can be categorised in three ways: reflexive, reactive and intentional.

As a summary, behaviour is:

- *reflexive* – the biological ability to manage the effect these factors have on my thoughts, feelings and behaviours
- *reactive* to internal factors – physiological (physical)/psychological (thoughts and feelings) or external factors (environment or human)
- *intentional* – the outcomes that I have learned come from my behaviour.

Or, using the bottle of Coke analogy: the things that shake up the bottle of Coke (reactive), the ability to keep the lid on (reflexive) and the benefit I get from releasing the pressure (intentional).

These causes never exist in isolation. All three causes interact in fairly complex ways to produce the behaviours that we see.

This complexity is a clear separation from the overly simplistic analysis of behaviour based on 'nature or nurture': 'Is it *who they are* or *how they were raised* that makes them good or bad?' The dominant factor in forming behaviour patterns has still not been agreed on.

Using the biopsychosocial model[49] of understanding people is a much more accurate way of understanding all aspects of the human condition and behaviour. Figure 16.1 uses the model to help understand mental wellbeing, but we could do similar Venn diagrams for all human attributes.

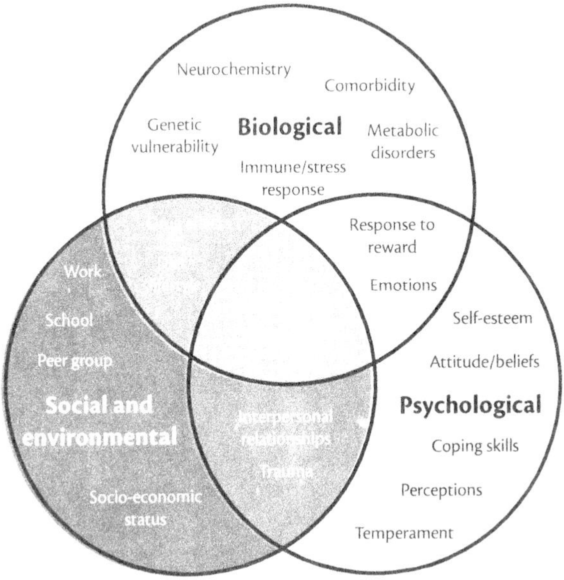

Figure 16.1 The Biopsychosocial Model

BIOLOGICAL

Our genes determine much of who we are, and our genes are passed from our biological parents. But genes are complex in their effects, and we know that environment and psychology can actually alter gene expression.[50] However, we cannot ignore our genes; they determine factors like height, skin pigmentation, and aspects of personality, development and abilities. There is evidence of some mental health conditions being hereditary.

However, our biology is more than our genes. Not every person with physical, sensory or intellectual disabilities was born with them, and yet those biological attributes will still impact on how a person interacts with the world and how the world may interact with them.

Even as we progress through life, events can happen that alter our biology, such as disease, drug abuse, accidents, trauma. For example, we have seen how trauma leading to PTSD can change how our brain reacts to stimulus biologically. Similarly, the onset of dementia can change our biology.

So what shakes our bottle, how well we can keep the lid on and how we experience the benefit of opening the lid have biological factors.

SOCIAL AND ENVIRONMENTAL

We have seen that 'HELP' stressors can affect the way we behave.

H – Human (example: feeling bullied)
E – Emotional and cognitive (example: fear)
L – Location (example: excessive noise)
P – Physical (example: hunger)

We have also explored that no matter how good we are biologically at keeping the lid on our bottle, the environment can take us over the edge. Or social pressures may encourage us to open the lid.

PSYCHOLOGICAL

However, as we saw with the window of tolerance, even though a person may be born with a small container (biological) of emotional resilience, and their environment may add 'marbles' of stress, threatening to overwhelm it, the container can be expanded by the person changing their thinking or strategy. (See 'Case Study 10.2 The Window of Tolerance', page 97.)

We may have amazing strategies to release the pressure from our bottle of Coke in socially appropriate ways, or our strategies can make it worse.

THE INTERACTIONS

As is shown in Figure 16.1, the three parts of the model come together at any moment to mould our mental health. For example, a person may have a 'glass half empty' outlook built in; there may even be a family history of depression. But luckily for that person, his life is rich and full and nothing bad happens, so he avoids depression.

However, changes in any one sphere can affect the others.

For example, if circumstances change (social), the psychological response could change. In the above example, if the 'glass-half-empty' person loses his job, then depression could follow.

Understanding the biopsychosocial model is useful because not only is it a way to understand behaviour, but it also includes the factors we may consider in managing it. The more factors a behavioural plan can hit, the stronger the impact.

For example, in 'Case Study 15.3 The Smoker':

- John is addicted to nicotine – biological
- John also smokes to cope with boredom – social/environmental or psychological (is there nothing to do, or does John not have ways to engage in the environment?).

The factors involved in overcoming the habit/behaviour are:

- gum – biological and psychological
- a game – social/environmental and psychological
- money – a mix of biopsychosocial benefits.

UNDERSTANDING HISTORY

As discussed at numerous points throughout the book, understanding a person's history can be a useful way of understanding the person as they are now, although it should never be used as the sole focus of who an individual is.

Professor Tom Kitwood introduced in his 1997 book *Dementia Reconsidered: The Person Comes First*[51] a formula or equation to illustrate the concept of person-centred dementia care. Below is an adapted and expanded version to cover all individuals.

> The Individual = G + B + P + SP + H + NI + E
> The Individual = Genetics + Biography + Personality + Social psychology + Health + Neurological impairments + Environment

There could be many additional factors that could be added to the equation; the idea behind it is that we are all more than any label, circumstance or history, but the more we know about a person, the better we can understand them.

CHILDHOOD

There is an analogy that comes from therapeutic parenting, a deeply nurturing parenting style, especially effective for children who have experienced childhood trauma.[52]

Imagine a room. In this room is an individual's early life experiences. We'll call this room one.

It contains how they were treated, talked to, cared for. It includes the environmental conditions of love, nurture, structure, play, routine, fun, hygiene, diet and health. It contains the experiences they had, good and bad. It was where their models of the world developed. This is my life, this is how things should be, how I should be treated and who other people are.

For some individuals, the experiences in this room may have been extremely negative, but it's what they know.

Now, let's say we have built a new room for them – that we try to create experiences and an environment that is better than they have ever had before. We'll call this room two. We fill it with all the things we believe are good and positive in the world, and then we stick them in this room too.

How should they feel? Happy? Grateful? Relieved?

Well, let's imagine that tomorrow you were abducted from the street and taken to another land. In this land the people behave and speak differently to anything you have experienced before. The environment is different; the way things are done is different.

How would you feel to start with? Happy? Grateful? Relieved?

Or would you feel scared? Angry? Resentful? Unsettled?

Even if someone told you that this new place was better, it is doubtful that anyone would feel safe or better to start with. Over time, you may see the benefits, the improvements and the advantages, but that may take some time.

The 'room one/room two' analogy is a brilliant way of understanding the experience of many looked-after children: their initial experience of care and the lack of trust they have towards it. It also explains why they often behave in ways to make where they are now feel like home.

> When staff shout, it feels like home. When there is chaos, it feels like home. When I have nothing, it feels like home. When I am bad, it feels like home and home is where the heart is.

It is also worth considering the old-logic spectrum that was explored on page 56. This looked at how early life experiences of behaviour management have a huge impact on how an individual sees themselves, which in turn can affect their interpretation of the behaviour of others.

So a caregiver shouting and criticising may be perceived as abusive, and removing attention or privileges may be perceived as neglectful or abandonment. These perceptions don't result in an improvement in behaviour but rather a deterioration.

BIOGRAPHY

CASE STUDY 16.1 | REMEMBER

What were you doing on 7 November 2014?

It is very unlikely you remember unless this day has significance for you personally.

If you were asked what you were doing on 11 September 2001, you may be able to recall where you were and even how you felt on the day of the attack on the Twin Towers.

The emotional memories you associated with the event are connected to the logical memories of the event and so are easier to recall.

Flashbulb memories are vivid, enduring memories associated with a personally significant and emotional event, often including such details as where the individual was or what they were doing at the time of the event. Flashbulb memories are more likely to be retained than the memory of an everyday event. Between the ages of 5 and 30, people are more likely to have flashbulb memories, as this is the period in their lives when a lot of 'firsts' happen – the first day of school, first boyfriend/girlfriend, first bereavement, first house, first job, etc. – experiences that hold high emotional value. These firsts in life are also talked about and thought about repeatedly, which results in them having a stronger imprint on our memory. This is referred to as the reminiscence bump.[53]

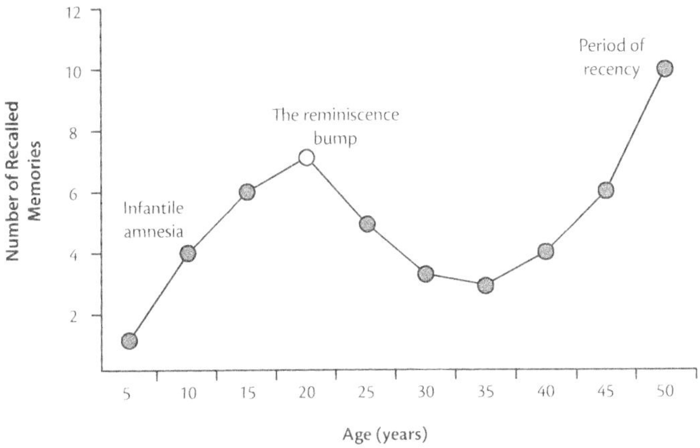

Figure 16.2 The Reminiscence Bump

Emotional memories endure for longer than logical memories in both old age and dementias.

Knowing an individual's history in the following areas can help us to understand behaviours in the present that may be linked to events and memories in the past.

- **Childhood**: Family, school, adverse experiences.
- **Adolescence**: School, work, adverse experiences, achievements, special memories.
- **Adulthood**: Relationships, work, residence, pets.
- **Retirement**: Hobbies and interests, hopes.
- **Likes and dislikes**: Colours, food, music, activities.
- **Habits, routines, skills and preferences.**

As discussed earlier in the book, trauma may play a factor in this, but all aspects of a person's past may impact on habits, reactions or engagement in the present.

CASE STUDY 16.2 HISTORY LESSONS

Joseph

After Joseph retired, he enjoyed gardening and used to go to his allotment early every morning. On his return home, his wife used to have a coffee ready for him and make him a bacon or sausage sandwich. Since the time when Joseph moved into a care home as he became poorly with dementia, he has had porridge every day and no longer gets to do any gardening. He doesn't want to say anything as he doesn't want to be a burden, but Joseph feels sad.

Harry

Harry's dad used to take Harry to a local football game every other Sunday. Harry loves football, but since his parents were killed in a car accident, he hasn't been to a single game.

Omar

When Omar was taken from his home by social services at age four, it was due to significant neglect. His mum struggled with mental health and drugs and unfortunately couldn't look after herself let alone a young child. Omar didn't like his foster home. The people were nice, but it smelt wrong. It smelt of flowers and chemicals, not old food and urine. Omar couldn't sleep in the bed as it was too soft and high off the ground. Omar was often found in the morning lying in wet clothes on the floor, lying on just the rug.

Bill

Bill was a plumber; he had been a plumber since he left school at 15. Bill often found work to do and sorted out all kinds of issues – radiators, sinks, leaking taps, whatever was needed. Unfortunately, the staff at the care home didn't appreciate Bill's work, as often the plumbing he dismantled was working fine to begin with. Bill was a challenging client, as he often got disorientated because of his dementia.

Knowing these histories can improve the planning process for care and behavioural management, as well as enabling understanding and empathising with the person as they are.

Caregivers deducing and learning more about the causes and categories of an individual's behaviour and history not only helps to raise understanding, but also leads to empathy.

EMPATHY

One of the most important aspects of the 6STM is 'understand and empathise'. So far, we have explored the causes of behaviour, and now we will move forwards in bringing those factors together and creating a hypothesis of what triggers a behaviour or what benefit is gained from the behaviour. We also need to be very aware that causes cannot always be discovered.

As we explored in Chapter 12, triggers can be extremely difficult to pinpoint. For example, what if whatever is shaking the bottle of Coke is something from the past, not the present.

It can also be easy to focus so much on a person's behaviour that challenges, its causes and even the labels/diagnoses a person may have, that we forget to connect with the person.

Whether we successfully discover causes or benefits of behaviours, the one area we should keep aiming to discover is the *feelings* the individual is experiencing. Also, with many individuals who are potentially feeling disjoined from reality, whether due to psychosis, dementia or trauma, the facts of the situation may be blurred – but the feelings are always true.

Empathy has been and will be mentioned throughout the process, as it should underpin everything we do. In proactive behavioural analysis, the behavioural plans we create and the responsive strategies we use to teach or de-escalate, we must never forget that we are working with a person.

As well as behavioural management, human connection should be included as an outcome on any behavioural or care plan.

Within the 6STM, empathy should be used as a proactive planning tool, a dynamic response tool and a reflective tool, so it will be covered in all stages of the system in different ways.

CONCLUSION

We need to become better detectives than judges.

The big shift in approach to help us *understand* an individual's behaviour is shown by the difference in the following questions that we might ask:

- 'What is wrong with you?' = being a judge.
- 'What's wrong for you, what are you feeling right now? And what has happened to you in the past that is affecting the present?' = being a detective.

The first question raises the notion that the person is in the wrong for their behaviour, and the emphasis for change is on them.

The second question begins to use a detective's toolkit, one of curiosity and investigation. A detective is not there to pass judgement or administer punishment; they are there solely to explore, understand and even empathise with the motives.

CHAPTER 17

BEHAVIOURAL ANALYSIS

In the previous chapters, we have explored lots of aspects of behavioural causes, increasing our knowledge of the complexity of human behaviour.

As mentioned, this benefits us for a number of reasons: it shifts us to a detective mindset, where we see the *individual* as a whole, not just a *behaviour*.

A person to be understood, not a problem to solve.

It also forces us to engage with our logic, reason and empathy (frontal lobe), which can allow us to better manage our own feelings, values, attitudes and reactions to behaviours.

This next section combines all of the factors discussed and brings the process into a more analytical form.

HUMAN MOTIVATION

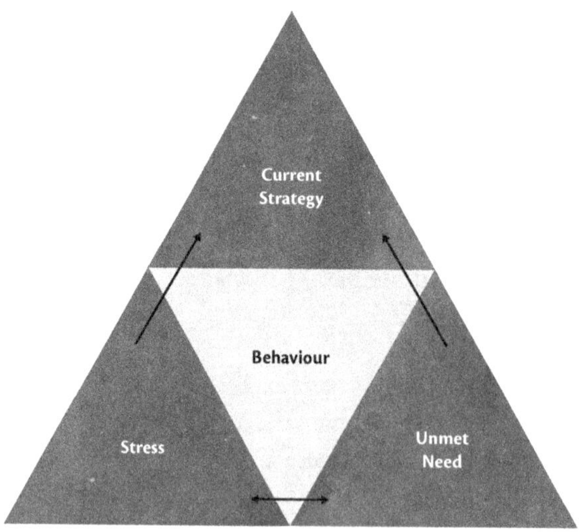

Figure 17.1 The Motivational Triangle

Figure 17.1 brings together the three causes of behaviour – reflexive, reactive and intentional – as well as being a model for creating a plan. The model can be used as a functional tool as well as an empathic tool, as will be explained.

Imagine a box. On the lid it says 'Aggression' or 'Pestering' or 'Rudeness' (this is the label we have given to a behaviour).

Inside the box is a triangle showing that the behaviour we see (the behaviour that challenges) is a strategy to meet a need or to cope with stress. These are the two factors we need to explore and identify by looking for clues and being a world-class detective.

The diagram shows that the behaviour (the behaviour we want to understand) is a result of the three elements coming together.

The summary of the diagram is:

- an unmet need stimulates stress

and/or:

- stress creates an unmet need.

These causes or reasons lead to a behaviour or strategy. The strategy has a purpose or function to allow the person to meet the need or eliminate/cope with the stress.

For example:

- You haven't eaten (unmet need), which leads to hunger (stress). Stress burns calories, which increases the need, and so you go to the fridge and get food (strategy).
- Work gets really busy and you are getting overwhelmed (stress) – you don't have the time or resources to meet deadlines (unmet need). You speak to your manager about additional support or redirecting some workload elsewhere (strategy).

In both of these examples, we were able to recognise the different elements of the triangle in ourselves, and the strategy was appropriate and adaptive.

However, not everyone can meet their needs, manage/recognise stress and have positive, socially acceptable, adaptive strategies to meet them, as has been explored in the last four chapters. As discussed, these 'behavioural deficits' lead to 'excess behaviours', which may be experienced as 'behaviours that challenge'. These behaviours can then become ingrained habits as discussed in Chapter 15, page 137. Once we have identified the behaviour as not just challenging but 'maladaptive', it now becomes the target behaviour we need to understand and empathise with; we also need to create a plan to manage, extinguish or change the behaviour.

The aim of the plan will be to meet the need, reduce the stress and manage the strategy. So, can we, the carers, achieve this goal, or can we teach the individual to meet their own need, recognise and manage their own stress or learn new strategies?

We have already explored a lot around stress factors using the HELP acronym in Chapter 14, page 125.

In Chapters 1 and 8 we explored the different excess behaviours that may be classed as challenging, but we also need to explore the direct link between the unmet need and the strategy.

UNMET NEEDS

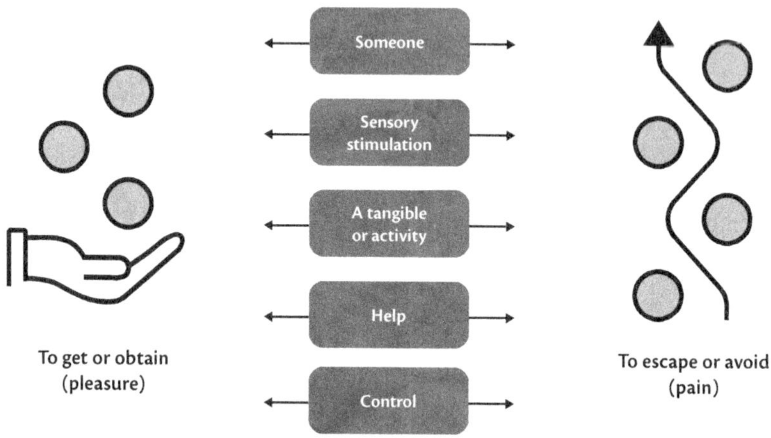

Figure 17.2 Unmet Needs

It is human nature to seek pleasure and avoid pain.

The diagram shows motivators that will trigger one reaction or another:

- **'Someone'**: The individual wants to get away from someone they fear or don't like or to get near to someone they love or respect.
- **'Sensory'**: To avoid pain or to gain satisfaction.
- **'Tangible/activity'**: To avoid discomfort or get an object; to cease an unpleasant activity or begin a pleasant one.
- **'Help'**: To stop being helped ('that's enough, thank you') or to seek help.
- **'Control'**: To gain a feeling of control or to avoid a situation where the individual feels they are being controlled.

This pleasure/pain model is a very simple principle and is often used in numerous behaviour management strategies to address behaviour. What it is potentially missing, which the triangle model adds, is the 'stress' acknowledgement, which is the emotional experience and why the empathy tool is so important.

Humans do not always follow pleasure/pain in a simplistic sense.

Take tattoos, bodybuilding and fitness, studying for exams – humans are very capable of going against their basic biological impulses in search of long-term benefits but are also capable of choosing behaviours triggered by emotions such as pride, fear, ego, envy, malice, etc.

Take the example of an individual who actively seeks reprimand because in his world that shows that someone cares. Or an individual who seeks to be restrained because that gives a feeling of safety. An observer would see a reprimand or a restraint as an inhibitor (something to extinguish a behaviour) but in fact, for the individual, the behaviour is positive and will act as a reinforcer.

By expanding our view to understand the need and the stress, we are trying to get to the root of an individual's behaviour – to look from the individual's point of view, not from our own.

CASE STUDY 17.1 I CAN DO IT MYSELF

Kamala has dementia; she has to be assisted with some elements of dressing and personal care. Kamala is a mum of five children and used to both run the household and work. She was a very independent woman, who was very house-proud, always well kept and efficient.

Kamala is being assisted with her personal care, but she becomes aggressive towards the caregivers. The caregivers ask Kamala to be kind, but Kamala is snatching, pinching and growling at the caregivers.

One of the caregivers says, 'Right Kamala, I am not going to help you while you are behaving like this. We are going to leave you alone to calm down and we will try again in a bit.' The caregivers leave Kamala.

Initially Kamala feels happy, as she wanted them gone – she wants to get dressed herself, she doesn't want fussing over. Unfortunately, Kamala can't manage it herself. Kamala feels useless and sad.

Commentary: Kamala is experiencing stress.

- **Human**: She isn't liking the way the caregivers are supporting her.
- **Emotional/cognitive**: She is feeling proud and defensive – she should be able to do this herself.

Her unmet need is to avoid people, escape activity and escape help.

Her strategy is aggression. Which works – the staff have actually reinforced her strategy. (They were meaning to inhibit the behaviour with: 'You behave like that, we don't help.' This is because they didn't explore the stress; they made an assumption about the feelings: 'She is just being difficult.')

> **CASE STUDY 17.2** SHE'S JUST DOING IT FOR ATTENTION
>
> Chelsea had come from an abusive environment. She had been neglected and hurt by many adults in positions of authority in her life. Chelsea now lives in a care home; she displays many behaviours that the staff find challenging. She engages in self-harm, suicidal ideation and other antisocial behaviours.
>
> Chelsea has a preference for female staff and often takes a dislike to certain staff (mostly older male staff).
>
> Chelsea demonstrates one behaviour that the staff often moan about, where she hyperfixates on who is working the night shift.
>
> Sometimes, when she finds out certain staff are on, Chelsea will threaten to hurt herself if certain staff don't work instead.
>
> Staff feel that Chelsea is being manipulative and attention-seeking.
>
> When Chelsea behaves like this, they warn her that she will not be allowed her weekend treat if she hurts herself and that she can't choose which staff work when.

Commentary: Chelsea is potentially terrified. Her unmet need is a lack of control, which stems from the stress of fear. If Chelsea felt safe and connected with all staff, why would it matter who was working at night? Her strategy is extreme, but the staff are using the tactic of removing more control to manage her behaviour, which will most likely escalate behaviours.

Let's look at two other examples.

> **CASE STUDY 17.3** THE FOOD HOARDER
>
> Clare comes from a neglectful background where food was scarce. She is now in care. She often only eats half of her meals and stashes the rest in her room. She steals from the fridge, she takes discarded food from waste bins, she shoplifts.
>
> The staff feel at a loss. They are providing regular meals and she is offered snacks. They are struggling to understand why Clare continues to behave in this way.

Commentary: Clare has a habit of food hoarding that is triggered by a fear of food not being available tomorrow. That the staff expect Clare to no longer hoard as they are providing food is a focus on the need and not the stress. Using the arm-folding analogy again, they are almost telling Clare, 'You don't need to fold your arms as you have always done – you can fold them the other way now!' So they haven't spotted the correct unmet need. The strategy is not to meet the need of hunger now... it's the need for guaranteed food tomorrow. It is a matter of control.

CASE STUDY 17.4 PANIC ABOUT PANICKING

Rachel has had a number of panic attacks at school. If Rachel finds classwork hard or finds the classroom environment overstimulating, or sometimes for no reason, she can recognise that she begins to feel anxious and overwhelmed. Her heart starts racing and she can struggle to catch her breath. She has tried to bury the feelings – to hide them and cope – but the feelings get stronger and worse, and she has now had a number of episodes where she has ended up hyperventilating and disrupting the lesson, with everyone looking at her. This has resulted in her becoming terrified to go to school at all, as she is worrying about having another panic attack.

Rachel has been removed from the class while the staff try to figure out what to do. This is making Rachel feel very excluded and she's worried about what the other children will think of her.

(This case study is revisited later in the book where the staff's approach is shown. See 'Case Study 20.4 Panic About Panicking – Revisited', page 184.)

Commentary: In this example, Rachel has not developed a functional strategy. Her strategy of just trying to cope has failed her and caused her more problems. Rachel will need support to meet her need to escape the stressful activity, environment or people that are contributing to her anxiety and get help. In the long term, she will need tools to cope with and manage her anxiety and find better strategies to achieve self-calming.

For each of these case studies, we could create a behavioural hypothesis:

> [**Individual's name**] engages in [**behaviour**] when they feel [**stressor**] or when [**antecedent**] because when they do, they [**typical consequence**] or want [**aimed consequence**]. This is more likely to happen during [**context**] and/or when [**setting events**] have occurred.

This hypothesis, like that of a scientific enquiry, is not yet fact but a starting point to explore its validity and accuracy. It may prove wrong or at least not 100% correct, and therefore it may get reviewed and adjusted as we move through the 6STM.

In the case studies we have just explored, there is enough information to create a starting hypothesis; for example:

> Kamala engages in aggressive behaviour towards staff when they provide personal care because when she does the staff leave her alone. This is more likely to happen in the evening and when the staff don't allow Kamala to do as much for herself as she can.

Chelsea engages in controlling behaviour when she is feeling unsafe because she may not know how to feel safe. This is more likely to happen when male staff are working, and taking control away seems to make it worse.

Clare hoards and steals food when food is available because when she does, she feels in control of her food. This seems to happen more when the staff notice Clare seeming anxious or agitated. (Increased disengagement or hyperactivity behaviours.)

Rachel experiences panic attacks when she feels emotionally overwhelmed or overwhelmed by the environment because she doesn't seem to know how else to cope or communicate her emotions, and the panic attack invites staff support and she is removed from the setting. This is more likely to happen in the classroom when it is noisy and busy and is more regular during maths classes.

Some of these case studies will be revisited in Stage 3: Proactive Planning, where possible adjustments to parts of the triangle are discussed.

However, it may not be easy to reach a hypothesis and then a plan. In such cases, we can try brainstorming to come up with suggestions that can be tried and tested or we can do more analysis.

FUNCTIONAL BEHAVIOURAL ANALYSIS

As has been shown, behaviour is complex, as are the people who display it. We need to be very aware of managing our limitations. For complex behaviours and cases, a competent trained consultant should be involved in assessment, analysis and planning programmes.

However, the list of principles described below is something we can all use with the aim of being objective, quantitative and evidence based; this can help us to move away from a purely opinion-based approach.

In summary, the Functional Behaviour Analysis works as follows:

1. Making use of the recorded occurrences of an individual's behaviour (details of how to record incidents are given in Stage 6: Learn from Incident).
2. Improving our understanding of an individual by exploring their history and known behavioural deficits.
3. Once sufficient examples have been collected, looking for patterns across the incidents.

4. Using these insights to create a plan to adjust the behaviour.

Making Use of Incident Records

Stage 6: Learn from Incident describes the ABC chart method for recording incidents. These detailed records are vital documents for the Functional Behaviour Analysis. The basic premise is that we are looking for what led up to the behaviour and what happened after the behaviour to create a hypothesis of the cause/trigger/stressor of the behaviour and/or the gain/benefit/met need/function of the behaviour.

In Chapter 39 there are a number of examples of ABC incident records (see 'Keeping Accurate Records: ABC Analysis', Chapter 39, page 397).

The last line of each of these shows the potential stressors or unmet needs that can be deduced from the single incident, as follows:

- Jessica felt distressed or lonely and wanted either attention, help or sensory input.
- Sam was feeling bored or overwhelmed. He needed sensory input and/or to stop the activity.
- Tim was feeling, low, angry or depressed. Tim wanted to avoid people, gain control.
- Margaret was distressed and upset. Margaret needed a person, 'Molly', or a drink.

From one incident, the initial idea may or may not give us a full hypothesis; that is why ongoing incident recording is so important.

Process of Elimination

Initially we may need to start with every conceivable cause of a behaviour or stressor/unmet need and then eliminate each one step by step. Using knowledge of a person's condition, history and previous habits, we may not need to explore every possibility in one go. However, it's a great exercise to perform about a behaviour to avoid falling into a negative assumption trap; for example, 'Ignore them, they are just doing it for attention.' This exercise may jolt thinking into other possibilities or reduce judgement by examining history, stressors and functions.

Let's look at the example of smearing behaviour.

Table 17.1 Sample Reason/Stressor/Unmet Need Matrix

Reason – cause/ history	Reason – stress	Purpose – need to gain	Purpose – need to avoid
Neglect – lack of skills to use paper	Physical discomfort	Sensory – comfort	Sensory – discomfort
Abuse	Emotional/cognitive: 'My bottom is not my own'	Control	
Sensory issues	Physical discomfort of paper on bottom		Sensory
Reaction	Emotional/cognitive: 'I feel invisible'	Control	
Reaction	Human: 'I want this person gone'		Human
Attachment	Human: 'I want connection'	Human	
Sensory	Physical – sensory pleasure, 'I like the feel'	Sensory	
Reaction	Emotional/cognitive: 'I feel angry so dirty protest'	Control	

This list could go on further, but as mentioned, by examining patterns of behaviour, we can start to notice potential functions or causes.

Look for Patterns

We also want to explore what makes the behaviour both more and less likely to happen.

Once a sufficient number of incidents have been recorded, the goal is to find patterns and trends.

For example, this behaviour often happens on Wednesdays. What is it about Wednesdays that can trigger this behaviour?

It seems to happen less with staff A but more with staff B.

Or this behaviour tends to happen when Janet is in the room, or after a request has been made of them, etc.

Or this behaviour is occurring more frequently now; has anything changed to cause that?

There may also be patterns of consequences (what happens straight after an event?).

This behaviour tends to result in attention, or a removal of attention, or a change in activity, etc.

From patterns we can improve our hypothesis.

When it Doesn't Happen

We can often learn as much about behaviour through identifying when the behaviour *doesn't* happen as when it does. This works especially well when the behaviour is particularly high in frequency.

If we notice a pattern in behaviour such as 'This always happens every day at breakfast', of course we can explore the triggers and needs. However, we could look at any day the behaviour *doesn't* happen at breakfast and look at what worked rather than what didn't.

We can also do an exercise called 'the perfect day'.

Imagine an individual had a perfect day where they didn't display any of the maladaptive behaviours we are concerned about. Imagine what might happen in this person's perfect day; for example:

- How much sleep did they get?
- What did they have for breakfast?
- What activities did they do?
- Who were they working with?

By creating the perfect day that we know would reduce the likelihood of behaviours that challenge, we can start to create a plan to create this day (or as close as is appropriate) more regularly.

EMOTION CHARTS

This process is similar to the ABC chart, but rather than ad hoc recording as incidents occur, we try to look at patterns of moods and emotions of the individual throughout the day. This can help to further develop an understanding of causal factors or the emotional effects of various routines – set events that commonly occur throughout a person's day; for example, breakfast, getting ready, bedtime, etc.

This is useful for the staff to complete, but it can also be useful for the individual themselves to monitor their own moods.

This emotion log can help to pick up causes that may not directly trigger events but can 'shake up the bottle of Coke'.

The process is described in 'Mood Monitoring', Chapter 39, page 406.

CONCLUSION

The process of understanding and empathising is the most important step in the process before we start creating proactive plans.

If we don't know why a behaviour occurs, or at least when it's most likely to occur, it is almost impossible to create a consistent plan of how it can be managed.

The process described in this section is also ongoing and dynamic. We should be constantly curious about the individual and encourage them to be curious about themselves, and we should promote positive person-centred care, environments and plans.

It is also worth noting that our main focus should never be on the individual's behaviour; it should be on the individual themselves.

PART 5

THE 6-STAGE TARGET MODEL STAGE 3

Proactive Planning

CHAPTER 18

INTRODUCTION TO STAGE 3

PREAMBLE

As we move into Stage 3 of the 6STM, 'Proactive Planning', the behaviour that challenges will have been identified, assessed as maladaptive and selected as a priority to be managed or changed within the setting. The process of being a detective rather than a judge will have begun.

The question changes from:

> What's wrong with you?

to:

> What's wrong *for* you, how are you *feeling* and what *happened* to you in the past?

Using previous history, an understanding of the individual's behavioural deficits and diagnosis, Functional Behaviour Analysis on any previous incidents, mood monitoring and even talking to the individual post-incident, we should have started to understand and empathise with the causes or function of the behaviour, with the aim of creating a behavioural hypothesis, as discussed in the last chapter.

Even if all the information has not yet been gathered about the maladaptive behaviour, a simple proactive plan can still be adopted as soon as the behaviour is identified.

STARTING WITH THE POSITIVE

CASE STUDY 18.1 RED BRAIN, GREEN POTENTIAL

Most people have at least some negative core beliefs about themselves. For example, 'I'm no good at languages,' or 'I'm always clumsy.' For some people, the narratives of their lives have created core beliefs of being worthless, stupid, bad or all of these. These core beliefs impact on what they feel they can achieve, how they should behave and how other people are going to treat them. The core aim of the care system should be to help an individual to see their potential and improve their outcomes.

So... the individual's brain is full of red negative liquid; we want to fill their brain with green positive liquid. How can we get the green liquid into their head? We have to keep pouring it. If we try to remove the red first by trying to teach the individual, through consequences alone, that red thinking is bad, all we are doing is adding more red liquid. We are telling them, 'You messed up again, you weren't good enough again.'

We need to change our philosophy to focus on the positive and pouring the green. We want to catch and reinforce the person behaving in ways that promote their wellbeing and improve their outcomes by teaching them new skills and celebrating successes. We want them to see that the red isn't true by creating an environment, plans and responses that build their sense of worth, value and self-esteem.

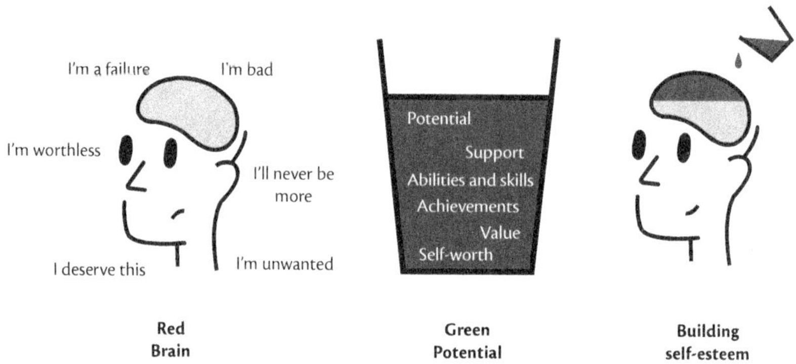

Figure 18.1 Red Brain, Green Potential

When we first begin the process of behavioural change, it is easy to focus on the negative, as discussed in Chapter 5, page 36.

A useful first step in creating a behavioural plan is to begin with the behaviour we *want* rather than the behaviour we don't want. If we don't know what behaviour we do want, how is the individual supposed to work towards it?

If we look at some of our previous case studies, we can explore some of the negatively framed questions that may be created:

- **Kamala, page 155**: How can we stop her getting aggressive? What do we do when she gets aggressive?
- **Janet, page 135**: How can we stop her banging her head?
- **Rachel, page 157**: How can we stop her panic attacks?

There may be a point where we have the information and understanding of the behaviour to try to explore and answer these questions, and it may well be an important step required to address the behaviour as a whole.

- **Kamala**: Why is Kamala getting aggressive?
- **Janet**: Why is Janet banging her head?
- **Rachel**: What is causing Rachel's panic attacks?

Any information we have to these questions can help inform on the further questions shown below, but initially we can change these questions into a positive viewpoint.

Then we can look at the opposite behaviour to the behaviour we don't want and create a question around that behaviour:

- **Kamala**: How can we help Kamala stay calm? What do we do when Kamala doesn't get aggressive?
- **Janet**: How do we want Janet to manage her sensory need?
- **Rachel**: How can we support Rachel with her emotions? What do we want Rachel to do when she feels overwhelmed?

This may seem like a very small adjustment that may come out with similar strategies to those emerging from negative questions. However, as discussed, we want to create an environment where we catch the good rather than the bad and we want to increase self-esteem. So we want to create opportunities to succeed rather than fail. But to create success, we first need to define the good behaviour and the goal.

We naturally use this strategy with young children. We tend to set behavioural goals in a positive frame. For example:

- We don't tend to ask the question: How can we stop her from messing her nappy? We automatically start creating a plan for: How can we teach her to use the potty/toilet?
- We don't tend to ask: How can we stop him from just lying there? We create a plan for: How can we encourage him to walk?

The Benefits

As explained in Chapter 9, humans typically have a bias towards noticing information that reinforces their view, and once something is drawn to our attention, we are more likely to notice it – as described in 'Case Study 9.1 Cognitive Bias – the New Car', page 82 (a variation of which is repeated in Case Study 18.2, page 168).

CASE STUDY 18.2 THE NEW CAR

Have you ever bought a new car and suddenly you start to notice the same make and model of your car everywhere you go? It appears to be more common than you ever noticed before. You have developed an awareness bias. There are not more of that car on the road than before... you are just noticing them.

When we ask the negative question around a behaviour, for example:

> What can we do about 'X' being abusive to caregivers?

we are most likely to notice when 'X' is abusive. Which means the staff will want to address this behaviour and potentially want to instigate criticism, lectures and consequences in reaction to the behaviour.

However, if we pose the question:

> How can we get 'X' to be respectful to caregivers?

we now want the caregivers to notice and catch when 'X' is respectful, with the aim of them reinforcing this behaviour, flooding the individual's brain with the green positive liquid rather than reinforcing the red negative liquid described earlier.

This is also much nicer and more positive for the caregivers; for example:

> I caught 'X' being respectful seven times today!

The big factor in this, which is why it is such an important first step, is that we are now reinforcing the behaviour we want. The law of effect from behaviourism is that 'rewarded behaviour will tend to be repeated'.

If being respectful is now more rewarding, being respectful should increase in regularity. If respectful behaviour goes up... abusive behaviour has to go down.

A person cannot be respectful and abusive at the same time.

Let's look at a few other simple examples:

Table 18.1 Negative and Positive Questions

Negative question	Target positive question
What are we going to do about him lying in bed all morning?	How can we get him up in the morning?
How do we stop her smelling bad?	How can we promote good hygiene?
What do we do when he breaks the TV?	What do we do when he treats property with respect?
What do we do when she threatens to harm herself?	What do we do when she shows self-love?
How can we stop him getting aggressive?	How can we help him to stay calm?

Example 1: What Are We Going to Do About Him Lying in Bed All Morning?

The next section of this chapter will expand on why looking for the cause of a behaviour is a useful strategy to help us empathise with and understand a person's motivation towards a potentially maladaptive behaviour, such as staying in bed all morning. It's easy to *surmise* that he stays in bed because he's depressed, ill or tired, and we may go on to explore and create plans around this information.

But are there days when he wants to get up, when he's more motivated? If so, let's find out why. Maybe he gets up on days when there's a cooked breakfast, or when he's going into town, or when particular staff are in. Can we use these motivators to our advantage? What similar procedures can we institute for each day?

CASE STUDY 18.3 WHY SHOULD HE?!

Suppose that an individual's desired behaviour occurs because of influences that can be regarded as a treat or that they have control over. And that to encourage the behaviour, the treat or control is given more often.

There have been a number of occasions where this principle of giving individuals whatever they want (viewed as a treat by caregivers) has encountered resistance from caregivers.

'Why should he get a cooked breakfast every day?' 'Why are we letting him dictate who he works with?' 'Why should he get treats every day?'

As we have discussed in multiple locations in the book, we need to be extremely mindful of our own values, biases and prejudices when we are creating behavioural plans to increase wellbeing and positive outcomes.

In Chapter 5, we saw that not every person has the same motivators.

For example, not every person goes to the gym for the same reason. Some go for social reasons, others for health, others for fitness goals and others for vanity. We can't assume that what motivates *us* should and will motivate everyone. However, let's say a person goes to the gym to lose weight initially. That's their original motivation, but over time, going to the gym becomes a habit, they enjoy the experience and they make friends. It also has a knock-on effect. Their self-esteem improves, and they start improving their diet.

What's happened is that the motivation has changed because the person has had an opportunity to explore additional benefits, and these will help to sustain the habit over the long term. It's important to note that the new benefits they are experiencing would probably never have driven the person to go to the gym in the first place.

So let's start with a cooked breakfast to get him up, and then give him other reasons to get up.

Example 2: How Do We Stop Her Smelling Bad?

Immediately the question introduces cognitive bias – caregivers will recognise when the individual smells, not when they don't. 'Oh, you smell a bit today... have you had a shower/washed your clothes?' Picking at the negative, constantly putting down, criticising.

Rather, to promote good hygiene, praise when the individual smells fine. 'Is that a new perfume? Looks like you enjoyed your shower...' Allow them to choose their preferred products, etc.

> **CASE STUDY 18.4** STEPHEN LUBY AND SOAP
>
> In *Atomic Habits*,[54] James Clear describes how Stephen Luby travelled to Karachi in Pakistan as a public health worker to try and address the unsanitary living conditions and associated disease spread in the overpopulated slums.
>
> His initial intent was to promote and educate the people about handwashing. However, he soon discovered that people knew the importance of handwashing; they just didn't have the behaviour as a habit.
>
> Stephen asked the right question: What would encourage people to wash their hands more?
>
> Stephen and the team supplied the neighbourhood with a popular premium soap product that smelled great and provided a nice-feeling lather and suds. The soap was quickly adopted by the community.
>
> Within a few months, rates of diarrhoea fell by 52%.

Example 3: What Do We Do When He Breaks the TV?

In this example, we could explore the answers to these two questions:

- What did we do when he broke the TV? Criticised the behaviour, informed him of the consequences, took his TV privileges away. If a new TV were to be bought for him, staff may perceive this as rewarding the behaviour, which could easily lead to comments such as: 'You're lucky you have that,' or 'You don't deserve that.' This would all be feeding the negative core beliefs.
- So, what do we do when he doesn't break the TV? Nothing.

Let's look at another example of this same type of question switch.

> **CASE STUDY 18.5** THE SCHOOL BOY
>
> Pavan was a looked-after child with an abusive past; he was diagnosed with autism.
>
> Pavan sometimes became overwhelmed before school and just couldn't cope with going in at normal time on some days. The school were very understanding that Pavan needed additional support, and so on the days he came in later they

would nurture and support him to join his classes. This worked well for Pavan. However, the school and Pavan's foster parents really wanted to help Pavan to go into school on time.

What happens when Pavan goes in late? Nurturing, support, one-to-one time.

What happens when Pavan goes in on time? Nothing.

Let's make going in on time at least as rewarding as going in later.

By looking at what happens for the individual when they meet our expectation of what 'should' happen, we can look to make that behaviour more rewarding rather than punishing what we feel is the wrong behaviour.

In Example 3, caregivers' typical reactions to an act of destruction means negative behaviour gets more attention (potentially reinforcing it or just acting to remind the individual that they are bad, feeding into their negative self-beliefs, lowering self-esteem and triggering shame shields). The positive behaviour of not breaking the TV almost certainly is not acknowledged or recognised. But when the TV gets broken, it becomes a big issue. This is where we need to be very aware of our expectations – 'He should know not to break things... he should respect property' – and maybe these are true, but maybe, due to this individual's history and experiences, he doesn't know or understand that principle. So do we punish... or teach?

We are not suggesting that every person who doesn't break the TV should be rewarded, but our expectations and assumptions must be questioned when the TV is broken.

CASE STUDY 18.6 DESTROYER

Tabatha's foster parents are confused. Every time Tabatha is given anything, like a new toy, she immediately damages it, despite seeming to want to keep the toy. When exploring Tabatha's history, they discover that her biological mum used to take any new item given to Tabatha away from her and proceed to give it to her two younger siblings. Tabatha was not allowed her own possessions... unless they were broken. The foster parents realised they needed to drop their expectations of what Tabatha should know about how to react and instead teach her and build her belief that her old reality was no longer going to happen.

In Example 3, it may be worth expanding the opposite question to encompass a more general positive behaviour. So the question could be: 'What do we do when he treats property with respect?' And then staff could take pains to catch him when he's respecting valuable objects or give opportunities for him to handle such things. We may also look at what he was feeling at the time and at emotional management (see Example 5).

CASE STUDY 18.7 THE UNBROKEN CUP

An individual had a tendency to get into a temper and smash the nearest objects. One day, in the kitchen, he went into a rage and picked up a cup, ready to throw it to the floor. Instead, he ranted a stream of abuse, put the cup down and stormed out.

- **Negative response**: Focusing on his ranting and raving.
- **Positive response**: Speaking to him: 'I noticed you wanted to throw the cup, but you didn't. That was so great to see!'

Example 4: What Do We Do When She Threatens to Harm Herself?

Here, we turned the question to self-love: 'What do we do when she shows self-love?' There will be times when this person doesn't self-harm despite feeling emotionally overwhelmed. Do we know what strategies she already uses, and can we build on these? We can see an approach to this self-harm question in 'Case Study 20.5 Tania, the Survivor'.

Example 5: How Can We Stop Him Getting Aggressive?

Sometimes multiple questions may come out of this exercise, especially if we are working in a team. For example, 'How can we stop him getting aggressive?' may become: 'How can we make him happier? How do we want him to communicate his anger? Can we support him to stay calm? How can we encourage him to be kind? How can we teach him to be self-aware and manage his emotions?'

We do not need to limit our plan to one question. If we write a plan that looks to answer all these questions and reinforce the appropriate behaviours and we succeed, then we have achieved our primary target, as aggressive behaviour will reduce!

Table 18.2 Example Questions and Answers

How can we make him happier?	Add more activities that make him happy to his schedule. Cognitive behavioural therapy (CBT).
How do we want him to communicate his anger?	Teach assertion skills, conflict management tools and alternative ways to vent feelings.
Can we support him to stay calm?	Create a calmer environment, give calming tools (meditation, calm space). Provide exercise opportunities.
How can we encourage him to be kind?	Role model, reward kindness by all.
How can we teach him to be self-aware and manage his emotions?	Mood monitoring, CBT, introspection work.

Positive outcomes for all!

Note: This process does not mean we ignore the negative question completely, but we have to start by finding the positive outcome we want rather than focusing on what we don't want. This is a simple starting point for improving outcomes. Exploring the negative question will take more time and detective work but that process may still be necessary in order to create a plan.

CHAPTER 19

DEVELOPING A STRATEGY

As we develop an understanding of why a behaviour occurs, we need to develop a strategy to manage or work towards the changing of maladaptive behaviours.

As discussed in Stage 2: Understand/Empathise, there can be multiple causes of a behaviour, and different plans may be required to manage each of these.

In Chapter 17, we used smearing as an example to create a list of all the possible causes/reasons or potential function/purpose for smearing. Let's just take a sample of these:

CASE STUDY 19.1 SMEARING (EXCREMENT)

Why might smearing occur?

- The individual evacuates and needs to get rid of it somewhere. Potentially, they've never been taught how to deal with excrement properly.
- It's attachment-seeking, because when they make themself dirty, people come over and clean them up.
- It's reaction-seeking, because they enjoy the faces, animation and behaviour of the caregivers when they smear. This may be a control, attention or sensory-seeking behaviour.
- It's sensory – toilet paper hurts their bottom, or they enjoy playing with this particular material.

By exploring all the evidence (incidents, history, ABC charts, etc.), we would aim to deduce the most likely cause or purpose/function of the behaviour.

If we jump to the conclusion without evidence, we may create an ineffective plan.

For example, let's say we *assume* a person is smearing for attention, so we create a plan around that function. However, if the cause is sensory discomfort, for example toilet paper is uncomfortable, the behaviour will continue because the cause has been misdiagnosed.

We must recognise though that sometimes one behaviour can have multiple functions and causes, as we saw in the example of Amir, one of the subjects of 'Case Study 15.1 Attention-Needing', page 135.

Amir engages in purging behaviour (making himself sick) as a way to get attachment and a way to cope with distress.

Table 19.1 Amir's Reason/Stressor/Unmet Need Matrix

Reason – cause/ history	Reason – stress	Purpose – need to gain	Purpose – need to avoid
Known physical and sexual abuse from history	Anxiety/distress	Sensory (physical purging)	Sensory (emotional pain)
	Anxiety/isolation	Human (need for hug)	

Strategies would need to be created for both functions, and ideally caregivers would need to recognise the difference in the function in the moment to respond appropriately.

This is similar to when a parent learns to recognise different cries from an infant to be able to respond and meet their needs appropriately. The one behaviour is a cry but there are differences that communicate the different needs.

The aim of informing staff of the way to recognise the communication of the behaviour in the moment works on the same principle.

For example, when Amir is distressed and is aiming to harm himself, he will put his hand in his mouth and keep pushing it to the back of his throat. He will continue to do this until he vomits. (Plan response: Staff should get some water ready and stay very calm with Amir. If they can, they should prompt an incompatible behaviour (e.g., beanbag, sensory lights and music) and try to calm Amir. But, if unable to prevent the vomiting, afterwards he will need staff support and calming – redirecting to a quiet spot and putting on some music helps Amir to settle; encourage Amir to drink the water any time he does not have his hand in his mouth.)

When Amir is needing physical connection, he will put his hand in his mouth and approach the staff making retching noises. (Plan response: Staff should stay calm and say, 'Amir, when your hand is by your side, we can hug.' Repeat this calmly until Amir complies and then staff should place their arm around Amir's shoulders and gently apply pressure.)

As discussed earlier, as well as understanding the purpose and cause of a behaviour that challenges, we need to decide, 'What behaviour do we want?' Without a defined goal, a plan is not much use.

The plan should also contain two strategies:

- Proactive: What are we going to change to reduce the chances of this behaviour? E.g., teaching the individual a new skill or changing the environment.

- Responsive: What are we going to do when this behaviour happens? E.g., changes in how caregivers respond to a behaviour.

Let's return to the smearing example and consider proactive and responsive strategies if the smearing is caused by the sensory issue of pain – we could provide baby wipes to see if this is more comfortable and changes the behaviour. Other plans for the different underlying causes could include:

- for a sensory cause (liking the feel of excrement), providing an alternative, such as plasticine (proactive)
- for an attachment-seeking/attention-seeking cause, teaching the individual ways to get attention (a new skill, proactive)
- ensuring that caregivers respond to the new triggers and minimising their reaction to smearing incidents (responsive)
- if the individual simply has never been taught what to do, introducing some toilet training (a new skill, proactive).

Let's now use the human motivation triangle to develop more in-depth plans.

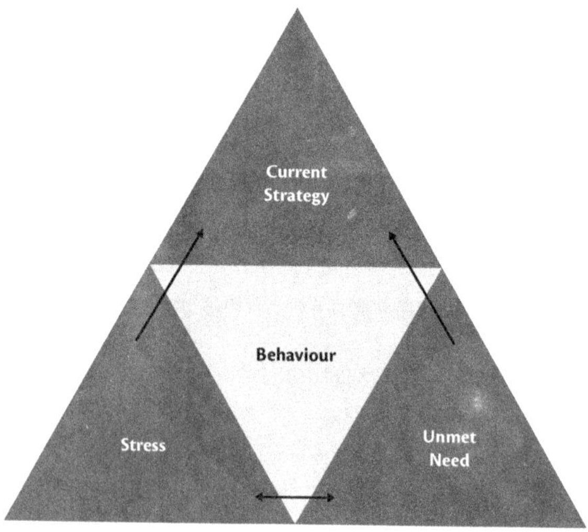

Figure 19.1 The Motivational Triangle

The diagram above has already been presented in Chapter 17, where it was used to demonstrate the need for discovering underlying causes of behaviours that challenge.

The diagram shows that the central maladaptive behaviour to be targeted is made up of three elements:

1. Stress
2. Unmet needs
3. The current strategy (items 1 and 2 are the reason or cause of the individual's current strategy that acts as a purpose or function to meet the need or cope with the stress)

We have already shown that we cannot change an individual's behaviour just by asking or telling them to change. Therefore, our aim is to adjust the three outer elements, resulting in an effect on the central behaviour.

The aim of the plan will be: can we meet the need, or reduce the stress, or do we need to manage the strategy (accept the strategy but manage the risk or people's reaction to it); or can we teach the individual to meet their own need, and recognise and manage their own stress by using a new strategy (that is safer or more socially acceptable)?

With all behaviour, there is very rarely one answer and only one section of the triangle that is targeted. Generally, a combination of the three elements of the triangle is causing the behaviour, and so tactics may address all three elements of the triangle within the behavioural plan.

The motivation triangle is a tool used to explore behaviour and see what different environmental or social adaptations or alternative skills can be introduced to address a maladaptive behaviour.

Let's revisit some earlier case studies. The original problem is reshown, followed by possible results from using the motivation triangle technique.

CASE STUDY 19.2 I CAN DO IT MYSELF (PAGE 155) – REVISITED

Kamala has dementia; she has to be assisted with some elements of dressing and personal care. Kamala is a mum of five children and used to both run the household and work. She was a very independent woman, who was very houseproud, always well kept and efficient.

Kamala is being assisted with her personal care, but she becomes aggressive towards the caregivers. The caregivers ask Kamala to be kind, but Kamala is snatching, pinching and growling at the caregivers.

One of the caregivers says, 'Right Kamala, I am not going to help you while you are behaving like this. We are going to leave you alone to calm down and we will try again in a bit.' The caregivers leave Kamala.

Initially Kamala feels happy, as she wanted them gone – she wants to get dressed herself, she doesn't want fussing over. Unfortunately, Kamala can't manage it herself. Kamala feels useless and sad.

Motivational Triangle Results

Caregivers could reduce stress by allowing Kamala to meet her own needs by exploring the process for dressing and personal care. Are there any technological aids that may help Kamala to get dressed herself or adaptions to her clothing like Velcro rather than buttons (special adapted clothing is available)? Are the clothes laid out in the right order to get dressed and the right way round? The need may be met by making reasonable adjustments to Kamala's environment to allow her to do as much herself as she can.

The staff may also be able to reduce the stress by changing their approach. Are they being person-centred or are they focused on the task? Are there times, situations or certain staff that Kamala copes better with? Can these be explored and learnt from to ensure a consistency in positive approaches?

Finally, rather than waiting for Kamala to use her aggressive strategy to avoid help, the caregivers can look for early communicators that Kamala is starting to get overwhelmed or irritated. The caregivers can then stop the activity, switch with another staff member or redirect Kamala to something different until she is calmer; then the activity can be resumed.

CASE STUDY 19.3 SHE'S JUST DOING IT FOR ATTENTION (PAGE 156) – REVISITED

Chelsea had come from an abusive environment. She had been neglected and hurt by many adults in positions of authority in her life. Chelsea now lives in a care home; she displays many behaviours that the staff find challenging. She engages in self-harm, suicidal ideation and other antisocial behaviours.

Chelsea has a preference for female staff and often takes a dislike to certain staff (mostly older male staff).

Chelsea demonstrates one behaviour that the staff often moan about, where she hyperfixates on who is working the night shift.

Sometimes, when she finds out certain staff are on, Chelsea will threaten to hurt herself if certain staff don't work instead.

Staff feel that Chelsea is being manipulative and attention-seeking.

When Chelsea behaves like this, they warn her that she will not be allowed her weekend treat if she hurts herself and that she can't choose which staff work when.

Motivational Triangle Results

Chelsea's stress of fear is going to take time to overcome. This will require building trust with the staff and the setting to manage her anxiety. One way this can be achieved more successfully is to help her meet her need for control in a safe way and slowly expose her to situations where she can learn that not having control over everything isn't necessarily dangerous.

This may involve letting Chelsea have more control over her care, situation and circumstances; this should allow her to feel safe and powerful in more of her life.

This should be done when Chelsea is calm, not when she is already panicking and using maladaptive strategies.

Tactics may include:

- scheduling planned one-to-one time with preferred staff for Chelsea
- having rotas decided in advance to allow Chelsea to know who is coming in and when
- creating opportunities for Chelsea to build attachments with all staff, and all staff responding in consistent ways to her emotions and her behaviour
- using empathy and empathic commentary to help Chelsea know that the staff accept her and care about her. (Empathic commentary is a technique described later in the book; see Chapter 34, page 328.)

The strategy will also involve ensuring that clear boundaries, routines and consequences for actions are maintained within the setting. This consistency and predictability will help Chelsea feel safer and reduce the need for her to manipulate situations to help her feel safe.

Her current strategy of threatening self-harm should be approached too. There should be a plan developed with Chelsea for how she can cope with her anxiety in better ways and to help her to recognise other tools that are available to her rather than self-harming or threatening self-harm.

CASE STUDY 19.4 THE FOOD HOARDER (PAGE 156) – REVISITED

Clare comes from a neglectful background where food was scarce. She is now in care. She often only eats half of her meals and stashes the rest in her room. She steals from the fridge, she takes discarded food from waste bins, she shoplifts.

The staff feel at a loss. They are providing regular meals and she is offered snacks. They are struggling to understand why Clare continues to behave in this way.

Motivational Triangle Results

The bonus chapter 'Clare and Margaret – Behavioural Plans' (which can be downloaded at https://library.jkp.com/redeem using the code ESGBAKQ) shows in Clare's behavioural plan that multiple tactics are involved in initially managing her food hoarding behaviour and, over time, changing it. See also Chapter 26, page 250.

Clare's stress is reduced by supporting her to know that food will come later and tomorrow through meal planning, having a snack box in her room and providing a structured meal routine.

Her unmet need is now being managed through the snack box she keeps in her room rather than stolen food. Over time, Clare's maladaptive strategy for stealing and hiding food should subside as she builds trust in her new environment through her experiences of food now always being available.

Clare's current strategy (taking food) is also inhibited in the plan by removing the bins after meals and providing multiple smaller portions rather than large platefuls. These add friction to Clare's current strategy.

The next few chapters will explore in more detail the three approaches: managing the current strategy, managing stress and meeting the need.

It is worth noting that as we create a plan, we may recognise limitations in our abilities to effect change in one or more of the elements of the triangle, and so we may need to develop a team around the person. Ideally, the individual should be included in this process.

Additional support may be required from speech and language therapists, occupational therapists, psychologists and therapists, and medical professionals.

It is also worth gaining support from and collaborating with other people who may be involved, such as family members, other caregivers, teachers and of course the individual themselves.

CHAPTER 20

STEP 1: THE CURRENT STRATEGY

When we are looking at the strategy and creating a plan, we need to explore the individual's deficits and why this is the behaviour they are using to meet their need or manage their stress rather than using more socially acceptable or beneficial (adaptive) options.

One example is communication – is this person using their behaviour to meet their need or manage their stress because they do not have another way to communicate due to a deficit in communication skills?

This is a great starting point, as we can start to explore the behaviour from the concept of communication. We will begin by asking three questions.

- What communication skills do they have?
- Do we need to learn theirs?
- Do we need to teach them one?

COMMUNICATION

(How we communicate)
Speech and writings

Non-verbal
Signs
Symbols
Gestures
Body language
Facial expressions
Pointing
Objects and pictures
'Behaviours'

Paralinguistic
Volume
Intonation
Rate
Tone
Fluency

(Why we communicate)
Attention
Greetings
Wants/needs
Request information
Give information
Ask questions
Protest/deny
Feelings
Choices
Preferences

(Where, when and with whom we communicate)
Partner
Time and place
Shared language
Shared communication system
Shared interests

Figure 20.1 Means, Reasons and Opportunities Model

The diagram displays the Means, Reasons and Opportunities Model.

The *means* are the skills the person currently uses to communicate. These are made up of multiple tools that all of us use in various ways. We have already seen that all behaviour is a form of communication, so all individuals have some communication abilities. Understanding an individual's existing communication skills and abilities can inform us of what potential strategies could be available for them.

The *reasons* are why we communicate, which is made up of a significant list of functions for communication.

Opportunities refers to the fact that the *way* we communicate will vary according to the circumstances. I may speak to my friend in a certain way but speak differently to work colleagues. When I'm at home, I speak in a certain way, but maybe I speak differently if I'm in a restaurant. I may have private jargon and private jokes with some people that mean nothing to others. I might watch my language in some circumstances but be less restrained in others (because of my inhibitors; see Chapter 10, page 93).

So, one answer to the first question – 'What communication skills do they have?' – is potentially the 'behaviour that challenges at the moment'.

The second question – 'Do we need to learn theirs?' – is where we explore incident reports to see if there are any pre-communicators (behaviour or language that tends to precede a behaviour). Some of these may be explicit – the individual is actually communicating their need but in a way that caregivers don't understand.

CASE STUDY 20.1 PRE-COMMUNICATORS

Alex is non-verbal autistic; he also experiences hypersensitivity. Sometimes, when staff are helping Alex dress, he will start to verbalise and make a moaning sound and begin rocking. This is Alex asking caregivers to stop, as he is experiencing pain. If they do not stop, Alex will hit out.

Mabel is living with dementia and experiences hypersensitivity. Sometimes, when the caregivers are helping Mabel with personal care, she will shout out, 'Ow, you are hurting me,' even though the caregivers are being gentle. Mabel is genuinely experiencing pain, so staff should stop the task (if safe) and allow Mabel to calm. If they do not stop, Mabel will pinch and scratch.

Magda is living with dementia. Magda is originally from Poland and despite knowing English, she is now only able to speak in Polish. Sometimes Magda will shout '*jestem głodna*' ('I'm hungry'). If Magda cannot get food, she will start walking around the room and taking biscuits and sweets from other residents in the home.

Rajani has learning disabilities and limited communication skills. When Rajani says 'Home soon', staff say 'No' to Rajani, as he is not going home. This makes Rajani very agitated, and he will withdraw from engaging for the rest of the day. Rajani is feeling homesick and missing his family. When Rajani says 'Home soon', staff should organise a phone call or Zoom meeting with either his mum or his brother for ten minutes. This helps Rajani feel better.

During the 'understand and empathise' process, the use of the ABC analysis may reveal these communication keys; they should be recognised, and a plan should be created around them.

The last question is: 'Do we need to teach them one?'

It may be appropriate to teach new communication skills to support the individual to better engage in their world. This could include:

- **Language education**: English, British Sign Language, Makaton, Picture Exchange Communication System (PECS) or picture charts.
- **Terms, phrases or tools**: Single words or phrases to enable the individual to express themselves or a card, object or symbol to act as a communicator.

CASE STUDY 20.2 AMIR (PAGE 135) – REVISITED

Amir pretends to make himself sick and makes a vomiting noise at staff to get connection and affection from caregivers.

Caregivers teach Amir to use either a card saying 'Hug' or a toy bear to communicate his need. If he gives the card or the toy bear to a caregiver, they know he needs a hug.

CASE STUDY 20.3 THERE'S NO NEED TO HIT, BERTIE

Sometimes Bertie would approach his foster father, Steve, and start slapping and pushing. If no attention was given, these hits could escalate. One day Steve realised something, and next time Bertie started hitting him, Steve just said in a soft, kind and nurturing tone, 'I'm wondering if you hit me because you need my attention but you don't know how to get it. Maybe in the past you *had* to hit people to get attention. But here, you can just ask for a hug and you know you'll get one!' Steve nodded to the space next to him on the sofa. Bertie jumped up and sat there, and Steve put an arm around him. (This is an example of empathic commentary, which is in Stage 5: Respond Appropriately; see Chapter 34, page 328.)

Note: Please be cautious and risk assess hugging, especially with vulnerable and abused children. Hugging is positive if it is managed safely and appropriately for both the individual and the caregiver. (Please use safer caring principles and maintain appropriate professional boundaries.)

The above examples all include a deficit in communication skills involving an inability in communication to express a stress or need to others.

Communication skills and improving communication are part of Stage 3: Proactive Planning but are also vital at the point of responding to behaviours.

Other examples of behavioural deficits are covered at various points throughout the book and should be considered. They may include the following:

- **Learning difficulties and disabilities:** Do we need to make reasonable adjustments for how this person can learn, do they need more time or repetition to develop a skill?
- **Memory impairments:** Can we add reminders to the environment or use tools to help this person with their memory?
- **Difficulties with sensory processing:** Can we get occupational therapy support and help them with managing their senses? Can we make environmental adjustments to make a sensory safe environment that's right for this person?
- **Difficulties with emotional regulation:** As shown in the following case study.

CASE STUDY 20.4 PANIC ABOUT PANICKING (PAGE 157) – REVISITED

In 'Unmet Needs', Chapter 17, page 154, we met Rachel, the schoolgirl who suffers panic attacks. Here, we revisit that case study to show how staff addressed the problem.

Rachel has had several panic attacks at school. The cause seems to be getting overwhelmed by certain work or when there is too much stimulus.

After an episode, Rachel has to be helped to calm by being guided to a safe, quiet space away from the classroom.

Rachel's keyworker wants to teach Rachel better ways to cope with her stress and build her resilience, but the decision is taken to start by teaching Rachel a better way to communicate her stress.

It is recognised that Rachel finds it difficult to ask for help when she is becoming overwhelmed, so a plan is created. Rachel is given three coloured cards: green, orange and red.

If Rachel recognises that she is finding something hard and needs help, she puts the green card on her desk. The teacher is instructed to acknowledge the card if it is noticed and let Rachel know that she will get some help in a few moments.

If Rachel puts the orange card on the desk, the teacher recognises and acknowledges that Rachel needs immediate support. The teacher can then either offer help or prompt Rachel to go to her safe space for a few moments.

However, if Rachel is feeling overwhelmed, she can stand up, show the teacher the red card and go straight to her safe space.

If Rachel goes to her safe space, someone will come to her within five minutes to help her to re-regulate and then bring her back to the class.

Having a way to communicate her needs means Rachel's confidence begins to grow. Other work is then done with Rachel for her to be able to self-regulate when she is still in class, and the need for the red card decreases.

Commentary: Rachel did not have a strategy to cope with her stress or meet her need and so was just becoming overwhelmed and making herself ill. As we explored in Stage 2: Understand/Empathise, often individuals develop intentional strategies with purpose and function to manage their stress and needs, but these strategies may be maladaptive.

LEARNED RESPONSE

Learned responses, as discussed in Chapter 15, page 135, may develop from innate behaviours (e.g., eating could lead to eating disorders), modelled behaviours (modelled by parents, peers or role models, e.g., peer pressure) or invasive thoughts/fixed ideas (e.g., OCD – obsessive compulsive disorder. This is an anxiety-based disorder associated with invasive thoughts, where a person engages in obsessional rituals to relieve distress. The invasive thoughts usually have themes of either contamination, e.g., fear of germs, handwashing, etc., or the desire for symmetry, danger or forbidden desires).

The learning and outcome of these strategies may be conscious or unconscious, but essentially, they are learned through reinforcement by external forces, 'I did this, and it triggered this response from others,' or internal reinforcers, 'I did this, and I felt better or felt less distress.'

CASE STUDY 20.5 TANIA, THE SURVIVOR

Tania had been cutting herself for three years. She describes the need to cut as being like the need to take a breath when you've been swimming underwater. She started cutting because she couldn't cope with her emotional pain. It helped; it took away the pain.

It allowed her to survive.

Now, though, Tania doesn't know how she can live without cutting. When she feels overwhelmed, she craves it like a drug.

After Tania cuts, she feels shame, she knows she shouldn't do it. The staff at her last placement used to tell her how naughty she was when she cut or tell her how she upset people with her behaviour. They also tried to hide all the knives to stop her. So she tried to hide her cutting and would use anything she could find to cut.

This new home is different. The staff seem to understand why she cuts; they don't tell her off. They just seem to want to help her not to feel so bad that she needs to cut.

They are working with her on a plan of other things to try before cutting. Tania now has a list of five things to do before she resorts to cutting.

1. Talk to staff.
2. Watch an episode of *The Big Bang Theory*.
3. Listen to her happy playlist on Spotify.
4. Go for a run.
5. Place a red coloured (food dye) ice cube in the crook of her elbow and hold it there until it's melted.

If any of those work, she tells the staff and they share in her pride. If they don't work and she ends up still needing to cut, she is encouraged to tell the staff afterwards so they can check she is okay and provide first aid if she needs it.

Commentary: Tania's cutting was a maladaptive strategy to manage her stress of anxiety and shame. The short-term relief she felt reinforced the need to cut to the point that it became an addiction. She needed a safer tactic. Working with her to find a new strategy will take time, but we always focus on the need, not the speed.

Note: It is important to recognise that before a plan was even created for Tania, she already occasionally engaged in these other tactics to manage her stress; she just hadn't made the connection and realised her successes. So staff could say, 'The other day you were feeling bad but you watched an episode of Big Bang and you didn't cut.'

With these learned responses, the plan created will be to teach the individual that other strategies can also work to meet their needs or manage their stress and may be more effective, improve their social inclusion and outcomes, or be safer and more appropriate.

When looking at Step 1, 'The Current Strategy', we need to know if we are teaching the individual a new strategy or skills, or changing their current strategy by helping them to use existing skills more effectively and consciously.

CHAPTER 21

STEP 2: MANAGE THE STRESS – RECOVERY FROM TRAUMA

Special terms used in this chapter:

Metabolisation: Metabolism is the sum total of all the chemical reactions in the body – for example, those used in digestion – but it applies to all chemical processes in the body. These chemical interactions are affected by biological, environmental and psychological factors. Stress, relaxation, pleasure, depression and even social interactions affect our metabolism. Simply put, mind influences chemistry. Metabolisation is the process of using experiences and changing thoughts, feelings and beliefs to alter brain chemistry. It's like changing diet or exercising to change the digestive metabolism.

Integration: This refers to the basic definition, which is the intermixing of people who were previously segregated. Many individuals who display behaviour that challenges can become segregated from others. Integration is about helping them to belong.

In Stage 2: Understand/Empathise, we explored many causes of potential stress and where they come from. This chapter and the next will explore what we can do to reduce stress and support someone to better manage their stressors.

If we can reduce the things that shake up the bottle of Coke, we have a chance to learn how to keep the lid on. If the lid is always off, no learning can occur.

Throughout the book, there are a number of sections and tools that look at reducing stress. They come from a variety of disciplines, such as trauma-informed care, CBT and therapeutic parenting. These include the way that we 'respond to behaviour' (see Chapter 32, page 311), but also teaching self-awareness and self-management, which are included in multiple areas of the book.

This chapter and the next explore specific approaches. This chapter describes the process for recovery from trauma. The next chapter describes the use of the HELP principle.

Note: Recovery from trauma has certain specialised requirements, but we can identify certain underlying principles that would apply to planning for any type of maladaptive behaviour. Tania's case study is revisited at the end of this chapter as an example.

We introduced the principle of Maslow's Hierarchy of Needs and trauma-informed recovery in Stage 1: Identify. It is worth exploring this principle as part of the planning approach.

Recovery from trauma is not a top-down process, meaning it doesn't only involve getting a person to think, feel and behave differently. It is a bottom-up process that is trying to change a person's very neurobiology.

There are three stages:

1. **Stabilisation**: Making safe (this can be a useful stage for anyone in a high stress state).
2. **Metabolisation and integration**: Making safe changes (changing thoughts, feelings and behaviour in a way that doesn't make the person feel overwhelmed, judged or unsafe. Need, not speed).
3. **Adaptation**: Moving forwards with a new sense of identity.

STABILISATION

- **Neutralising sources of traumatisation**: Do all that we can to eliminate any triggers that will cause invading thoughts to return; try to give the individual time and space to heal.
- **Finding a 'good enough' secure attachment figure**: Caregiver/s whom the individual can trust in a therapeutic relationship.
- **Psychoeducation**: It isn't always easy for someone who is in a traumatic state, but the idea is to try to help them understand that certain things they do are related to their trauma – to things that have happened in the past. Following from that, help them come to terms with: 'The past is the past, the present is the present.'

- **Developing coping strategies to manage symptoms:** In a nutshell, expanding the 'window of tolerance' (page 117). This may include: therapies such as Eye Movement Desensitisation and Reprocessing (EMDR), trauma-informed CBT; positive activities such as yoga and meditation; learning new skills.
- **Boosting brain resilience:** Sufficient exercise, sleep, diet and water consumption.
- **Safe environment:** One that is structured and predictable. Predictability and routine tend to be a little boring but also tend to be more comforting because the individual knows what will happen and when. Caregivers should be consistent in responses to the individual to reduce the anxiety of having different reactions from different people.

  Examples may include:
  - set mealtimes and mealtime routines
  - limited visitors or set staff teams
  - a clear care/support plan that staff follow
  - structured bedtime/morning routines
  - allow the environment to feel as similar to their normal environment as is appropriate. Allow familiarity, which may include familiar objects, smells and layout. (Remember the room one/room two analogy from page 147 – some of the things in room one may seem wrong to us but may feel safer to an individual.)
- **Stabilising self-destructive behaviours:** Trying to minimise or manage hazardous behaviours like self-harm and eating disorders to reduce the chances of worsening or increasing risks.

CASE STUDY 21.1 STABILISATION IN TRAUMA

The staff felt that Mathew's bedroom should be tidy. Mathew would leave clothes on the floor; food would be left lying around. His room was chaotic, and some staff felt it was unhygienic. Based on Mathew's past, it was decided that this was the wrong battle for now. Mathew came from mess and so initially his room was allowed to be his own. It was agreed that staff would go in every two days and help Mathew clear any food, and once a week just to clear dirty clothes, but otherwise it would be left alone.

As Mathew become more trusting in the setting, he began to do the food and clothes chores independently. One day he asked a staff member if they would help him tidy his room as he fancied having it redecorated.

CASE STUDY 21.2 STABILISATION IN DELIRIUM

Ellen was in hospital with a severe infection. She was really struggling with paranoid delusions that the doctors were scientists who were trying to experiment on her. She would be very aggressive to staff and refuse the medication that she needed to get better. The family were contacted and asked if they could bring in some familiar items from Ellen's room, especially photographs and her bedside clock and lamp. The family were also asked to try and arrange additional visits to Ellen while in hospital or even Zoom meetings to help her to feel more settled.

METABOLISATION (BIOLOGICAL CHANGE) AND INTEGRATION

Over time, the stabilisation techniques have begun to make the individual feel safe and that the environment is steady and reliable, and they have started to change their very core beliefs and brain wiring to believe they are safe (the acceptance of room two). We can then build on this foundation to ensure that the individual feels that this is the 'new normal'. The underlying causes of the trauma are still there, and at this stage it's possible to progress to methods to handle the trauma, as shown in the following list. This is also the stage that other habits of behaviour may be explored and managed. So, we can now start introducing changes in a way that focuses on need rather than speed and allows the individual to still feel safe.

- **Uncovering trauma and coming to terms with it and grieving through guided therapy**: Note: This is *not* done by caregivers simply getting people to talk about the problems without guidance and training.
- **Developing physiological and psychological self-management by teaching the individual new strategies to manage difficult emotions and flashbacks:** Teaching new self-care skills, such as those listed in 'Coping Strategies', Chapter 22, page 197.
- **Processing**: Acting out to talking out – at this stage, an individual may be able to reflect on their behaviour (acting out), recognise that their behaviour may cause negative consequences and explore whether there may be better ways. Now that trust is developing, the individual may be able to explore any shame or negative thinking patterns and accept that their self is not fixed. They may be able to accept praise if they haven't before, as trust and self-worth may be developing.
- **Cognitive restructuring**: Teaching the individual new ways of thinking. Many people have negative thought patterns that come from core beliefs (who we are) and scripts (who we think we should be) and the idea is to get the individual to realise that just because they think something doesn't mean it's true. An example of that is what we call catastrophic thinking, which is an automatic negative thought.

  For example, a person may be on a diet but one day get really hungry and have a chocolate bar. Catastrophic thinking is: 'I failed my diet. I've messed up. I never manage to do diets. I always do it wrong.' But, just because that's the thinking doesn't mean it's true. They just had a chocolate bar, and that doesn't mean they've failed.

ADAPTATION

As the individual progresses through the healing of past experiences, they begin to feel comfortable with their new personality. New opportunities now arise to do the following things.

- **Explore their changed personality, perceptions and relationships**: They may now need guidance to help them cope with the new world that faces them – to maintain positive thinking or maybe develop new relationships or build confidence to develop new relationships.
- **Increase engagement and social interaction**: E.g., taking up a hobby or socialising in any appropriate and enjoyable way.
- **Develop self-esteem**: Typically, self-esteem can grow through achievements and successes, a growing self-worth; e.g., a person might enjoy equestrian therapy – looking after a horse. The person sees that the horse looks beautiful after grooming and that the horse is staying alive and alert because of the person's work and care. And the person can think, 'I'm worth something.'
- **Handle emotional challenges in a better way**: An individual may need teaching about conflict management; e.g., how to deal with a friend who disagrees with them and how to cope when they feel they're in danger of losing control.
- **Enjoy life**: Many individuals with a traumatic background seem to lose all joy in life. So find opportunities for the individual to find the joy in their life that they've missed for several years.

As mentioned, these strategies can be used in a multitude of circumstances; there does not have to be historic trauma that has been diagnosed.

CASE STUDY 21.3 TANIA, THE SURVIVOR (PAGE 185) – REVISITED

In the earlier case study about Tania, we saw how certain plans had been made for how Tania could be helped to stay away from self-harm.

This version of the case study reviews the problem through the lens of recovery from trauma. The assumption is that Tania is not necessarily suffering from trauma but from a maladaptive behaviour. Let's see how the principles of recovery from trauma could be applied.

1. **Stabilisation**: Implement a low-stress setting, minimise change, create

predictable routines and boundaries to help Tania feel safe. Make sure she feels accepted and can start to develop some good enough attachments with a few key staff. Teach her about her feelings and what's going on in her brain that causes her to need to cut.

2. **Metabolisation (biological change) and integration**: Start to explore other strategies she could use instead of cutting. Maintain acceptance of her and her problem, but encourage a change to promote self-care. Help Tania to change her negative thinking and build her self-esteem. Now that she feels safe, she may accept praise.
3. **Adaptation**: Tania may now have some new strategies that she uses to manage her emotions; she may now be able to work to continue to build her self-esteem and start to expand her horizons. Keep building on self-awareness and self-management.

Being familiar with these stages can allow caregivers to ensure they can adapt their plan to focus on the right stage with an individual to best support them. We may not always be aware of an individual's history or challenges, so being sensitive and adaptable during planning and the implementation of the plan, and being willing to re-explore identification and understanding, is important. We may find we start to implement a plan but realise that we are picking the wrong battles and/or that an individual is not ready to address some behaviours.

At this point, it is worth revisiting 'Case Study 12.1 The Row with Your Partner – Revisited', page 106. This shows the three stages in action:

1. **Stabilisation**: We feel safe.
2. **Metabolisation and integration**: We adapt our understanding of the other person and the experience changes either how we feel about them or how we feel about ourselves; we then reintegrate with the person.
3. **Adaption**: The new understanding of ourselves and the other person allows us to adapt our behaviour and future interactions.

CHAPTER 22

STEP 2: MANAGE THE STRESS – USING THE HELP PRINCIPLE

In Stage 2: Understand/Empathise, we used the acronym HELP to understand stressors. We can use this again in planning. Here is the acronym written out in full:

- **Human**: Unhealthy or unbalanced relationships, lack of trust or a need for connection.
- **Emotional/cognitive**: Mental/emotional wellbeing, resilience, self-esteem and flexibility of thinking.
- **Location**: The environment itself is stressful.
- **Physical**: Physical health and basic needs.

We will explore potential short-term and long-term strategies to reduce and cope with stress in each of these areas.

HUMAN STRESSORS

It is vital that caregivers develop therapeutic relationships with individuals in their care.

In relation to behavioural change and management, who are you more likely to listen to, accept feedback from and work with? Someone you trust or someone you don't?

It is easier to break trust than it is to make trust!

Throughout this book, we have described caregivers' personal beliefs, attitudes and values as being fundamental to successful behaviour management and improved outcomes, and we know that building trust is one of the most important aims of a caring relationship.

Several aspects combine to create a therapeutic relationship. Details of these are covered in Chapter 27 and Chapter 28, starting at page 256.

EMOTIONAL/COGNITIVE STRESSORS

A big part of proactive planning should consider an individual's emotions and thoughts. In Stage 2: Understand/Empathise, we explored the concept of reflex behaviours and how we don't act on impulse but are constrained by inhibitors.

It is so important that we see the brain as adaptable and recognise that it's not that a person *can't* change their behaviour, it's that they find it difficult and they may not realise that help and tools are available. We will explore this more later when discussing habit change in Chapter 24, but part of our plan should include emotional self-awareness and self-management.

For example, to control your anger you must:

- realise you are getting angry
- want to control it
- have alternative strategies to both manage the anger and manage the situation.

The reason 'manage the situation' is included in that statement is important, because depending on context and circumstances, it could be right for us to be angry...

Is our anger justified? Anger is an indication that something is wrong for us. That's a good thing... feelings are good. However, the emotion does not mean we are correct. Do we need to change the way we think or feel, or do we need to request a change in the situation?

CASE STUDY 22.1 THE NOISE IN THE ALLEY

You are walking home alone on a dark night, in an unfamiliar place. You find yourself walking down an alley and you are feeling slightly apprehensive. All of a sudden, you hear a noise behind you. Your thoughts race. Is someone there? Was it an animal? Was it the wind? You think it's danger, you feel scared, so you don't wait for evidence; you react and run out of the alley without looking back. You run straight over to the other side of the road and into an open shop to collect your thoughts and feel safe.

Was that the right thing to do? The immediate answer may feel like 'yes'. If it was something dangerous, then maybe running was the best option, and if it wasn't dangerous, then running didn't result in anything bad – so isn't it better to be safe than sorry? However, this narrative doesn't mean that *objectively* it was the best action to take. Just because you felt it was right at the time, just because you can justify it to yourself afterwards and it meant that nothing bad happened to you, doesn't confirm that there was something bad in the alley or that your reaction was the best action to take. The feelings don't make the thought true!

What if it wasn't anything bad – it was just a cat – but you ran out of the alley and in your panicked state didn't look before you ran across the road, which resulted in you being hit by a car. That this was not the outcome indicates that you were lucky rather than indicating that you were accurate. What if the noise down the alley was a person who was ill or injured and desperately needed your help? That would mean your feelings were wrong and your action was more detrimental than beneficial!

However, unfortunately we can't rewind and see what would have happened if we had stayed in the alley. (Unless you happened to read in the news the following day about a person having a heart attack in that alley at the same time you were in there, you'd be unaware of the opposing evidence so you may still believe your actions were for the best.)

Commentary: This case study is intended to raise an understanding that thoughts and feelings are not a reliable pathway to truth. This is a principle often used in therapy to address automatic negative thoughts. For example, just because you *think* that a person hates you doesn't mean they do. Just because you *feel* unlovable doesn't mean you are unlovable. Being angry doesn't make you right.

Getting people to explore the evidence for their thoughts and feelings can help individuals to recognise unhealthy and detrimental thoughts and feelings that could be holding them back from positive outcomes.

Skills that are beneficial in developing emotional self-awareness and self-management that we should encourage in others and ourselves include:

- labelling and recognising emotions
- identifying what triggers emotions
- analysing emotions and how they affect others
- understanding the relationship between emotions, thoughts and behaviours
- recognising personal needs, values, judgements and biases
- recognising and managing unhealthy thought patterns
- identifying personal strengths and areas for growth
- practising self-compassion
- cultivating self-confidence, positive self-regard, a 'growth' mindset and optimism.[55]

Self-management is the ability to navigate and shift our thoughts, emotions and behaviours in a healthy way in order to make decisions and reach goals that benefit ourselves and others.

There is plenty of information in this book that can be used to support this process.

In Chapter 31 we will explore an *introspection* process, which is the process of supporting individuals to recognise their own feelings and triggers and to begin exploring what they and others can do to help them recognise escalation.

One of our aims throughout the whole behavioural management process is to improve outcomes, and one outcome we would like to achieve is positive mental wellbeing.

The mental health continuum means that regardless of labels and diagnosis, mental wellbeing is a spectrum that is separate from mental illness, and both make up a person's overall mental health. In the way that a person may have a condition like diabetes but manage their condition well overall and actually have really good physical health, this principle can also apply to mental health.

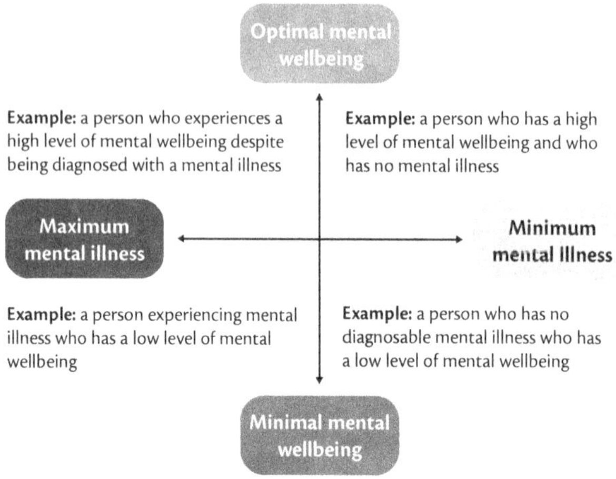

Figure 22.1 Mental Health Continuum[56]

To achieve mental wellbeing, let's return to the biopsychosocial model described earlier.

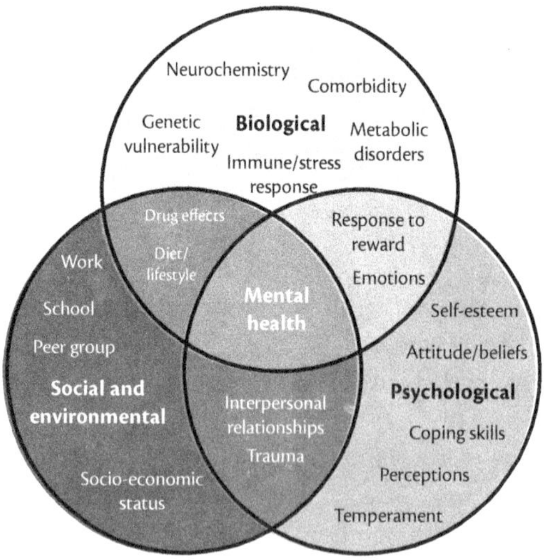

Figure 22.2 The Biopsychosocial Model

As in the mental health continuum, these three areas affect mental health and are all interconnected. We should examine all three areas in treating mental ill health and promoting positive mental wellbeing.

The following section looks at different approaches that address specific areas or that can be blended together to address several needs. One strategy is unlikely to provide a complete solution.

Coping Strategies

Here are some examples of coping strategies that can be presented to, and explored with, an individual for better self-management. There are any number of possibilities, sometimes depending on the nature of the problem, the person and environmental limits.

Distraction Techniques

- **Engage in a hobby:** Painting, knitting, gardening or any creative activity.
- **Watch a movie or TV show:** Choose something light-hearted or engaging.
- **Read a book:** Dive into a fictional world or learn something new.
- **Listen to music or a podcast:** Choose something soothing or uplifting.
- **Play a game:** Board games, video games or puzzles.
- **Exercise:** Go for a walk, run or practice yoga.
- **Cook or bake:** Try a new recipe or make a favourite dish.
- **Socialise:** Call or meet up with friends or family.

Grounding Techniques

- **5-4-3-2-1 technique:** Identify 5 things you see, 4 things you can touch, 3 things you hear, 2 things you can smell and 1 thing you can taste.
- **Deep breathing:** Practice slow, deep breaths, inhaling through the nose and exhaling through the mouth.
- **Body scan:** Focus on each part of your body, starting from your toes and working up to your head.
- **Hold a grounding object:** Keep a smooth stone, stress ball or any tactile object to hold.
- **Cold water:** Splash cold water on your face or hold an ice cube.
- **Describe your surroundings:** Verbally describe everything you see around you.

Mindfulness

- **Meditation:** Practice guided or unguided meditation.
- **Mindful eating:** Focus on the taste, texture and aroma of your food.
- **Nature walk:** Observe the sights, sounds and smells of nature.
- **Mindful breathing:** Focus solely on your breath and its rhythm.

- **Gratitude journalling:** Write down things you are grateful for each day.
- **Yoga:** Practice yoga to connect your mind and body.

Emotional Release

- **Cry:** Allow yourself to cry and release pent-up emotions.
- **Scream into a pillow:** Release frustration or anger in a safe way.
- **Journal:** Write down your thoughts and feelings.
- **Art:** Paint, draw or sculpt to express your emotions.
- **Dance:** Move your body to release built-up energy.
- **Exercise:** Engage in physical activity to let out stress and anger.

Self-Love

- **Positive affirmations:** Repeat positive statements about yourself.
- **Self-care routine:** Pamper yourself with a bath, skincare or other self-care activities.
- **Set boundaries:** Learn to say no and protect your time and energy.
- **Celebrate achievements:** Acknowledge and celebrate your accomplishments, big or small.
- **Spend time alone:** Enjoy your own company doing something you love.
- **Nourish your body:** Eat healthy foods and stay hydrated.

Thought Challenging

- **Identify cognitive distortions:** Recognise and label distorted thinking patterns.
- **Evidence for and against:** Write down evidence supporting and contradicting a negative thought.
- **Alternative perspectives:** Consider different viewpoints or outcomes.
- **De-catastrophising:** Assess the actual likelihood of the worst-case scenario.
- **Reframe negative thoughts:** Turn negative thoughts into more positive or neutral ones.
- **Affirmations:** Replace negative thoughts with positive affirmations.

Accessing Higher Self

- **Volunteer:** Offer your time to a cause you care about.
- **Perform acts of kindness:** Do something nice for someone else.
- **Connect with nature:** Pet animals, visit nature, watch animals in nature.
- **Pray or meditate:** Connect with your spiritual beliefs.
- **Smile at strangers:** Spread positivity and notice the responses.
- **Join a community group**: Engage with others of similar values.

Talking Therapies

Caution: The following therapies should only be carried out by a qualified practitioner.

Some types of talking therapy are listed below:

- **Cognitive behavioural therapy (CBT)**: This is dedicated to changing negative thought patterns by addressing our behavioural responses to uncomfortable situations or emotional distress.
- **Dialectical behavioural therapy (DBT)**: This is a form of CBT tailored to help people cope with interpersonal issues. It was developed specifically to help patients struggling with personality disorders. It combines the practices of CBT with meditation and a focus on relationships.
- **Psychodynamic therapy**: This is a type of talking therapy focusing on examining a person's past experiences to better understand and interpret present behaviours and emotions.
- **Humanistic therapy**: This type of therapy's approaches include client-centred and existential therapy. Humanistic therapy addresses problems by inspecting multiple angles of a person's life. It may unpack a particular issue by examining thoughts, actions, relationships and physical feelings.
- **Eye movement desensitisation and reprocessing (EMDR) therapy**: This is an effective psychotherapy method proven to help people recover from trauma and other distressing life experiences, including PTSD, anxiety, depression and panic disorders.

Holistic Therapies

Some types of holistic therapy are listed below:

- **Aromatherapy**: Using smells to change moods and feelings.
- **Sensory rooms and objects**: Therapeutic spaces that stimulate the senses or objects that provide sensory stimulation.
- **Music therapy**: Listening to and/or playing music.
- **Doll and play therapy**: Child version: Engaging in play to safely act out stories from their past. Adult version: A person with dementia playing with a doll and re-enacting past stories.
- **Massage, meditation, yoga**.

Lifestyle Changes

We have all heard the phrases 'You are what you eat' and 'Healthy body, healthy mind'. These may seem like clichés but there's a lot of truth in them.

Lifestyle changes include encouraging the individual to take more exercise or see more of their friends and family.

We know that exercise is statistically as successful for reducing depression as talking therapies and medication. Exercise releases endorphins and lowers cortisol levels.

Careful exposure to the sun increases the level of vitamin D, which has been correlated to improved cognition and overall brain function.

Having enough water to drink and a healthy diet is vitally important.

Ensure that an individual engages in certain forms of activity throughout the week, like something social, something physical, something they really enjoy and something that has a sense of achievement to it. There are some activities that fulfil a number of goals. For example, for someone who enjoys nature, a group nature walk provides enjoyment, exercise, sunlight and social interaction. If the length of the walk is gradually increased and targets are added, a sense of achievement can follow.

Activity Scheduling

A common tool for improving mood and reducing depression is activity scheduling. Unfortunately, with a condition like depression and other mood/anxiety disorders, one of the symptoms is an inability to take pleasure from activities that were previously enjoyed, so it can be quite common for people with depression to withdraw and progressively become less active. This occurs without the realisation that activities, social engagement, achievement and fun are the very things that help to overcome depression, improve mood and promote wellbeing. An activity schedule can be completed in advance to review what level of activity and engagement an individual has already and then adjusted as part of the proactive plan.

Review

Over the course of a week, make a list of which activities a person engages in each day. Then look at how many activities they engaged in that provided satisfaction within the following four categories. Some activities may meet multiple categories.

- **Physical**: Movement and exercise (e.g., walking, jumping, sports, dancing).
- **Pleasurable**: Something they enjoy (e.g., taking a bath, listening to music, sitting and doing nothing).
- **Social**: Something involving other people (e.g., a group activity, eating a meal with others).
- **Achievement**: Something with a sense of accomplishment (e.g., completing a jigsaw, cooking a meal, tidying the wardrobe).

Once a baseline is established, we can see if there is an unbalance of the categories. If there is unbalance, we may work with the individual to start increasing some of the categories over each day to give their lives better balance.

Medication

Medication can have a beneficial effect for such cases as depression, hyperactivity, hallucinations and distress.

It's easy to prescribe medication, but it should not be seen as a 'silver bullet'. We should always be looking for other strategies to improve mental wellbeing overall. However, many people may need medication to balance emotions and therefore be able to consider other methods. This book does not cover or explore medication options; that does not mean they should not be used. However, they should definitely not be used as the sole solution.

For example, someone who suffers badly from depression may not even be able to leave the house. It may be that medication will stabilise their mood enough for them to be able to access psychological and social measures. Over time, the non-medication therapies may allow the medication to be stopped.

Reducing Anxiety

Fear of the unknown and the stress of change and transitions fall into both the emotional/cognitive and environmental stressor categories. There are actions that we can take that reduce stress and anxiety for these factors.

Staged Desensitisation

CASE STUDY 22.2 'ALONG CAME A SPIDER AND SAT DOWN BESIDE HER, AND FRIGHTENED MISS MUFFET AWAY'

Beth has been scared of spiders for as long as she can remember. Beth hates them, and she becomes completely overwhelmed by spiders.

Beth claims she cannot go out to pubs on Halloween because of the webs and fake spiders that people put up. If she sees one, she will either freeze or run; she was even physically sick after a spider landed on her once.

Do you think we would help Beth to overcome her arachnophobia by telling her it's silly and pointing out the fact that they can't hurt her? What do you think would happen if we just tried to get Beth to overcome her fear by holding a spider and just 'dealing with it'? It's possible Beth would just have a meltdown, be completely overwhelmed and not be able to even engage rationally as a result.

One way we may be able to help Beth is through staged desensitisation. We would try to find the closest interaction with spiders that Beth could cope with. We would introduce this situation on regular occasions until Beth no longer felt stressed by this level of interaction. Then we would move on to a new stage, which would involve a slightly closer interaction... and repeat until Beth could cope again and then keep progressing the stages forwards. How many stages there were would be dictated by Beth's ability to cope.

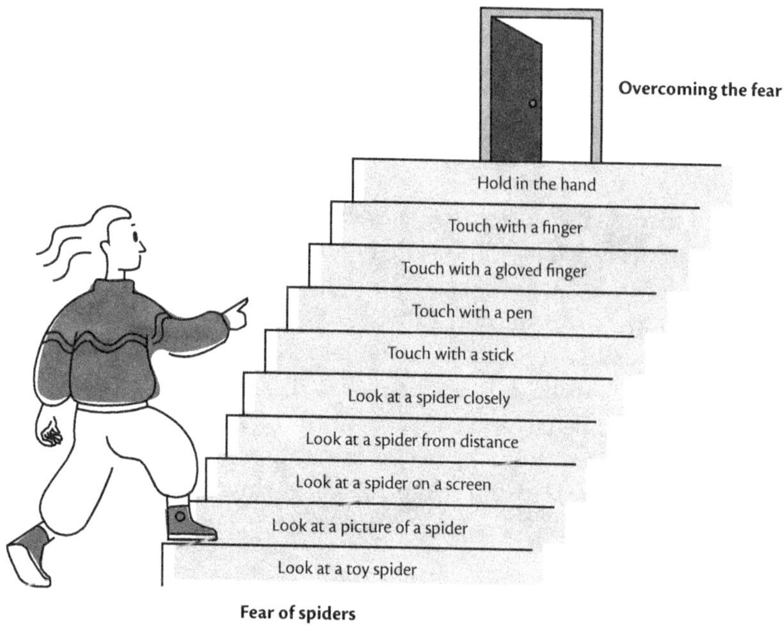

Figure 22.3 Staged Desensitisation

Commentary: The process above recognises that, for Beth, her ability to cope with spiders is not a rational choice, it's an emotional response. We need to recognise and understand that and create a plan of how to help.

> *I believe that anyone can conquer fear by doing the things they fear to do, provided they keep doing them until they get a record of successful experiences behind them.*
>
> ELEANOR ROOSEVELT

Predictability, Routine and Transitions

We all like predictability to some degree or another. Not knowing 'what's happening when' can create stress.

Having schedules, calendars and daily routines that are available and understandable to the individuals can reduce the stress of not knowing.

Any changes to this routine need to be managed and communicated as a plan. If something changes, then individuals need to know what is going to happen instead.

Individuals who find it hard to focus on a set routine due to memory or attention dysregulation and are easily distracted may benefit from having routines shown graphically or conveyed in some other medium.

CASE STUDY 22.3 EXAMPLE ROUTINES

Weekly schedule:

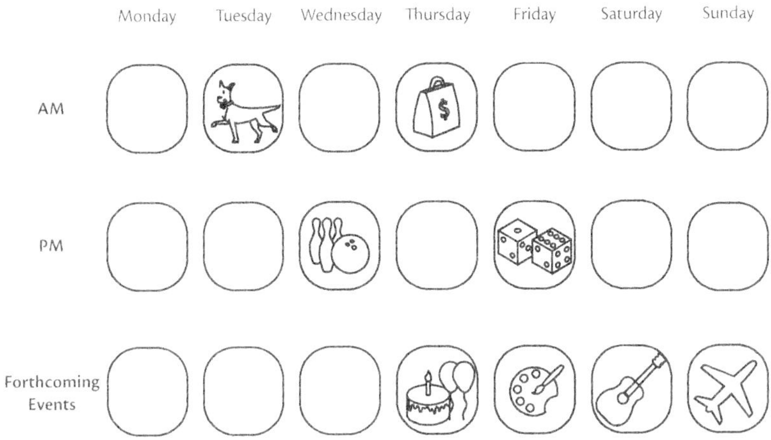
Monday
Tuesday
Wednesday
Thursday
Friday
Saturday
Sunday
AM
PM
Forthcoming Events

Brushing teeth steps:

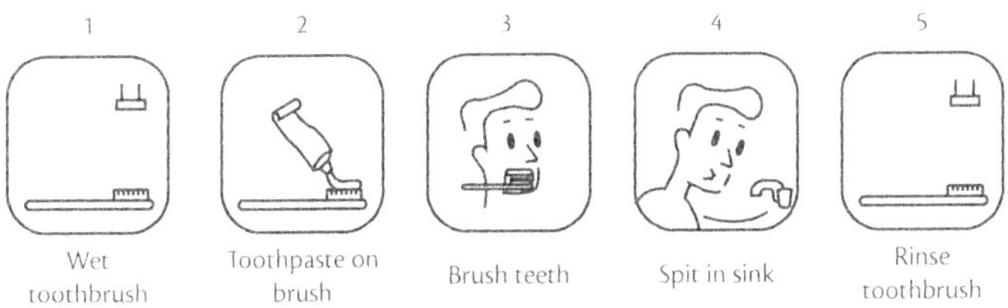

Daily routine:

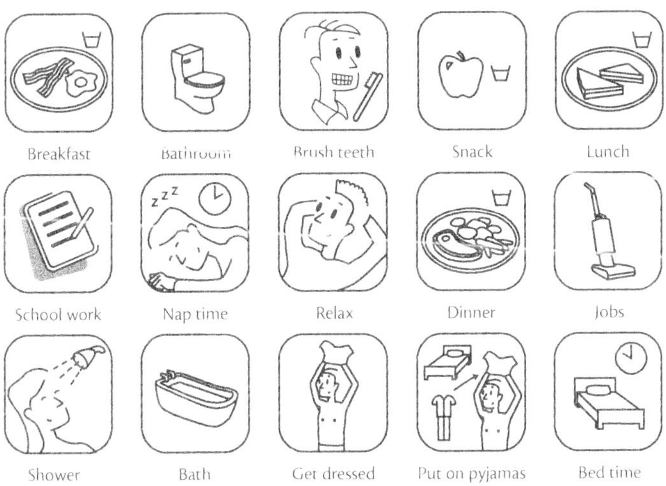
Breakfast
Bathroom
Brush teeth
Snack
Lunch
School work
Nap time
Relax
Dinner
Jobs
Shower
Bath
Get dressed
Put on pyjamas
Bed time

Daily task check sheet:

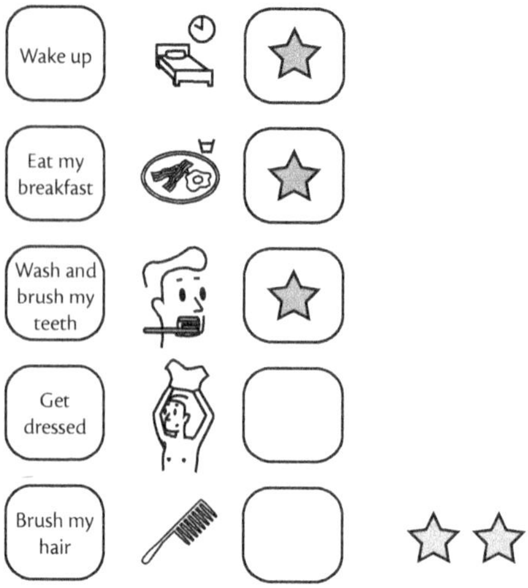

Morning routine set with playlist:

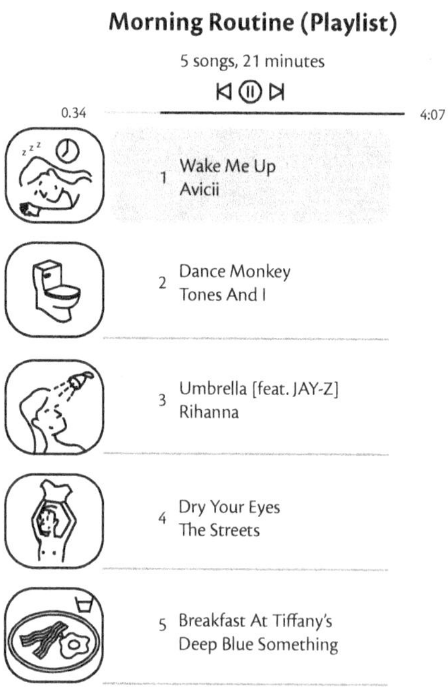

Figure 22.4 Example Routines

Transitions – moving from one place to another or even from one activity or routine to another – can create uncertainty and stress. When we are in control of other people's transitions, this can be amplified significantly.

CASE STUDY 22.4 FIRE ALARM

Imagine you are out at a shop, you have a loaded basket of clothes that you have been desperately trying to find time to buy and you are planning to get the bus in 15 minutes. Suddenly the fire alarm in the store goes off and people are moving to the exits. How do you feel? How many questions about what you should do are running through your head and how much confusion are you experiencing?

Commentary: The sudden transition of a fire evacuation feels highly emotive for most people. If there had been a warning of when the alarm would be going off, and then reminders and maybe a visual timer to let you know how long you had until the alarm, that would have a huge effect on the stress. We can't do that for a fire, unfortunately. We can often do it for transitions in care settings, though.

MANAGING CHANGES IN ROUTINE

In the next section on planning, it's worth mentioning that plans can go wrong, routines can be messed up and transitions may have to happen. The way we manage these is important. Typically, more warning about a change and more choice and control over a change will help us to cope with it and still feel safe.

CASE STUDY 22.5 MAKING LIFE EASIER

Wally's family usually visit him at the home every Thursday. Unfortunately, Wally's family have informed the home that they will not be able to come this Thursday due to a holiday. Although the staff find this out on the Monday, it is decided that they will not tell Wally until Thursday. The decision is made due to previous incidents where Wally struggled emotionally when he knew his family weren't visiting, which resulted in consecutive days of meltdowns, aggression and distress.

The staff feel that one day of these meltdowns is easier to manage than having episodes on Monday, Tuesday, Wednesday and Thursday.

However, in post-incident review, whether or not staff are acting in Wally's best interests is discussed. First, withholding the information from Wally about his family is restricting information, which may not be in line with Wally's human rights. Also, it is understood that Wally struggles with anxiety, and a common theme for those with anxiety is that:

- bad things happen suddenly
- I have no control over the bad things that happen.

By waiting till the day of the problem to tell Wally, the staff have reinforced these core beliefs.

So, although they may have to manage the fallout of telling Wally on the Monday, the fact that Wally would then have an opportunity to choose other options (something else that's fun to do instead on Thursday and the possibility of arranging other opportunities to see family such as a FaceTime call instead) will help to counter these core beliefs.

Over time, this change in approach helps Wally to build trust with staff and better cope with changes.

Commentary: As has been mentioned numerous times, need rather than speed should be the approach. We are always working towards strategies that have a long-term improvement in trust, resilience and outcomes. We are aiming to move towards prevention of behaviours occurring rather than 'firefighting' each incident.

Planning

> *Failing to plan is planning to fail.*

When we are supporting individuals who may struggle to emotionally regulate or manage their behaviours, we must adapt our expectations and create plans. Just a simple trip to the supermarket or park may create situations and circumstances where known behaviours that challenge may occur and create a greater cost due to the situation, or new behaviours may arise. We need to be prepared to manage these behaviours as they happen but we can also create a plan so we can better *respond* and not *react*.

CASE STUDY 22.6 THE THEME PARK OUTING

Mandy is autistic. A trip is being planned for her to visit a theme park. Rather than just turn up on the day, here is a list of things we might want to consider beforehand:

- How long are we planning to go for?
- How far is the journey?
- How many caregivers are going or should go?
- What rides are suitable for Mandy?
- Mandy struggles with waiting. So how can we keep her occupied in a queue? Can we pay to 'skip the line'? Are there peak times to be avoided?
- If Mandy can't cope, what will we do? Is there a safe space? Leave the park earlier than planned? What about transport if so?
- How will we end the trip, especially if Mandy doesn't want to leave?
- What about food (take it or buy it there), water, toilet arrangements?
- What's the plan for coming home?

These factors should be risk assessed and planned.

Commentary: By looking at all potential challenges for Mandy on the day, we can promote positive risk taking and allow Mandy to engage in new experiences and opportunities. These do create situations that may cause distress and therefore behaviours that challenge, but the benefits of expanding horizons usually outweigh the costs.

Priming

Priming is similar to the process described in 'Case Study 22.2 "Along Came a Spider and Sat Down Beside Her, and Frightened Miss Muffet Away"'.

It introduces change or new experiences slowly and in stages to help a person prepare and develop resilience. Priming can be used to help with managing changes or introducing new sensory experiences for those with sensory processing issues or new experiences for those with anxiety issues.

CASE STUDY 22.7 THE THEME PARK OUTING – CONTINUED

Mandy struggles with anxiety; new experiences and situations can lead to significant stress. Having planned well for the trip, the caregivers decide it will also be a good idea to prime Mandy for what she is going to experience. For example:

- visit the theme park website
- watch YouTube videos of the park and the rides
- walk her through the layout and a map
- ask Mandy what she would like to do there.

Create a plan with Mandy for times and food as appropriate (don't try to be too precise – you can't dictate the exact time you'll get on a ride, but you can decide on the order that Mandy prefers).

The following examples are all based on supporting those with autism in different scenarios.

CASE STUDY 22.8 A DIFFERENT DRIVER

A bus company had a contract to shuttle autistic children to and from school.

The children were very used to seeing David driving the bus, and they knew the route.

Some days, David was not available, and a different driver took over, sometimes even using a different bus and a different route. This change in routine upset some of the children; the change created uncertainty and increased anxiety.

To reduce the children's distress, the company created a book that parents could use to prime their children so that the person turning up to drive them to school wasn't a stranger.

The book had the names and pictures of all the drivers, plus a little information about them, their buses and their routes. So the kids knew, 'This driver is Bill, this is what his bus looks like and this is his route.'

This reduced some of the stress.

CASE STUDY 22.9 THE HAIRDRESSER

Sasha had never been to the hairdresser before. Sasha struggles with new places and people, so getting her hair cut would be extremely stressful for her.

A hairdresser was chosen one month before the planned haircut. The hairdresser had experience of cutting autistic children's hair and was informed of the plan. The hairdresser lent Sasha's caregivers an apron. Scissors and a comb and spray bottle were purchased.

Sasha needed priming for the environment and the haircut.

Environment

To start with, Sasha was taken for a walk past the hairdresser's salon and encouraged to look in.

Next, she was taken in to sit in the salon for a while without getting a haircut.

Next, she sat in the chair for a few minutes but was allowed to get up and move.

Then the hairdresser pretended to do a bit of cutting and made the 'snip, snip' sound without touching Sasha's head.

Haircut

An apron was introduced and worn by Sasha while watching an iPad for ten minutes.

Snipping noises and head combing were introduced every day for short periods only, with a slight increase in duration.

Gradually Sasha was desensitised and grew in confidence, with the knowledge that 'I did that, and nothing bad happened to me'.

Keys to priming include:

- gradual introduction and staged desensitisation, as shown in the case studies
- making activities that are rare more common; e.g., instead of nail trimming, file nails every day
- ensuring that engagement with new objects, foods, clothes, etc. is fun and low pressure; e.g., food play or placing new clothes near to the individual for a while.

Summary

All of the examples and principles in this section about emotional and cognitive stressors fall under the biopsychosocial model and address different parts of the model with the aim of reducing stress and improving emotional and mental wellbeing.

LOCATION STRESSORS

If we understand a person's preferences and ability to regulate regarding noise, smells, colours, temperature and even lighting, we can make adjustments to the environment in ways to reduce stress. We can alter lighting, smells, colours and noise in many ways through changing decor, flooring or furniture, using infusers, providing music or at least providing areas that a person can access that meet their preferences.

CASE STUDY 22.10 LOW STIMULUS

You want to read a book. Imagine you are feeling stressed, your brain is busy and there is so much going on. There are people moving everywhere – it's noisy, chaotic. You can't concentrate. You crave calm. You go to your safe space; it is plain in colour, it is soft and comfortable, quiet; the lights are on but they are not too bright. There is nothing to distract you. *Reducing stimulus allows you to focus.*

CASE STUDY 22.11 HIGH STIMULUS

You have had a tough day. Your emotions are raw, and you can't switch off. It's too quiet where you are. There are noises – they may not be loud but they keep attacking your senses. You need to distract your brain to reduce the psychological noise and be able to calm. So you put on the TV. You can switch off everything else and just be absorbed by the TV. The TV could be replaced by a fireplace, a lava lamp, music, an audio book. *Creating stimulus allows regulation.*

Commentary: These two case studies allow us to relate to people who are over- or under-stimulated. The first example could be a child in class who is positioned near the door of the classroom and can't focus due to distractions. The second could be anyone who can use a sensory input to help regulate and calm; for example, there are forms of meditation that refer to fire gazing (staring into a fire) to assist calming.

CASE STUDY 22.12 THE BATHROOM

The Jacobs family were finding that their autistic son was distressed in the bathroom of their new house. They very quickly decided to make some alterations.

They bought soft mats for the floor to reduce the cold on the feet and reduce the echo. They bought a heated towel rail to ensure warm towels, and they bought a rubber toilet seat adapter to soften the feel of the toilet. They removed the blinds but added a frosted glass screen to allow more natural light in the room, and they added a dimmer bulb in the bathroom so they could soften the lighting. They also put an LED shower head in to make the shower more pleasurable, and they bought a sensory bathroom kit that included a projector to make the bathroom a positive sensory setting. The final step was that they only used low-odour products to clean the bathroom and used a specific air freshener that they knew their son was comfortable with.

These adjustments allowed their son to feel safe and comfortable in the bathroom, which allowed him to engage in positive hygiene.

Commentary: Recognising sensory challenges or just environmental preferences can allow us to alter the setting proactively to reduce stress for an individual. This can be challenging when we are meeting the needs of multiple individuals who need to be in one setting together.

It is worth considering using different rooms and outside spaces to provide a variety of areas where individuals can move to depending on their mood.

Using sensory rooms or sensory gardens can provide engaging and calming spaces. Having places to run, jump, hit, dance and generally release tension is useful.

Ensuring bedrooms are personalised allows individuals to feel safe and to know that they can de-stress by either decreasing or increasing stimulus as required. The bedroom should allow them to express their identity, or they should be able to identify it as their space through design or objects.

Low-stimulus rooms with minimal furniture may be perceived by some to be boring, clinical or even prison like, but for some individuals, this level of low stimulus can feel like a huge relief from the everyday world. Pop-up black-out tents that can either be left in situ or used as mobile safe spaces can also provide a similar relief.

Part of planning may also involve thinking about other environments that an individual may be entering and stressors that could occur in that setting. For example, thinking about timing (choosing quieter times), allowing someone to familiarise themselves with a location to get their bearings or ensuring they know where to go if they need a break or even the toilet.

Special Note: Sunlight

Many people are aware of SAD (seasonal affective disorder) and that sunlight produces vitamin D in the body, but the benefits of safe exposure to sunlight stretch past this. There is evidence that it improves many areas of mental and physical health. Here are some benefits of sunlight for your health:

- Better sleep
- Uplifting mood
- Improved cognition and mental processing
- Increased energy
- Improved symptoms of mental health conditions, including ADHD and bipolar disorder
- Lower blood pressure
- Lower risk of metabolic syndrome
- Reduced inflammation in joints and skin conditions
- Stronger bones
- Extended life expectancy

Exposure to sunlight through being outside, near windows or in conservatories should be ideally scheduled into people's daily routines if possible. Alternatives can include light therapy using artificial lights that emit the same light wavelength.

Dementia-Friendly Setting

People living with dementia often have deficits in their sensory processing due to the condition, which affects all the senses. Ensuring an environment is dementia friendly through design and adaption can reduce distress, improve orientation and promote independence and wellbeing. Below are a few examples of things to consider whether in an individual's own home or in a residential setting.

Designing Dementia-Friendly Environments

Living with dementia often results in sensory processing difficulties that affect all senses. Creating a dementia-friendly environment through thoughtful design and adaptation can significantly reduce anxiety, improve orientation and enhance independence and well-being. Here are several considerations for both personal homes and residential care settings:

- **Simplify the space:** Remove excess clutter to ensure that essential items are easy to find. Keeping only frequently used objects in sight helps individuals with dementia navigate their space more efficiently.
- **Use distinct colours:** Avoid complex patterns and opt for high-contrast colour schemes to help individuals differentiate between objects and surfaces. For example, using a red plate on a white tablecloth, a brightly coloured toilet seat, or contrasting colours between floors and walls can enhance visibility and depth perception. Highlight key items like light switches with bright colours or frames.

- **Keep doors open and use clear labels:** To reduce confusion, keep doors open or consider removing them. Label rooms and cabinets with simple, clear signs or pictures to indicate their contents or purpose. For instance, use words like 'food' or 'bathroom,' or pictorial cues such as a toilet or a bed. Directional arrows can also aid in navigation.
- **Incorporate time and date reminders:** Place easy-to-read clocks and calendars in prominent locations to help individuals stay oriented to time and date. Digital clocks that display the time, part of the day and date can be particularly helpful. Additionally, large-print calendars can assist in keeping track of daily events and appointments.
- **Display personal mementos:** Position photos and keepsakes that evoke positive memories in visible spots to encourage reminiscing and create a familiar, comforting environment.
- **Clearly identify bedrooms:** Mark the individual's bedroom with distinct signs or personal items to help them recognise it easily among other rooms.
- **Label fixtures:** Clearly label taps and showers with 'hot' and 'cold' indicators to prevent confusion and ensure safety.
- **Enhance lighting:** Ensure bright, even lighting throughout the space to reduce shadows, which can be misinterpreted and cause anxiety or accidents. Adequate lighting improves visibility and reduces the risk of falls.
- **Utilise familiar scents:** Incorporate familiar and soothing scents, such as lavender or vanilla, to create a calming atmosphere. Scents can trigger positive memories and provide comfort.
- **Introduce nature elements:** Include indoor plants or access to outdoor gardens to bring nature into the living space. Natural elements can have a calming effect and provide sensory stimulation.
- **Designate quiet areas:** Create quiet, low-stimulation areas where individuals can retreat to reduce stress and overstimulation. These spaces should be comfortable and free from loud noises or bright lights.
- **Implement safe flooring:** Use non-slip, even flooring to prevent falls. Avoid busy patterns that can cause visual confusion and ensure there are no abrupt changes in floor levels.

By incorporating these additional ideas and strategies, you can create a dementia-friendly environment that supports the needs of individuals living with dementia, promoting their safety, comfort and quality of life.

PHYSICAL STRESSORS

Physical stressors include such things as hunger, thirst, pain and illness, and problems with sleeping, excreting, sex and so on.

Many ways to manage these are already referred to in other areas of stressors and other areas of the motivation triangle.

Routines, activity scheduling and medication may all be tools that can be used to encourage healthy lifestyles and reduce physical stressors.

Many individuals are able to meet their physical needs to some degree. Also, many care settings are very aware of meeting people's physical needs.

Many neurological disorders (like dementia, severe learning disabilities, etc.) can sometimes create barriers to meeting these basic needs due to the way the conditions affect an individual's ability to recognise or communicate their physical stressors.

Let's look at some case studies to give this some context.

CASE STUDY 22.13 BIG JERRY

Jerry is 79 years old and is living with dementia. He is 6' 3" tall and used to be very athletic when he was younger. Jerry can be extremely aggressive, but it is not always clear what Jerry needs. It happens most often at lunchtime in the dining room. The staff are finding Jerry so difficult that they don't know whether they can manage him at the home anymore.

However, a behavioural analysis is done for Jerry that looks at patterns to his behaviour, and there seems to be a theme.

At lunchtimes when Jerry gets his food first, the staff don't experience negative behaviour, but if Jerry has to wait, Jerry gets angry.

Some staff feel that if they give Jerry his food first, they may be rewarding his negative behaviour. It is pointed out that Jerry is a big guy, and he is just hungry – his dementia is affecting his inhibitors and so he isn't going to learn to be patient. The staff are best off just feeding Jerry first.

Jerry is also generally less challenging when he gets two puddings rather than one. It is noticed when the 'detectives' step in that Jerry is being given similar-sized servings to other clients despite his bigger frame. Jerry's main issue is hunger.

CASE STUDY 22.14 EDNA'S BROKEN HIP

Edna had dementia, and despite usually being a lovely lady, the staff noticed a change. She had become aggressive and depressed, and had lost all of her spark. Some thought it was down to the progression of her illness. One staff member noticed that Edna kept swiping at staff during certain personal care activities, something she hadn't done before. It was always when her left side was being done. The staff member had also recently attended a course in understanding pain and pain management in dementia care, and noticed some of Edna's grimaces and faces that the trainer had referred to.

The staff called a doctor and Edna was taken for a check at the hospital, where it was discovered that Edna had actually fractured her hip.

CASE STUDY 22.15 DEATH BY INDIFFERENCE

In March 2007, Mencap published *Death by Indifference*,[57] which reported the appalling deaths of six people with a learning disability – deaths that the six families involved and Mencap believe were the result of failings in the NHS. These accounts communicated concerns that the NHS is too often failing to provide the most basic nursing care, such as nutrition, hydration and pain relief, for people with a learning disability.

In 2016, the death of a young disabled woman (Laura Booth, 21) following a routine eye operation at the Royal Hallamshire Hospital in Sheffield was partly caused by malnutrition as a result of neglect, a coroner ruled. Her mother, Patricia Booth, told the inquest that her daughter stopped eating shortly after she was admitted to hospital and that doctors ignored Laura's attempts to communicate with them.

Settings should always ensure that basic needs are met and recognise that behaviours that challenge may be ways to communicate these basic physiological needs.

Food

Individuals should have access to appropriate nutrition, preferred foods and a safe diet. Food should also be enjoyable.

Even if people are on specialist diets, pureed foods can be nicely presented.

With careful planning, diabetic diets can still include the food a person likes.

Individuals with specific challenges with textures or tastes may have limited diets, but they can still achieve nutrition in other ways; for example, by fortifying meals with vitamins. Priming may help to introduce new food types; breaking dishes down into separate ingredients can work better for some people.

If people struggle to engage in sitting and eating, environmental adjustments can be made. (If a person spends all their time walking, provide food they can eat on the move; if they struggle to sit still, provide sensory stimulation (such as a wobble stool) to help keep them engaged; if they find mealtimes too intense, let them sit in front of the TV snacking if that works better for them.)

It is important that mealtimes should be calm, as anxiety (fight/flight) is the opposite to rest and digest. A stressful environment does not promote healthy eating habits.

Drink

People are often poor at recognising thirst, so monitoring and providing appropriate levels of fluids may sometimes fall to the responsibility of caregivers in providing prompting, reminders and access.

Pain Relief

Recognising and ensuring individuals are pain free can make a big difference to reducing stress. Some individuals can't express pain or may not consciously be aware of pain (like Edna above), so caregivers need to have strategies to examine and identify indicators of pain and then provide the appropriate medical support or referral.

Excretion

Nutrition and fluids are a big factor in excretion, and providing a balanced diet that includes fibre and plenty of water can make a difference.

Comfort

Provide warmth, coolness and fresh air depending on an individual's preference and the setting.

Rest/Sleep

People's ability to rest and sleep can be affected by multiple factors. Some may be environmental, linked to noise, light or discomfort. Some may be based on the person's natural circadian rhythms, which can vary from person to person. Sleep is vital for wellbeing, but not every person has the same sleep cycle. Learning what works best for the individual, creating routines and ensuring positive diet and exercise can help a person's sleep patterns be healthy.

CHAPTER 23

STEP 3: MEET THE NEED

The causes and functions of a behaviour that challenges can be summarised as follows:

> The need to get/obtain – *or* – avoid/escape an item or items from the following list: person/sensory stimulus/activity/something tangible/help/control.

As we look at these causes and functions of behaviour, we want to look at two points. Should we meet the individual's need for them? Or can we support and teach them how to meet their own need?

Let's look at why this person is not able to meet their needs and see if, instead, they are using the behaviour that challenges as a strategy to meet their needs:

- Do they not understand their own need?
- Have they never been taught other ways?
- Is it just a habit?
- Is it a communication issue as discussed earlier?
- Is the need restricted for some reason?
- Do they know how to meet the need?
- Does the environment or staff provide opportunities to satisfy the need easily?

The following table shows specific approaches to these questions.

Table 23.1 Sample of Meeting Needs

Need	Get/obtain	Avoid/escape
Person	How do we want them to get time with a person? Can we arrange and manage that time for them? Can we create other positive relationships?	Can we reduce contact with the person they don't like? Can we improve the relationship? How would we like them to communicate that they would like time alone?

Activity/ tangible	Can we provide and schedule this activity? Can we adjust the environment to allow access? Can we provide safe alternatives?	Does the person need to do the activity or engage with the tangible? Is there a replacement preferred option available?
Sensory	What sensory input do they want? Can we provide the sensory need safely?	Do we need to change the environment to avoid this sensory stress? Is there any tool or strategy to reduce the sensory stress? Can we help them to cope? (This is covered more in Chapter 36.)
Help	How can they communicate this need? Can we provide ways for them to help themselves?	What can they do for themselves? Can we provide tools or adjustments so they can do it themselves more easily? Can we teach better communication?
Control	Can we give them more control in other areas? Can we allow more control over this in a safe way?	Can we reduce the demands on them when they are struggling? Can we give them more autonomy?

Notice that in the above questions we are consistently asking positively framed questions. As we move further through the process, we will sometimes look to ask certain questions about how we may be able to add friction to performing the maladaptive behaviour or at least reduce reinforcement of it. (Friction: a resistant force applied to make the current strategy harder to perform or less likely to be reinforced.) Then we can start to create a plan for how we can answer these questions. Now that we have explored managing the stress, we will look at teaching strategies and how we can change habits. Remember from the arm-folding exercise in 'Case Study 15.2 Exercise: Arm Folding', page 136, that behaviours don't tend to change just because someone tells us to change them.

CHAPTER 24

CREATING THE PLAN

Let's revisit the motivation triangle:

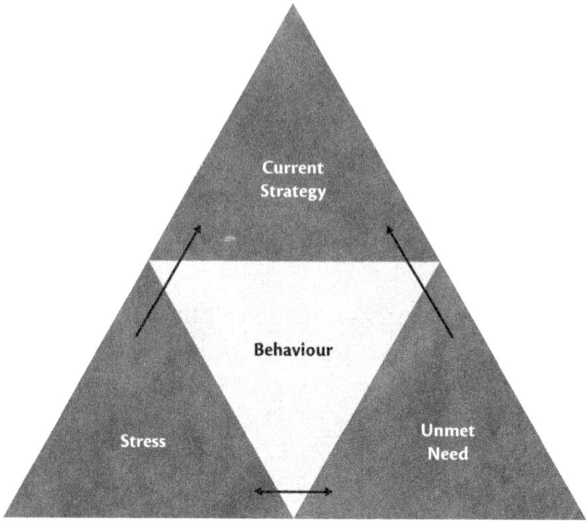

Figure 24.1 The Motivation Triangle

We have explored each section individually and focused on changing the environment to reduce stress and meet the needs.

We have also introduced the concept of teaching new skills and changing habits. As discussed in Stage 2: Understand/Empathise, habits are often subconscious, they are hard to change and are rarely changed by just telling a person to change them. It can take anywhere from 18 to 254 days for a person to form a new habit and an average of 66 days for a new behaviour to become automatic.[58]

We have already seen in 'The Actor-Observer Bias', Chapter 15, page 138, that to change a habit the alternative must be:

- obvious – they can see the alternative
- easy – it's achievable for them
- attractive – they can see the benefits
- rewarding – they experience a benefit from the alternative.[59]

When making a plan, we must first address the barrier of change both biologically and psychologically.

CASE STUDY 24.1 THE BRAIN IS A WILDERNESS

Brain plasticity

The brain is like a wilderness. When we are young, the environment and activities we experience lay down neurons in the brain like paths through a grass meadow. The paths are easy to make, because it's only grass, and if the path is continually walked, it doesn't take long for the grass to stop growing and the paths to become fixed. We make lots of paths as children as we run all over, learn and engage. Adults guide us along paths of rights and wrongs. Friends lay other paths for better or for worse. Lots of things draw us down paths, connecting our thoughts to our actions and our senses with our understanding.

As we grow up, the plants around the paths grow and the meadow becomes wilder. Unused paths may disappear; the paths that are used endure. New paths are easy to make as we move into adolescence, but the old paths are still the easiest to walk. Old paths, like old habits, can feel safer, more familiar. If we don't concentrate and work at it, old paths feel so comfortable that we can stop making new ones and end up losing access to areas of the forest that are wondrous. Skills, abilities and experiences that we could have developed are never discovered, because old paths feel easier to walk or maybe we feel that this new path is too hard to make. Nonetheless, during adolescence, we may make some brand-new paths and forget old ones, and we slowly make the paths organised, laying down gravel to fix the paths we use the most.

The older we get, the wilder the meadow grows until it becomes a jungle. The paths of skills, memories and abilities that we walk regularly are here to stay. New paths are not as easy to make now; it feels like we need a machete sometimes to change a path or create a new one. Sometimes we find an old path that we haven't used for a while, and with only a little work, we can have that path up and accessible again (like riding a bike – we never forget; or like being a former smoker – the habit can be only one cigarette away).

At times, despite being older, we feel distressed, and we run blindly. We end up on one of our childhood paths by mistake, where we behave in childlike ways.

As we get old, so does the jungle; paths are hard to make now. Branches sometimes fall and block the paths; we can sometimes get round them but sometimes we get lost and can't find where we wanted to get to.

This analogy is a simple way of understanding the ever-changeable brain. The brain is never fixed; neuron pathways can always be created and lost. Habits are just a pathway of neurons that are hard to step off, and, as mentioned, new habits can take some time to become automatic.

To change a behavioural habit, the ideal situation would be to recruit the individual themselves into the process. This will obviously depend on the individual's mental capacity and the nature of the maladaptive behaviour. We need to be aware of the cycle of change model to allow us to recognise where an individual is within the process of change.

THE CYCLE OF CHANGE[60]

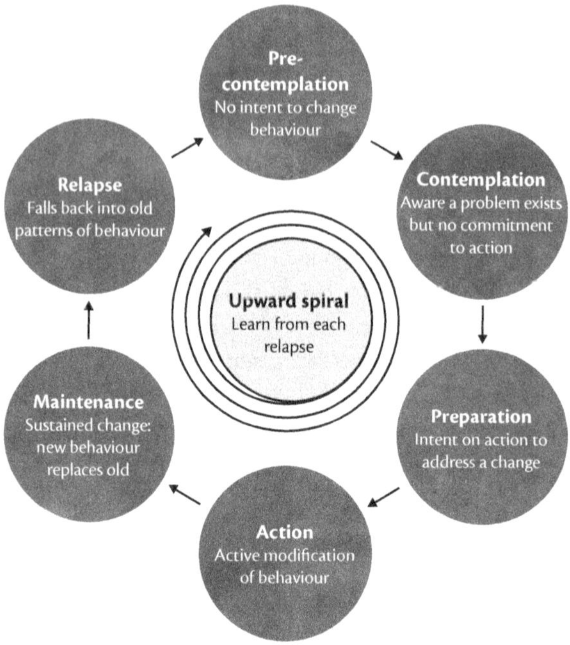

Figure 24.2 The Cycle of Change

Changing behaviour is a process, as shown in the diagram.

Changing behaviour takes time.

Whatever plan is created for an individual, it must always take into account that the plan must be focused on *need*, not *speed*.

Take a closer look at the diagram and bear in mind the following:

- A person's behaviour will not change just because someone tells them to change.
- A person must have some involvement – to actively want to participate in changing behaviour.
- Helpers can support the individual to change.

Let's look at each item in some detail.

Pre-contemplation

The individual has no intent to change their behaviour. The individual can only see the benefit of their behaviour and either cannot see the cost of it or, on assessment, cannot see the costs of change outweighing the benefit of change at this time.

Helper's role: Raise doubts and increase perception of the risks by pointing them out in a non-judgemental, reflective way.

For example, maybe the problem is self-harming. Risks associated with sexually transmitted diseases (STDs) or blood poisoning could be raised. Maybe there's a dietary problem – the individual is overweight. It could be pointed out that because of their weight, the individual's participation in certain activities that they might like could be prevented.

Suggest how things could be different.

The objective is to plant a seed of doubt.

However, at this stage, although we may not be able to change the behaviour, we might just need to *manage the risk* of that behaviour. So, if it is a case of self-harming, well, that isn't suddenly going to stop. However, we can manage it by reducing risk; for example, making sure they've got clean equipment or they do it where they are supervised so somebody can help them if it goes wrong, or making sure they know how to do it in the safest and lowest risk way possible. See 'Case Study 20.5 Tania, the Survivor', page 185.

Contemplation

The individual is starting to wonder if a change will be worthwhile – weighing up the pros and cons. If the individual eventually decides that the benefits outweigh the costs, they will move on. This process isn't necessarily conscious; there's constant internal analysis.

Helper's role: Support the individual to weigh up the pros and cons of change and work on helping them tip the balance by exploring ambivalence ('I want to quit for my health but I enjoy it') and alternatives (see 'Case Study 15.3 The Smoker', page 139).

The helper can also reinforce the individual's motivation – to add reasons for change and risks of not changing. The helper can boost the individual's confidence perhaps by exploring previous successes achieved by the individual and focusing on the individual's skills, not their weaknesses.

Preparation

Here an action plan is created, with some clear goal setting, even if it's quite informal, such as: 'Let's try to reduce this by that much by then.'

Helper's role: Encourage the individual to set goals, possibly remembering SMART goals, which means they meet the following criteria:

- **Specific**: Be specific in what you want to accomplish and the action steps you will take.
- **Measurable**: Determine how you will track your progress: think how much, how many and when will I know my goal is accomplished?
- **Action-oriented**: Select an action for your goal – identify what you will do to reach your goal.
- **Reasonable**: Set goals you can realistically accomplish in a few weeks or months.
- **Timeline-based**: Set time expectations. Have a start date and finish date by which you expect to reach your goal. This gives you a clear target to work towards.

The helper should not create the plan, just assist. The individual must own the plan.

CASE STUDY 24.2 I DON'T SMOKE

Specific: I will quit smoking one month from today.
Measurable: Each day I'll track my smoking and my triggers to smoking in my planner or journal.
Action-oriented: I'll sign up to a quit smoking app on my phone, buy vegetables and chewing gum for when I get the urge to smoke and avoid smoking breaks with other smokers.
Reasonable: Tell my sister I'm quitting and ask for her support. Each week I'll check in with my app and my sister.
Timeline: In one month I'll quit smoking and adjust my ongoing action plan as needed to be successful.

Action

The individual starts to modify their behaviour following their plan.

Maintenance

The individual tries to sustain the changed behaviour.

Helper's role: On signs of relapse, suggest strategies to avoid it. For example, alternative pleasurable things to do instead of grabbing a snack or smoking a cigarette. Encourage successes.

Relapse

The individual stops working towards the goals.

Helper's role: Do not be judgemental. Explain that relapse is quite expected. ('Giving up smoking is easy; I've done it many times.')

But try and learn why there was failure. Was the timescale too aggressive, for example?

Look at what worked; congratulate the achievements.

Respond to remarks such as 'See, I'll never be able to do it' by explaining that there's the cycle of change, and if a new attempt is started, with new ideas about what worked and what didn't, it may start from a better place and achieve more success.

Being a Helper

The cycle of change model is a structure to bear in mind when a person is involved in changing their own behaviours and habits. Individuals may need help through this process, and models like Motivational Interviewing (MI) techniques can work very effectively in a helping relationship. Here are a few techniques taken from MI.

Establish how important the change is for them with an 'importance ruler'.

- Example: Think of how important it is for you to lose weight on a scale of 0–10. On this scale, 0 is not important at all and 10 is extremely important. Where would you be on this scale?
  - Why are you at 'X' and not 0?
  - What would it take for you to go from 'X' to (a higher number)?

This identifies the discrepancy between their current situation and where they would like to be. This can be followed by asking the person to elaborate further on this discrepancy and then summarising this discrepancy and reflecting it back.

Next, it is important to build confidence in their ability to change. This involves focusing on strengths and past experiences of success. Again, a 'confidence ruler' could be employed.

- Example: Think of how confident you are that you can cut back the amount you are drinking on a scale of 0–10. On this scale, 0 is not confident at all and 10 is extremely confident. Where would you be on this scale?
  - Why are you at 'X' and not zero?
  - What would it take for you to go from 'X' to (a higher number)?'

Finally, decide on a 'change plan' together. This involves standard goal-setting techniques, eliciting from the person what they plan to do (rather than instructing or advising). Examples of key questions used to build a 'change plan' include the following:

- It sounds like things can't stay the same as they are. What do you think you might do?
- What changes were you thinking about making?
- Where do we go from here?
- What do you want to do at this point?
- How would you like things to turn out?
- After reviewing all of this, what's the next step for you?

It is common for individuals to want 'quick fixes'. A simple phrase reminding them of their autonomy is useful: 'You are the expert on you, so I'm not sure I'm the best person to judge what will work for you. But I can give you an idea of what has worked for other people.'

CASE STUDY 24.3 SNAIL – TALKING TO A CHILD WHO DISSOCIATES (FREEZE)

'I notice sometimes when you are feeling overwhelmed, you seem to disappear into your shell like a snail. When you are in your shell, we don't get to talk to you, but I understand you are not doing it on purpose and I'm wondering if it feels safer when you are in there.'

'How does it feel when you are in your shell?'

'What do you like about being in your shell?'

'Is there anything bad about being in the shell?' (E.g., 'Do you remember the other day when the house all had the movie night but you needed to be in your shell in your room – do you feel like you were missing out?')

'Is there room for anyone to join you inside the shell?'

'Are there times where you need to go into your shell more than others?'

Commentary: It is important that such a conversation is carried out in Stage 3: Proactive Planning. This may also be performed during Stage 6: Learn from Incident as part of the reflection process; see 'Reflection', Chapter 39, page 394, which includes many suggestions of phrases and questions that can be used.

CHAPTER 25

TEACHING METHODS

The term 'learning' is often misunderstood as being a purely conscious process where we gain new knowledge, skills and understanding, but it also involves acquiring new behaviours, values, attitudes and preferences, and can occur without any conscious awareness. Some learning is immediate, induced by a single event (e.g., being burned by a hot surface), but usually repetition is required.

Learning may occur as a result of classical conditioning, operant conditioning or habituation (an innate response to a stimulus that decreases after multiple exposures, e.g., staged desensitisation: 'This stimulus scared me and it made me scream but I kept experiencing it and it didn't hurt me so it must be safe') or as a result of more complex activities, such as play.

Any plan created for managing and changing behaviour will involve an individual learning a new or alternative behaviour, skill or strategy to manage their stress or meet their need. Preferably, the plan has been made with assistance and input from the individual.

Caregivers and individuals can adjust the environment, interactions and circumstances that direct the learning in a certain way. If the caregivers are managing this process, it is referred to as teaching.

This chapter explains strategies for how that teaching can be done.

TEACHING TECHNIQUE: ROLE MODELLING

The first method of teaching that should be referenced before we move into more traditional teaching methods is role modelling.

A role model is a person or group serving as an exemplar for the goals, attitudes or behaviour of an individual, who identifies with and seeks to imitate the role model.

The understanding of the impact of role modelling is based on Social Learning Theory, proposed by Albert Bandura.[61] Social Learning Theory emphasises the impact of observing, modelling and imitating the behaviours, attitudes and emotional reactions of others. The theory considers how both environmental and cognitive factors interact to influence human learning and behaviour. As we look at the impact of reinforcers and punishment in the follow-up sections of this chapter (see 'Reinforcers', page 228), we will see that the behaviourist principle of pleasure and pain influencing actions still applies in social learning, but the rewards or inhibitors are less obvious. The pleasure comes from acceptance by individuals or groups within an environment of the fact that we behave in similar ways to them.

CASE STUDY 25.1 BOBO DOLL STUDY[62]

The Bobo Doll experiment, conducted by psychologist Albert Bandura, sought to explore how children learn aggression through observation. In the study, children were divided into three groups: one witnessed an adult acting aggressively toward a Bobo doll, another observed a non-aggressive adult, and a control group had no adult model. The aggressive model exhibited behaviours such as hitting the doll with a hammer and throwing it while yelling 'Pow, Boom'. In contrast, the non-aggressive model played quietly and ignored the Bobo doll.

The results indicated that children exposed to the aggressive model were significantly more likely to imitate aggressive behaviours themselves than those who observed the non-aggressive model or were in the control group. This study provided strong evidence for the theory of observational learning, suggesting that children learn and replicate social behaviours by watching the actions of others, highlighting the impact of role models on child behaviour development.

Commentary: From early childhood we begin to imitate those around us, which begins to set up the scripts of how we should and shouldn't behave. This is why the phrase 'It's not "Do as I do," it's "Do as I say"' from parents is so inappropriate, as kids will do what they see.

Understanding this principle and applying it to the setting is an important step in shaping behaviour that we feel is and isn't appropriate.

Let's say we want to increase respectful behaviour, which we used as an example question in 'Starting with the Positive', Chapter 18, page 165.

We are looking to decrease abuse and so we want to encourage respect.

How can we encourage respect? Well, as we will explore in the following sections, we could reward or reinforce it whenever we observe it. But let's start with the role modelling.

If we role model respect, we are acting like the models with the Bobo doll except we are not modelling aggression to be socially learned, we are demonstrating *respect* to be socially learned. So we start with the premise, 'I treat people with respect and no matter how disrespectfully they may treat me, I still respond with respect (I may still assert my boundaries and not allow abuse, but I still do it in a respectful way).' That may seem like a very small step for one caregiver to take but...

CASE STUDY 25.2 DARYL DAVIS

Daryl Davis is a black blues musician who, for the past 30 years, has spent time befriending members of the Ku Klux Klan. He starts from a position of listening rather than confronting, he shows complete respect to people who 'hate him without knowing him'. Over time spent listening, respecting and gently introducing alternative viewpoints, friendships start to develop. Once the friendships develop, the Klansmen realise that their hate may be misguided. Since Davis started his one-man crusade of talking with these members, over 200 Klansmen have given up their robes.

To find out more about Daryl's story, you can watch the film *Accidental Courtesy: Daryl Davis, Race & America*.

For some individuals, their early-life role models may have set up very different scripts of how they should behave (as described in the 'room one/room two' analogy, page 147). So, overcoming these models of the world that may involve aggression, violence and drug use may take significant time. This is not an overnight strategy.

The above case study shows the effect of one person's actions to make social change. When we add the power of a group into this, the effect is amplified. We saw a good example of this in 'Case Study 5.6 The Waiting Room', page 40, where group actions were echoed until nobody knew why they were standing up each time a buzzer sounded.

There is a good real-world example of this in an elderly care setting:

CASE STUDY 25.3 IT MUST BE WHAT THEY DO HERE

Mavis was new in the residential home; she was still fairly independent and was very capable of feeding herself despite her dementia and cognitive impairments.

At mealtimes Mavis would sit at a table with a number of other individuals. The other three individuals at the table were less able than Mavis and needed assistance to eat.

Two caregivers came and sat by two of the other individuals and helped them to eat, leaving Mavis and one other. The other lady was waiting for assistance and did not engage with her meal. So neither did Mavis. After the two caregivers had finished, one of them moved to support the last lady but Mavis's meal was taken away, as they assumed she wasn't hungry.

Mavis's nutrition deteriorated until the circumstances were noticed. Mavis was moved to another table with other independent eaters and began to feed herself once more.

In Chapter 9, we made an initial list of positive attributes and behaviours we may want to promote and encourage in the environment. This is a great starting point for establishing what actions caregivers should role model.

It also worth being aware of another social learning factor:

Vicarious Reinforcement

We will be looking at reinforcers in the next section but it is worth referencing a variation of the Bobo doll experiment, as it highlights a connection between role modelling and more traditional teaching strategies.

The variant of the Bobo doll experiment involved the actors receiving either a reinforcement for being violent towards the doll or a negative consequence for their aggression. This significantly impacted on the behaviour of the children. Those who saw the aggression being punished did not repeat the aggressive behaviour when given the opportunity, whereas those who saw the behaviour reinforced were more likely to engage in it. This version of the experiment demonstrates that seeing others rewarded increases the likelihood of the behaviour occurring.

Let's apply this to respectful behaviour again. Let's say the staff started catching and reinforcing any respectful behaviour displayed by anyone in the setting. This acts to further condition the script that respectful behaviour is really rewarding and therefore, over time, increases the likelihood of that behaviour being repeated.

REINFORCERS

A reinforcer is any stimulus (such as a reward or the removal of something unpleasant) that increases the probability of a desired response.

Setting reinforcers is an important part of the planning process. If they are presented correctly, at the right time, they can act to encourage a person to repeat a behaviour, and, as mentioned in the learning and habit-creation discussion in Chapter 15, repetition is vital to make a new behaviour a habit. For reinforcers to be effective, their nature should be informed by Stages 1 (Identify) and 2 (Understand/Empathise) of the 6STM as they will need to be based on an individual's preferences.

There are three types of reinforcers:

1. Noncontingent
2. Negative
3. Positive

Noncontingent Reinforcers

A noncontingent reinforcer is not earned, it's just given as a positive for that person without the presence of any specific behaviour. Young children commonly experience noncontingent reinforcers. An infant can just be lying there, and without needing to cry, they get attention and a cuddle (especially the first born). Young children typically get parents playing with them or giving them food and treats without having to ask or act out any specific behaviours. The benefit of a noncontingent reinforcement is that it can build trust and develop a sense of positive self-worth: 'I must be good because good things just happened to me.'

By creating a sense of value for being *who they are* rather than *how they behave*, we can counter an individual's self-perceptions that they are not good enough, not worthy: 'Wow, someone is doing something nice for me for no reason. Maybe I'm not as bad as I thought. Maybe they like me and I matter to them.'

Noncontingent reinforcers can affect an individual's core beliefs.

Warning: Initially, noncontingent reinforcers and positive reinforcers can be viewed with mistrust from some people. They may view them as a control method, or they may have experienced grooming (nice things were offered first and then there came a price). This is where habituation is important for learning: 'Rewards are bad, as they mean this person wants something from me... but they keep giving me nice things and attention without wanting anything... maybe this belief (path in the forest) isn't correct.'

Negative Reinforcers

This is not the same as punishment, which is the introduction of a negative stimulus to reduce a behaviour (explored later). A negative reinforcer is the *removal* of a stimulus to encourage a behaviour. Negative reinforcement is not a bad thing... it is the removal of the bad thing.

For example, an individual may react badly to a lot of noise. The plan for the individual could include removing the noise by offering ear defenders. The individual learns that by asking for ear defenders, the problem can be overcome.

Similarly, at times, an individual may be overwhelmed by people and just want time alone. Instead of exhibiting some unwanted behaviour, the individual can learn that if they ask to be left alone, people will move away.

You drive to work every day; the traffic is awful and stressful. One day you take a different route, and it takes you less time and causes less stress. This new behaviour will now repeat.

Infants use negative reinforcers all the time to control their parents: the baby cries... the mother doesn't like the sound so comes to the baby, feeds her and rocks her to sleep... and stops the sound. The baby is conditioning the parent.

Positive Reinforcers

A positive reinforcement is any stimulus that is presented to an individual before, during or after the desired behaviour has been shown that increases the likelihood of that behaviour's presentation. It could be a treat or giving attention. For example, if an individual comes over and says 'Hello' and they are then engaged with and attended to, the individual learns that a good way of getting attention is to say, 'Hello.'

Reinforcers may be presented immediately or after a delay, depending on an individual's ability to connect the two events.

CASE STUDY 25.4 WHEN TO APPLY A REINFORCER

1. The Toddler

When Ralph says please:

- we smile and say well done – effective
- we inform him that he will get to go to the park on Thursday – ineffective.

2. The Neurotypical Adult

When Andrew does well at work:

- we smile and say well done – *maybe* effective
- we say if he keeps up the good work, he is line for a promotion – effective.

Commentary: One difference between the two examples may be age, but the difference being referred to is actually cognitive ability – the ability to retain the concept of the reward to repeat the behaviour, and at the time of the reward, the ability to connect the causality.

The other factor in the example is motivation – a toddler wouldn't care about a promotion and Andrew wouldn't care about going to the park.

There are two types of positive reinforcer:

- Unconditioned (primary)
- Conditioned (secondary)

Unconditioned (primary) reinforcers don't need to be learned. They are *typically innate drivers* such as food, water, warmth, touch, attachment, connection, joy, pride, pleasure and so on – the basic human needs. If an individual has been deprived of these for some reason, then gaining access to them is very motivating and an overall reinforcer of the new regime.

Conditioned (secondary) reinforcers have to be learned by experience.

A conditioned reinforcer is a previously neutral stimulus (it isn't a reinforcer). If the neutral stimulus is paired with a primary reinforcer, it acquires the same reinforcement properties that are associated with the primary reinforcer.

An example of a conditioned reinforcer is money. Money by itself is technically worthless, but what money can buy tends to be a primary, unconditioned reinforcer. Over time and by pairing the primary and secondary together, the conditioned reinforcer acts like a primary reinforcer.

CASE STUDY 25.5 PAVLOV'S DOGS

You may already know about this effect, identified by Ivan Pavlov, a Russian physiologist.

Pavlov noticed that every time food (a primary reinforcer) was presented, dogs would salivate on the arrival of the food before they even started eating. He then introduced the ringing of a bell every time that food was presented. Over a period of time, the mere ringing of the bell (with no food present) would cause the dogs to salivate.

This effect is known as 'classical conditioning'.

The food was the primary reinforcer, the bell the secondary reinforcer.

Over time, by pairing the two together, the secondary reinforcer produced the desired effect without providing the primary reinforcer.

CASE STUDY 25.6 THE GENT WITH THE SENSORY OBJECT

Bob suffered from bouts of severe stress. He had PRN* medication to relieve the symptoms.

However, it was noticed that the calming effect happened at the moment the tablet hit his tongue, long before any medicinal effect could have begun. Therefore, the calming effect was psychological, not physiological.

The medication was the primary reinforcer, but the *thought* of the medication became the secondary reinforcer.

Bob's care facility wanted to wean Bob off his medication, so an alternative pairing was introduced. Whenever Bob needed his medication, he was also given a sensory ball that he enjoyed fidgeting with, rolling over his skin or being massaged with. Over a period of time, Bob was able to significantly reduce his use of medication. The presence of the ball (the secondary reinforcer) relieved Bob's feelings of stress.

An individual must be able to connect three things: the behaviour, the primary reinforcer and the secondary reinforcer. Again, this will be dependent on their cognitive abilities, which in turn will affect how the reinforcers should be presented and for how long the pairing will need to continue before the conscious or unconscious connection is made.

* '*Pro re nata*' is a Latin phrase meaning 'in the circumstances' and refers to the administration of prescribed medication as the situation calls for it.

CASE STUDY 25.7 MONEY AS A REINFORCER

Money is an abstract concept. This means that money is just bits of paper or coins that represent value but are not valuable in themselves.

Ask a toddler if they would like a £1 coin or four 20p pieces. They are likely to want the 20p pieces because there are more of them.

What has more value – a mobile phone or a bar of chocolate? To someone with typical intelligence and neurotypical functioning, it's an obvious answer. The mobile phone has more value – you could buy hundreds of chocolate bars for the price of one mobile phone. But what if you live in the moment (you struggle to plan and see yourself in a future state) and you are not using your mobile phone right now... but you are feeling hungry? Which is more valuable?

> As an example, a child with foetal alcohol syndrome might say, 'I'll swap you my phone for that chocolate.'

Children with FASD conditions need supporting with financial literacy, and the teaching methods used to educate them must be adapted around their condition.

CASE STUDY 25.8 THE STAR CHART

Frankie's parents created a star chart for him. If he behaved well, he got a star. If he got five stars in a week, Frankie got a bag of sweets at the end of the week.

Frankie was always so happy when he got a star and so his parents thought the reinforcer was working. Unfortunately, it wasn't long before Frankie's parents realised that his behaviour was not actually improving, and he wasn't earning enough stars to get the treat.

The issue was that although Frankie loved the star, he just didn't connect the star to a particular aspect of his behaviour. He also didn't feel affected if he didn't get a star, as he wasn't connecting the stars to the sweets. Once Frankie's parents managed to get Frankie a diagnosis of FAS (foetal alcohol syndrome) and they underwent training to better understand their son and his condition, they changed their strategy. Frankie needs shorter term rewards, and although the parents liked using the star system, they changed the stars into little cards that had a picture that represented the positive behaviour. These were added to a happy board and referred to regularly and praised.

It was recognised that Frankie learnt better through ongoing role modelling of positive behaviour from parents (acting as they wanted Frankie to act) and that lots of repetition of immediate reinforcements worked better. There was also complete understanding that normal learning curves could not be expected and that the skills learnt today may not be there tomorrow; the parents had to just keep going and build on the positives.

We could ask: Why should we go to the trouble of implementing a regime of conditioned reinforcers and getting the individual to make the necessary connections? Why don't we simply use unconditioned reinforcers?

Unconditioned reinforcers only work if the subject is in a state of deprivation. A child is unlikely to clean their room to receive an edible treat if they have just finished eating lunch. Conditioned reinforcers are less likely to lead to satiation. Satiation is when our need is met or when we need progressively more of something to get the same effect – a case of 'too much of a good thing'. This can happen to all reinforcers. For example, an individual's favourite meal is shepherd's pie, but after four weeks of it being used as a reinforcer for having a successful week, they say they don't want shepherd's pie anymore.

Types of Conditioned Reinforcer

Reinforcers can be classified by their attributes, as follows:

- **Edible**: A highly preferred food item. A potential problem with this type of reinforcer is that it may create unhealthy eating habits as a way of coping with the targeted behaviour. If the individual receives a chocolate whenever they do something right, there could be issues with sugar levels and weight gain. So, edible reinforcers can be very useful but have to be used carefully.
- **Sensory reinforcer**: Things that give pleasure to one or more senses; e.g., music, massage, sensory rooms, head scratchers, sensory objects like weighted blankets, fidget toys and so on.
- **Tangible reinforcer**: Any item that the individual values. It could be money, stickers, tokens. This type of reinforcer can be perceived as being infantile, but most of us work for money because of what it can buy. We need to be mindful that for this type of reinforcer to be effective, the recipient must be able to make the connection between the tokens and what the tokens can be used to buy – 'I get this from that' – and that can take a long time.
- **Activity reinforcer**: Anything that the individual enjoys doing; e.g., going fishing, watching TV, jumping on a trampoline and so on.
- **Social reinforcer**: Getting the desired attention or interaction with another person.

Whatever reinforcer/s are selected, it must be something that suits the individual.[63]

Praise – a Secondary Reinforcer!

This section is relevant to 'Case Study 5.2 The Good, the Bad and the Ugly', page 36.

Praise is often seen as the default reinforcer that many people use to encourage a repeat of a certain behaviour. Parents and teachers praise children; a boss may praise an employee; the Oscars praise an actor. Praise only works as a motivator if the praise is desired, if the recipient likes, trusts or values the person who is offering it, if it is seen as genuine and if it is perceived as justified.

Praise is useless and potentially counterproductive if the recipient:

- doesn't care about praise
- sees praise as manipulative
- doesn't believe the praise
- perceives the praise as a judgement or a criticism
- experiences anxiety rather than pleasure due to feelings of increased expectations.

We should always praise the *behaviour* or the *process*, not the person or the outcome. Carol Dweck's famous study on 'growth mindset praise'[64] showed what a huge impact words have on our mindsets. The study showed that students who received praise that was focused on their *efforts and strategies* entered a growth mindset. These students worked harder, became more resilient, and performed better than students who were praised for their *talents and abilities* – these students will likely enter a fixed mindset.

Good behaviour doesn't make a person good, no more than bad behaviour makes a person bad. As described in 'Case Study 5.2 The Good, the Bad and the Ugly', we need to ensure we always praise growth mindset principles.

- Don't praise being clever, praise working hard.
- Don't praise being good, praise being thoughtful.
- Don't praise the work itself, praise the work or thinking that went into it.

CASE STUDY 25.9 THE CEO IN BED

Denise used to be a CEO (chief executive officer) responsible for a large company with over 50 employees. Now she's in a care home, suffering from a number of physical problems.

Denise is in bed, and the staff need her to roll onto her side so they can place the sling underneath her so she can be hoisted to the toilet. The staff ask if she can roll for them, and Denise manages to pull herself over.

One of the staff who is present says, 'Well done, Denise!' in a tone usually reserved for a child using the potty.

In the light of her life experience, Denise could well see this remark as condescending and patronising.

CASE STUDY 25.10 THE WASHING UP

A caregiver asks Ed to do the washing up. After a while, the caregiver goes into the kitchen and sees everything nicely washed, dried and stowed away.

The caregiver says, 'Oh my word, Ed, you've *actually done it!*'

There is an implied criticism there rather than praise: clearly, Ed doesn't always do the task successfully. We must expect good behaviour and respond accordingly.

CASE STUDY 25.11 DAMNING WITH FAINT PRAISE

Little Frances has often been a nuisance when going to the shops with Mum. But this time she's an angel.

Mum says, 'It was really nice going shopping with you today.'

But follows up with: 'Now why can't we do it like that every day?'

Again, there is an implied criticism.

The three case studies show how using praise may not always achieve the intended result of boosting an individual's self-esteem.

We have already seen that praise can also be seen as a judgement on an individual, evoking feelings of shame.

Instead of praising an individual, the following options may be better:

- Empathise with an individual's joys and successes ('You seem so pleased with your room now it's tidy, I am glad it's made you happy. You must be really proud').
- Use appreciation, thanks and acknowledgement ('I really appreciated your help with that job; thank you'). This is better for older children and adults anyway, who may find direct praise patronising (especially if they are being praised for something they themselves don't feel deserves praise).
- If an individual can't cope with praise because it's too much for them and it causes them to act out with behaviour that challenges, find other ways to offer it, such as:
  - post-it notes with praise or appreciation
  - text messages
  - letting them catch you praising them to someone else
  - making it indirect ('I love it when people do "X" for me,' or for younger kids, 'Mr Teddy says, "Well done for cleaning your teeth"').

We can also encourage the individual to learn to praise themselves. After the individual has successfully completed a task, we can ask, 'What was your favourite thing? How do you feel now it's all done?'

Unwittingly Reinforcing the Wrong Behaviour

CASE STUDY 25.12 OKAY, DO IT YOURSELF THEN

We are trying to help Rob to get ready for school.

Rob starts to get agitated – he lashes out, is verbally abusive.

The caregiver responds by saying, 'Right, fine. If you're gonna behave like that, I'm not going to help you.' The caregiver leaves the room, thinking that Rob will be chastened and will be better next time.

In fact, all Rob wanted was to be not fussed over, to be left alone. And his behaviour (agitation, lashing out) achieved that aim. So the caregiver leaving the room reinforced the unwanted behaviour.

CASE STUDY 25.13 SHOUTING BRINGS ME LOVE

Fran comes from an environment of domestic abuse. She has witnessed aggression, violence and abuse as a norm in her household. Shouting is the only form of attention that has made her feel noticed or important in the world. So shouting may be mistaken for a form of affection or love in her world view. She may welcome being shouted at – it's what she deserves and it helps her to feel acknowledged.

This may lead to her acting in ways to get shouted at, and she may try to manipulate a situation to provoke a shouted reaction.

The reinforcement is repeated.

Commentary: We have to put ourselves in the mind of the person that we're supporting rather than our own mind.

Reinforcers have to be based on the individual and on knowing the individual themselves.

When to Offer the Reinforcer

Part of the proactive plan is deciding on an appropriate reinforcement schedule.

The schedule will be updated based on progress and results. The aim is to maintain a behaviour, not just manage and change it.

The following table gives two examples for presenting reinforcers and gradually withdrawing them.

Table 25.1 Reinforcement Types and When to Use Them

Reinforcement type	Description	Advantage	When to use
Continuous	Reinforcement for every observed instance of the desired behaviour	Learning new behaviour occurs quickly	When starting a new skill

Intermittent	Reinforcement is provided in certain instances but not every time	Good for behaviour maintenance	To maintain a behaviour

There are four variations of reinforcement strategy.

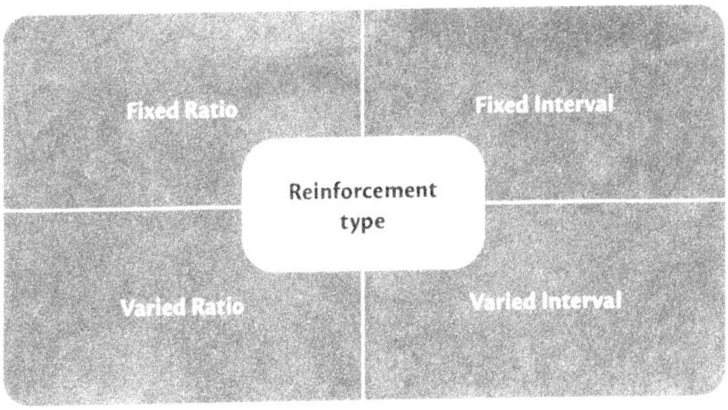

Figure 25.1 Reinforcement Strategies

Ratio Schedules

Ratio schedules are based on providing reinforcement after a set number of occurrences of the desired behaviour. They work well when there are defined actions performed by an individual, such as volunteering to help with clearing up or dressing themselves properly.

- **Fixed ratio**: The reinforcer can be applied at a fixed number of instances of the desired behaviour; e.g., 'every time' or 'every third time'. The interval can be changed as progress is made. A real-world example of this is a salesperson who gets a bonus after every third sale.
- **Variable ratio**: The reinforcer can be applied according to a caregiver's judgement based on 'every few times'. A real-world example of this is a gambling machine – it pays out just often enough to keep a person playing.

Ratio schedules, particularly of the variable type, are useful, as they are fairly 'extinction resistant', meaning that the desired behaviour is likely to be sustained. This is because the expectation of the reinforcer is slightly unpredictable, which creates anticipation; anticipation increases dopamine in the brain and acts as an additional reinforcer to the behaviour. This is why gambling addiction is so pervasive; 'I'm sure I'll get a reward on the next one' is a very powerful motivator.

If we are thinking about the process of linking primary reinforcers (unconditioned stimulus) and secondary reinforcers (conditioned stimulus), we may need to use ratio schedules to reinforce the link between the two stimuli. For example, in Pavlov's study, the bell (secondary) caused salivation, as it was originally paired with food (primary). However, when Pavlov stopped giving the food and only rang the bell, initially the dogs salivated at this secondary reinforcer, but over time, when food was no longer presented, the dogs no longer salivated. The salivation was now extinct as a behaviour. If Pavlov had used a variable ratio conditioning strategy – still presenting food with the bell every now and again – the behaviour would have been maintained for a lot longer.

The disadvantage of ratio schedules is the need for ongoing monitoring to catch and count instances of the good behaviour.

Interval Schedules

Interval schedules are based on providing a reinforcement after a set time has elapsed. These can work well when the desired behaviour is of an ongoing nature and the reinforcers are presented after a certain time; for example, after focusing on work in the classroom for 20 minutes or a personal trainer offering a 'well done' after you run on the treadmill for five minutes.

- **Fixed intervals**: The reinforcer can be applied after a set elapsed time; e.g., 'every five minutes' or 'every Friday'. A real-world example of this is a salesperson who gets a bonus every Friday based on the number of sales.
- **Variable intervals**: The reinforcer can be applied at random intervals as time passes. A real-world example of this is a person checking social media and seeing the new likes they have.

Variable intervals do not require as much individual monitoring, as reinforcements are based on the passage of time, not the number of times the behaviour occurs. With fixed intervals, there tends to be an increase in behaviour closer to the reinforcement time. For example, if a teacher gives students a weekly quiz every Monday, there is an increase in studying by the students over the weekend. On Monday, the students take the quiz and are reinforced for studying (positive reinforcement: they receive a good grade; negative reinforcement: they don't fail the quiz). For the next few days, they are likely to relax after finishing the stressful experience until the next quiz date draws too near for them to ignore.

Punishment

The previously mentioned reinforcers are based on strengthening desired behaviours. Punishment is designed to weaken undesired behaviours. Punishment can certainly do this, based on the principle that people will move away from pain to not-pain.

Punishment is the presentation of an adverse event or outcome that causes a decrease in the behaviour it follows. There are two kinds of punishment. In both cases, the behaviour decreases.

Positive punishment, sometimes referred to as punishment by application, presents an unfavourable event or outcome in order to weaken the behaviour it follows. Smacking a child for misbehaving is an example of punishment by application. Other examples include criticism, or sending them to a place that is uncomfortable, or the old school punishment of writing lines.

Negative punishment, also known as punishment by removal, occurs when a favourable event or outcome is removed after a behaviour occurs. Taking away a child's video game following misbehaviour is an example of negative punishment.

But punishment has numerous ethical and behavioural concerns.

- It can increase the likelihood of other negative behaviours and outcomes. As a result, it can lead to a negative spiral that could become abusive.
- Punishment may not be allowed under the Human Rights Act (1998) or under the Mental Capacity Act (2005).
- It can create a negative mindset in the staff, who come to feel that the individual is living up to their 'being difficult' label again.
- It can create a negative mindset in the individual: 'I want attention, but when I shout to get you to notice me, you either tell me off, ignore me or say you won't take me out if I don't stop.'

The individual may stop the behaviour, but they may feel bullied, unsupported and unworthy. In turn, this can lead to a lowering of their self-esteem, which in turn can lead to more or alternative negative behaviours, especially as the individual still doesn't know how to get the attention they crave. This diagram shows this cycle:

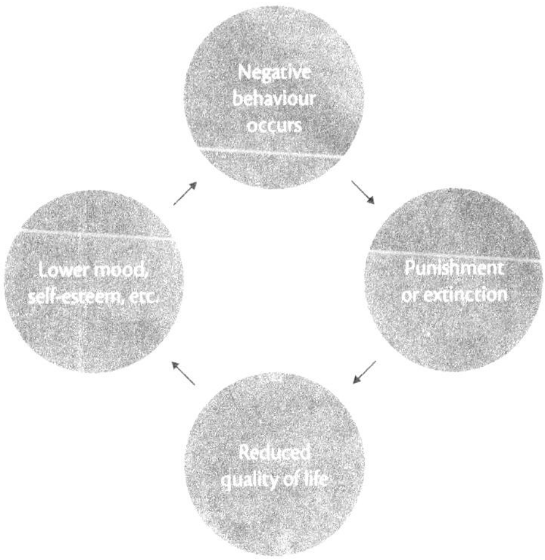

Figure 25.2 The Punishment Cycle

Extinction Procedures

Extinction is a reduction in a particular behaviour due to the lack of reinforcement it receives or the negative effect it elicits. For example, a company changes the flavour of a drink you used to love, but you don't like the new flavour as much, so you stop buying it. This is not the same as punishment.

Another technique to change behaviour is to inhibit any reinforcing stimulus or add friction to receiving that same reinforcing stimulus (as mentioned in 'Case Study 15.3 The Smoker' about John quitting smoking, page 139). *These should only be used alongside a positive reinforcement programme.*

Strategies include:

- ignoring the behaviour, not the person (while still ensuring safety)
- removing or minimising any reinforcement it may bring
- preventing sensory feedback
- not allowing escape or avoidance
- making it harder to get the reinforcement (adding friction)
- natural and balanced consequences.

Each of these is described in the following paragraphs.

Ignoring the Behaviour

Note that the strategy is to ignore the *behaviour*, not the individual. However, if the behaviour is harmful, then minimal, no-fuss intervention is the key.

Minimal response involves a person responding to the behaviour but in a way that offers minimal stimulus. For example, cleaning a person up after smearing but with minimal communication or facial expressions so the interaction is boring rather than exciting or stimulating. Or, if there is a case of headbanging, quietly placing a cushion on the table to prevent the physical harm. At the same time, the caregiver doesn't panic or beg the person to stop; instead, they may just calmly empathise with the individual and prompt a desired behaviour: 'I can see you're upset... When you rest your head still, we can find out what's wrong.'

Along with this, an appropriate positive reinforcer should follow any act of desired behaviour.

CONSISTENCY

If an 'ignoring' strategy is selected for the individual, it must be consistently applied among all staff. For example, suppose the problem is smearing, as above, and appears to be being used to gain attention. Part of the plan to change this behaviour is that staff should support with minimal stimulus, as above. But if one staff member breaks rank and shows disgust or anger at the individual, the behaviour has been reinforced again. These mixed messages will significantly impact on the effectiveness of the approach.

POSSIBILITY OF INCREASING THE UNDESIRED BEHAVIOUR

CASE STUDY 25.14 NO MORE SWEETS

Alfie always gets his way at the supermarket – he pesters to get sweets, and he gets them.

In an attempt to change this behaviour, it has been decided to ignore his pestering and not buy him sweets. This will be accompanied by a strategy to teach Alfie ways to get his desire met in an appropriate way. For example, maybe Alfie can earn his sweets or he gets sweets on a Friday if he doesn't pester for the rest of the week.

The immediate result will be that the pestering will go on and on, because the expected result of the behaviour, from past experience, hasn't worked this time for Alfie. Over time, the pestering may die down.

Caution: Planned ignoring and similar examples like 'the naughty step' (page 55) may be highly detrimental to individuals who can't regulate and who believe that no one wants them, etc. Minimal response/time in is often more appropriate: 'I ignore the behaviour, not you.' Time in is explained in Stage 5: Respond Appropriately, page 311.

Remove Reinforcement

This relates to removing the reinforcing item, activities or people. For example, if the behaviour is being used to get the attention of a particular person, ensure that the person is removed to extinguish the behaviour. Again, this approach should only be used with consistency and be accompanied by a positive reinforcer.

Preventing Sensory Feedback

In the earlier headbanging example, putting a cushion between the head and the object the individual bangs against means they're not getting the same feedback from it, so they may not bother. Another example would be putting long sleeves on a person who has an excessive scratching habit.

Not Allowing Escape or Avoidance

If the individual's functional aim of their behaviour is to avoid an activity or something they don't like, then once the individual has returned to a calm state, they must be returned to the task at hand. This will act as an inhibitor to that behaviour recurring.

Making it Harder to Get the Reinforcement (Adding Friction)

'Adding friction' refers to any strategy that makes getting the unwanted reinforcing stimulus harder to achieve. There are lots of general life examples that people may use themselves to alter their unwanted habits and behaviours. These include not having any biscuits in the house if they are on a diet, not having cigarettes in the house when quitting smoking and using a timed electronic safe to lock away their phone to avoid using it when they are meant to be working. In all these examples, the person could still get the biscuits, cigarettes or phone if they really wanted them, but it would require more effort, time or pain to access them. These same types of strategy can be used in a behavioural plan to make the unwanted or maladaptive strategy harder to achieve, so the target behaviour becomes the easier option for the individual.

Natural Consequences and Balanced Consequences

> *Newton's Third Law, 'Action and Reaction', states that for every action (force) in nature, there is an equal and opposite reaction.*

Despite the focus on reinforcing the behaviour we *do* want (rather than what we don't want) to elicit change, there are some circumstances where it is appropriate and important to allow a person to learn from the consequences of their actions. Natural consequences require the caregiver to take no action, as the consequences will naturally come from the environment or other people.

Balanced consequences are enacted by caregivers but should be based on the specific incident and be presented logically and not emotionally.

It may be the case that we are dealing with a behaviour that is repeated, and part of our proactive plan may include clearly defined examples of natural and balanced consequences that advise staff how to respond immediately after an incident of the behaviour. It is often the case that natural and balanced consequences may initially be received on an ad hoc (as the behaviour occurs) basis. For a full explanation and examples of what natural and balanced consequences may include, see 'Correction and Consequences', Chapter 39, page 388.

TEACHING TECHNIQUE: PROMPTING

When learning a new skill, an individual may need some prompting to help them to perform the task or steps within the task.

There are several types of prompts.

- **Physical assistance:** Hand-over-hand guidance – the teacher places their hands on the individual and moves the individual through the activity. Typically, this is hand-over-hand but not necessarily so; e.g., when teaching martial arts, it may be necessary to reposition an individual's arm or move their arm in the correct direction. The individual can then be invited to repeat the action unaided.

- **Modelling**: The teacher demonstrates and invites the individual to copy the teacher's actions.
- **Verbal**: The individual has reached a sticking point. Verbal prompts are of three types:
  - The individual is told what the end result should be.
  - The individual is guided to the desired action by question/answer.
  - The individual is guided verbally through the process.
- **Visual**: Use of a video, photographs and so on showing what to do or what the result should be.
- **Positioning**: Making it easy for the individual to progress from one step to another by the arrangement of the environment; e.g., when getting dressed, the items of clothing could be laid out in the sequence of use.
- **Gesture**: Pointing, nodding or shaking the head to help the individual move on; e.g., if a shirt has just been put on, a light gesture towards the buttons could prompt the individual about the next step.

TEACHING TECHNIQUE: CHAINING

CASE STUDY 25.15 LET'S MAKE A CAKE

Olivia has never baked a cake before. She is given the ingredients and told, 'Okay, Olivia, bake a cake.'

The result is guaranteed to be a failure. She has been set up to fail.

So we need to teach Olivia how to bake a cake. But where do we start?

What knowledge does Olivia already have?

Unlike the approach to Olivia, who was initially set up to fail, we try to set people up to succeed. We need to set our expectations based on their abilities, their pre-existing knowledge and their pre-existing skills, to slowly develop and promote completion and success.

Chaining is the process of breaking a task into small steps and then teaching the individual one step at a time.

There are variations on how to do this:

- **Forward chaining**: This is when the first step is taught (prompted or unprompted) and reinforced upon completion. Then the first and second steps are completed before reinforcement is provided. This is continued until completion of all steps is required before reinforcement is offered.

  So, when we're teaching Olivia to bake a cake, we might begin by showing her the first step – how to crack and beat the eggs. She succeeds and receives her reinforcement.

The next time, Olivia is shown how to fold in the flour, and she must successfully deal with the eggs *and* the flour before her reward.

Progress must not be forced; progress should be at the individual's pace.

- **Backward chaining**: This is the same as forward chaining, except teaching begins with the last step and works backwards as each step is successfully learned.

  E.g., if we were teaching an individual to dress themselves, the last process might be to put on socks. So we help them to that point and then teach them how to put on socks, giving reinforcement when they succeed.

  Next time, maybe it's trousers before socks. Both must be completed before reinforcement is offered. And so on.
- **Total task chaining**: The individual has sufficient pre-existing skills to be able to fully complete all steps of a task. Only upon completion is the reinforcer offered.
- **Behaviour chain interruption**: This is used to confirm that the subject has the skills to show appropriate alternative behaviour when one of the steps in the chain is interrupted.

  E.g., by using a behaviour chain, Sally has taught her brother Sam to make the bed. On this occasion, before he is finished, she hides the pillowcases. She waits for him to ask where the pillowcases are, or to look for them, or to go to the linen cupboard to get new ones, etc. Reinforcement is offered for an appropriate response.
- **Behaviour chain with limited time**: This is when a person has to complete the required task within a limited time in order to receive reinforcement.

  E.g., an individual has learned how to get ready for school, but we want them to take less time.

In this chapter, we have explored in detail a multitude of teaching strategies to help reinforce behaviours we want to develop and to potentially extinguish maladaptive behaviours.

Teaching is a dynamic process, as at every step of the process, if learning is achieved, the individual will be different as a result. This may trigger new reactions, challenges and behaviours. We must be flexible enough to adapt but consistent enough to allow skill development.

It is important to be realistic and recognise that sometimes we are not just teaching new skills/behaviours; we are also trying to unteach old ones. Some skills are more complex and will require more time or intensity in the teaching. We also need to be aware of the individual's capability to learn and how they learn best, not how we think they should learn. Teachers are often taught that some students learn visually, some through reading and writing, some through listening and some through doing, and so they must adapt their lessons to be inclusive of all. However, some people learn through reflection of a process, some learn as they go, some want to trial and error and others want to investigate everything theoretically before they act on it. It is not for us to decide how a person should learn. Teaching any new skill, habit or behaviour should still be person-centred.

We also need to acknowledge an individual's willingness to learn and engage. We are supporting autonomous human beings who have their own mind and may or may not choose to engage in a change. We can't care more about their behaviour than they do... remember the 'caring hand' analogy from Chapter 4, page 31.

CHAPTER 26

CREATING A COMPETING PATHWAY

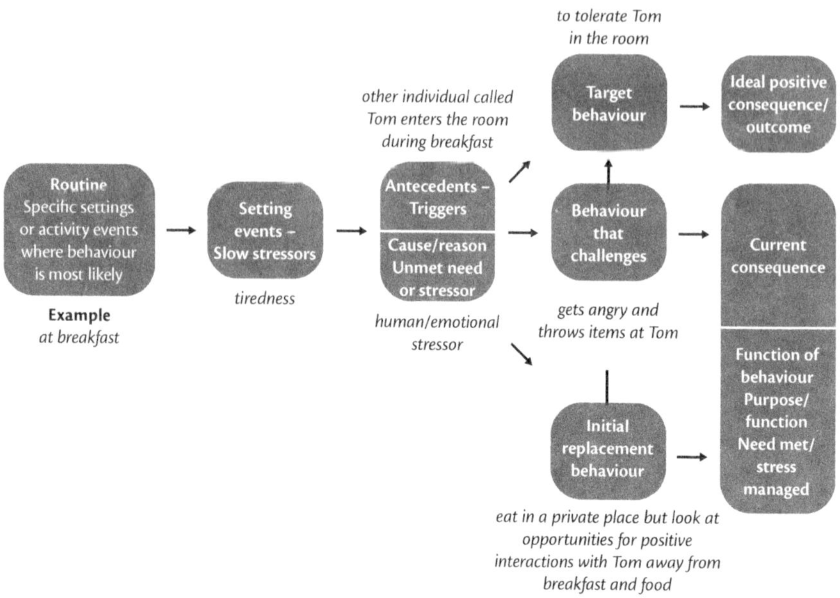

Figure 26.1 A Competing Pathway

Let's use the previous stages of the 6STM and what we have learned in this third stage to now improve our hypothesis and create a plan, using the diagram above as a structure.

- **Routine**: The settings and locations where, or activities when, the behaviour is most likely to occur; e.g., on the bus, at breakfast, at bedtime, when staff are providing personal care.
- **Setting events**: Slow stressors (things that we know make the likelihood of a behaviour stronger); e.g., when he's tired, when Sandra is working, when someone was late, when we run out of cereal.
- **Antecedents**: What happens before.

- **Reason/cause**: Stress or unmet need.
- **Behaviour that challenges**: The maladaptive behaviour being addressed.
- **Current consequence**: Current reaction or response.
- **Function of the behaviour**: Purpose/function (stress managed or need met).
- **Target behaviour**: What is our/their ideal outcome.
- **Ideal positive outcome**: What we want for the individual.
- **Replacement behaviour**: What strategy we would prefer.

Note: What follows is a series of forms that could be used in the creation of a plan to deal with the problems facing Sam.

Table 26.1 Background Information Form

Individual's name and brief info	Sam is a non-verbal autistic man. He can use picture charts and cards to communicate. He really enjoys head massages, haircuts, showers, anything that stimulates his head.
Routine	Anytime he's engaged in an activity that involves doing something. If Sam is engaged in a passive activity, the behaviour does not occur.
Setting events	When tired and with certain staff who respond inconsistently.
Antecedents – what happens before?	Sam engages with an activity like getting dressed, washing up dishes, gardening. But if the activity lasts longer than ten minutes, Sam becomes agitated.
Reason/cause (stress or unmet need)	Anxiety, overwhelmed, bored.
Behaviour that challenges	Sam hits his head repeatedly with his hand for about two minutes.
Current consequence	Some staff ignore Sam, some interrupt the activity and change the activity.
Function of the behaviour – purpose/function (stress managed or need met)	Sensory input and activity avoidance.
Target behaviour – what is our/their ideal outcome?	To meet sensory needs in a safe way himself and to communicate a request to either change activity or take a break. To increase resilience to activity duration.
Ideal positive outcome – what do we want for the individual?	To be able to cope with activities, especially activities that promote independence, social engagement and physical and mental stimulation. To feel confident to communicate needs.
Replacement behaviour – what strategy would we prefer for now?	To communicate a need to pause an activity or change an activity via staff-guided prompts. To meet sensory needs in a safe way via staff prompts.

Table 26.2 Planning Form

Question	Strategy	Implementation and monitoring method
What can we do to reduce the stress?	When Sam is tired, staff need to be mindful of Sam's ability to cope, and staff need to respond to Sam consistently based on this plan.	Care plan and behavioural plan update.
How do we want Sam to meet his need?	We want Sam to be able to communicate his need to pause activities he needs to complete or change activities that he wants to change. We want Sam to use a sensory head scratcher (HS) rather than hitting himself to meet his sensory need.	
What skills does Sam need to learn to achieve these?	Sam would benefit from being able to communicate to the staff the need, and staff need to respond by allowing a break, a change of activity and use of the HS.	
How can this be taught? **Step 1**	Step 1: Staff will start using a card with a picture of the HS on it. This will be shown to Sam, and Sam will be prompted to touch the card to get his HS for one minute. This will be taught over one week: Day 1: Fixed ratio activity – one action: one reinforcer for 30 minutes of teaching session Days 1 and 2: Fixed interval – one hour Day 3+: Variable interval – approx. one hour	A preferred member of staff will initially teach Sam that the card leads to the HS using a 30-minute teaching session on day 1. Random staff will then present the card at the fixed interval and the variable interval. Success will be recorded in Sam's behavioural plan.
How can this be taught? **Step 2**	Step 2: During an activity, staff will invite Sam after ten minutes to take a break and use his HS, but if Sam seems agitated before ten minutes (see response strategy), the invitation is offered. The staff will carry the card with a picture of the HS on it. When Sam indicates HS by touching the card, staff will direct Sam to a quiet place and Sam will get to use the HS for one minute. Afterwards, Sam should return to activities he needs to finish or choose a different activity using his picture charts.	A keyworker will be allocated to Sam during activities. The keyworker will perform the strategy. Sam's successes should be recorded in his behavioural plan, along with any incidents of head hitting. At the end of the day, if no head hitting has occurred, 'tingly shampoo' should be offered. Incidents and successes will be reviewed after two weeks to decide on next step.
How can this be taught? **Next steps**	Next steps: The duration before using the HS will be extended from ten minutes in increments of two minutes. Staff will also introduce choice cards of 'stop' or 'change' that Sam will carry himself and that he can use to approach the staff and communicate to them that he needs a break or wants to change the activity.	To be confirmed.

What are the individual's motivators, reinforcers?	HS is a preferred item. If Sam uses the HS rather than hitting his head for a full day, Sam gets to use the 'tingly shampoo' at night.		
Do we need to include any friction, extinction strategies or consequences?	Staff must maintain calm with Sam even if he makes the wrong choice. Sam should always return to activities that need to be completed, e.g., completing dressing if inappropriately dressed.		
Is the alternative...			
obvious?	**achievable?**	**attractive?**	**rewarding?**
Staff will offer the HS.	Sam uses picture cards for other activities.	Sam loves the HS for short periods.	Sam will get positive sensory input and pause or change an activity.
How should caregivers recognise escalation?	When Sam initially gets agitated, he will often stop the activity and initially start by rubbing his head before hitting it.		
How should caregivers respond?	When Sam is getting overwhelmed, offer Sam his communication chart and encourage him to use it. If Sam cannot engage with his cards, the HS card should be shown, and Sam should be redirected to a safe space and given his HS for one minute and then encouraged to return to the activity if needed or to choose a new activity if it isn't important to return. If Sam begins violently hitting his head with his hand and will not respond to verbal redirection, Sam may respond to a physical non-restrictive guiding technique to be moved to his safe space where he will continue to bang his head for usually no more than two minutes.		

As Sam is non-verbal, the staff need to teach Sam new ways to communicate his need. Over time, the hope will be that Sam can use cards to communicate more independently. Also, by giving Sam a method that he can use to control when he takes breaks and changes his routine, we hope his resilience to activities will increase over time until he can fully complete tasks.

The next example is very different, as Clare's behaviour is triggered by potential trauma rather than an event.

As discussed in 'Case Study 17.3 The Food Hoarder', page 156, Clare's need for food is not the problem; it's her fear of there being no food tomorrow. So although routine will need to be built into the plan and trust will take time to build, trust is the target outcome.

Table 26.3 Background Information Form

Individual's name and brief info	Clare is nine years old but functions at a lower emotional and cognitive age. She has come from a severely neglectful and abusive background.
Routine	Mealtimes are high stress and evening times and weekends are worse.
Setting events	Clare finds any change in the house stressful, particularly new children coming to live there.
Antecedents – what happens before?	n/a
Reason/cause (stress or unmet need)	Fear of hunger, need for control of food, unable to ask for snacks. Fear of abuse.
Behaviour that challenges	Clare takes food from her own plate, the bin, the fridge or shops and hides the food in her room.
Current consequence	Clare has access to food that she feels cannot be taken from her (despite it being unsafe). She feels in control of her food availability.
Function of the behaviour – purpose/ function (stress managed or need met)	To feel safe that there is food there for tomorrow, to have control over her food.
Target behaviour – what is our/their ideal outcome?	To enjoy her three meals a day, come and ask for a snack if hungry, ask for snack/treats in shops.
Ideal positive outcome – what do we want for the individual?	To feel safe and comfortable. To eat safely and healthily. To feel confident that meals will keep coming and that she can access more if she needs.
Replacement behaviour – what strategy would we prefer for now?	Managing with a snack box that she can hide in her room that is filled with safe/healthy snacks; eating all of her meals.

Table 26.4 Planning Form

Question	Strategy	Implementation and monitoring method
What can we do to reduce the stress?	Clare is in the stabilisation stage of trauma recovery – routine on meals is key. Also, staff must be building trust and safety, as well as confidence in basic needs being met: • Breakfast ready by 7.30am • Snack at 11am • Lunch at 12.30pm • Snack at 3.30pm • Dinner at 5pm • Bedtime snack at 7pm	All staff trained in PACE Model concepts. Ensure all staff read Clare's history and care plan. Ensure staff avoid punish/reward responses to behaviour.
How do we want Clare to meet this need?	Ask for food if needed. Manage her stress with a snack box.	
What skills does Clare need to learn to achieve these?	Trust and confidence that food is available here and it always will be. Trust that adults will help her get food when she is hungry. Alternative ways to cope when feeling anxious.	

cont.

Question	Strategy	Implementation and monitoring method
How can this be taught? **Step 1**	Step 1: Give Clare control over food in a safe way by providing her with a secret snack/stash box so that she can hide food in her room. Inform her that each day if she brings the box to the staff they will refill it with good foods that Clare can choose from a selection of options.	Five items in her box. Cereal bars, boxes of raisins, rice cakes, protein bars. Carrot sticks (changed daily). Maximum of one chocolate bar. Any regressions to food stealing should be logged to monitor for reduction. Keep a log of what food Clare eats at meals and snacks and what has been eaten from her box. This will need reviewing when Clare goes back to school in September (school needs to be aware and included in plans). Staff will participate in a daily morning routine with Clare as part of her daily schedule of meal planning.
How can this be taught? **Step 2**	Step 2: Create routine and confidence in her meal/snack routine. As Clare moves into the metabolisation/integration stage, introduce some slight delays in meals.	
How can this be taught? **Step 3**	Step 3: Work with Clare to recognise feelings and how she can feel better without using food. Additional: Meal planning and routine will also become a daily activity with Clare each morning. In that way, she can build trust that food is coming, and it gives her an alternative way to have control over her food.	
What are the individual's motivators, reinforcers?	Clare loves doing make-up and having pamper sessions. This should be offered as noncontingent reinforcers in the stabilisation stage.	Minimum of twice a week and allow Clare to choose with whom and when it happens – based on a schedule of who is free/when.

Do we need to include any friction, extinction strategies or consequences?	A room check should be completed daily to remove any inappropriate food and throw it away. If an item is stolen, that food will be removed and returned to the shop if appropriate. During meals, small portions should be provided but additional portions offered. Bins containing food waste should be emptied after each meal. No other consequences should be used while in the stabilisation stage.	Keep a log of found food.	
Is the alternative...			
obvious?	**achievable?**	**attractive?**	**rewarding?**
It's available and controlled by Clare.	It will be easier to access the food in her stash than the fridge or bins.	It is foods that taste better and are liked.	Clare has control.
How should caregivers recognise escalation?	n/a See other behavioural plans for other anxiety behaviours.		
How should caregivers respond?	Follow trauma recovery models and empathic responses. Do not praise, just share in Clare's emotions when she brings the box for refill.		

Commentary: These plans have been created around one specific behaviour that challenges for each person. These specific plans will then be integrated into the individual's full behavioural support plan, which will include all of the individual's 'target behaviours' we are looking to achieve to improve their outcomes and quality of life. The full behavioural plan for Sam (found in Chapter 38, page 379) will inform staff of the appropriate actions for prevention, proactive management and responses in all areas of a person's care.

TESTING THE SOCIAL VALIDITY OF INTERVENTIONS

We must ensure that any plans conform to appropriate practices of human rights and are socially appropriate.

Whatever plan is agreed, it must meet the following criteria:

- **'The supermarket test'**: If the plan involves using some kind of intervention when the behaviour happens, we should ask ourselves whether we would feel comfortable making that intervention in a crowded supermarket (or any public space).

CASE STUDY 26.1 THE PINCHER

Craig is an individual with autism, who, when anxious, sometimes pinches to get people to move away from him. Maybe the positive response for Craig is sensory or gaining a feeling of control.

A slap on the hand is suggested – it may stop Craig at that moment.

But within a care home, this would be considered assault. So it is inappropriate in the supermarket setting too.

- **'In their shoes test'**: In other words, would I feel comfortable if this intervention were being done to me? If the answer is 'no', then the intervention is not appropriate.

  Care must be taken with this test, because different people may give different views. We should also ensure that we consider the person as they *are*, not as they *were*, in the case of those with a condition like dementia or acquired brain injury.
- What evidence is there that shows a benefit for the individual themselves from the intervention as opposed to others' personal feelings being the sole factor considered?

  This is why it is beneficial to have a multidisciplinary team (multiple stakeholders) exploring what the right intervention is.

CASE STUDY 26.2 DOLL THERAPY

Doll therapy works well in elderly care settings. It involves getting individuals with dementia to engage with toy dolls – dressing them, looking after them, feeding them and things like that.

Some people may perceive this as infantilising: 'They are an adult.' But all the evidence shows that, for many people, doll therapy can significantly reduce distress, increase the individual's sense of worth and improve their mood.

So, the multidisciplinary team can take that decision.

- **The individual has given consent**: This is the most important test of all.

  The people involved in creating the plan have been making decisions about what's right and what's wrong for the individual.

  It is a basic human right for the individual to be involved in these decisions.

  Even a child can be made aware of what is being discussed.

The more the individual is involved in the plan, the better the outcome will be – it's a team working together.

The planning process is an ongoing journey through the 6STM and will involve constant review and improvement. It is worth ensuring that all opportunities are taken to include any people who have a stake in the individual's wellbeing – particularly the individual themselves – in the planning process.

CHAPTER 27

RELATIONSHIPS – PROFESSIONAL OR PERSONAL

This chapter will look at the importance of relationships in behavioural management, whether they are professional relationships (a paid caregiver or teacher) or personal relationships (a parent or family caregiver).

The opposite to anxiety is not calm... it's trust.

Trust – a firm belief in the reliability, truth or ability of someone or something.

Predictability is an important factor in the effects of stress and anxiety. For example, in an experiment where animals are given the opportunity to determine whether electric shocks delivered to them will be signalled or unsignalled, they typically choose to spend their time in the signalled conditions regardless of whether the shock is escapable or inescapable.[65] Knowing that something is coming allows us to prepare ourselves. This reinforces why routines and consistency are so useful and important in reducing stress.

The predictable becomes reliable. Trusting that a thing is going to happen, or that a person is going to be there when we need them, allows us to feel safer. Reliable environments, activities, people and met needs all help to reduce stress and build confidence.

CASE STUDY 27.1 ATTACHMENT INCREASES CONFIDENCE

A study was done on the different effects of nurturing and non-nurturing rat mothers on the behaviour of their pups. Some rat mothers spend lots of time licking their pups; other mothers don't.

The pups of nurturing rat mothers, rather than staying closer to their mother, were far more exploratory, confident and calm. This was the opposite to what was expected at the time, as it was believed that 'mollycoddling', heavily nurturing parents created timid and shy children.

Commentary: Having a safe, predictable, trusted base allows us to feel safer to explore the world. This is why part of the trauma recovery model mentions finding a 'good enough' attachment figure with whom to build trust (page 188).

We are social animals. From the moment we are born, we are reliant on other people for our very survival. Relationships and social engagement/connection are useful for reaching our full potential. There is evidence that social isolation is directly linked to 'adverse health consequences, including depression, poor sleep quality, impaired executive function, accelerated cognitive decline, poor cardiovascular function and impaired immunity at every stage of life'.[66,67]

These findings were based on perceived isolation – the subjects felt lonely. There are plenty of people who do not need others or friendships to feel content. They have perfectly satisfying lives and suffer no ill effects, despite a lack of relationships. For many of us, though, family, friends, colleagues, associates, role models and so on can give us a sense of purpose and help us to expand horizons and develop and add to our quality of life.

At the same time, if we have poor relationships that are negative, the effect can be the direct opposite and reduce our sense of wellbeing, belonging, value and worth. For people who have experienced bad relationships or been mistreated or who find relationships hard to understand and navigate, trusting people can be a real challenge.

Let's revisit the case study about Christine, who has a profound fear of being driven on a dangerous road ('Case Study 14.4 Fear of the Fall', page 129). There, we show that Christine needs to be in control...

CASE STUDY 27.2 FEAR OF THE FALL (PAGE 129) – REVISITED

Christine is terrified of heights; one of her biggest phobias is being in the car when it is on a road with a steep drop on one side.

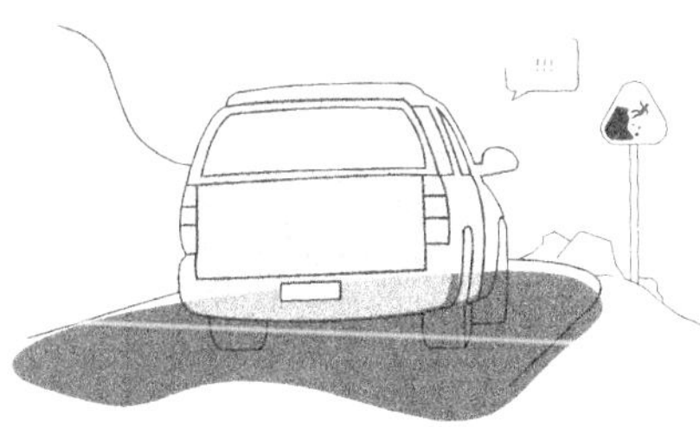

Figure 27.1 Driving at the Edge

She describes the feeling: 'I feel sick, my vision goes blurry, every part of me wants to leap from the car away from the drop, it's overwhelming. I can cope with it if I'm driving, but if someone else is driving, I close my eyes, hold my breath and pray for it to be over.'

Commentary: Most people in Christine's situation would not be so seriously affected. But while the car is on the mountain, Christine can barely function.

Why? She needs to be in control ('I can cope with it if I'm driving'). We all feel safer when we are in control.

However, if Christine truly trusted the person who was driving, wouldn't she feel safe?

This need for control may be stronger in individuals who have experienced harmful people or inconsistent or neglectful caregivers in their life; they are unlikely to trust and so will try to protect themselves from control or try to maintain control themselves.

GOOD ENOUGH ATTACHMENT FIGURES

'Good enough' is a subjective statement. We mean good enough as opposed to perfect.

The idea of a 'perfect' parent may be a caregiver who is there to meet a child's needs as soon as they call and do whatever the child needs doing for them to meet their needs and who protects the child from all fears and upsets.

Most people realise that this idea of perfection is perfectly inappropriate and impossible. A parent can never attain perfection or be able to maintain it, nor should they. They will ultimately create such a state of stress for themselves by trying to achieve the unachievable that they will be less able to meet the emotional needs of the child. They will also leave a child vulnerable to risks and limitations in independent skills as they grow older if they shelter them from everything and teach them nothing.

'Good enough' parenting is consistent, positive, nurturing, supportive and encouraging, promotes positive risk taking and, importantly, has boundaries.

These are actually the makings of any 'good enough' healthy relationship and attachment.

The extent to which each of these attributes may vary depends on the nature of the relationship – whether it is professional or personal in nature – and the appropriate boundaries required.

BOUNDARIES

The boundaries of any relationship are important to both parties. Clear boundaries allow us to feel more secure because we 'know where we stand'.

For the caregiver, developing healthy boundaries prevents or reduces:

- emotional burnout
- imbalances of power
- allegations or safeguarding issues
- shifts to unhealthy relationship dynamics.

For the individual, they also prevent or reduce:

- unhealthy dependency
- imbalances of power
- abuse.

There are various types of healthy boundaries, and they are described below.

Boundaries on Times

These include duration of support, times of availability, scope of role and support.

Any relationship can benefit from time apart, but for a caregiver, time is needed to meet their own needs that is separate from time spent meeting the needs of the individual. These boundaries work two ways: both the individual and the caregivers may want times of privacy. Even a five-minute break can allow us to self-care and switch off. It may also allow an individual to develop resilience by learning to cope without a caregiver for short periods (with intervals being increased over time if needed). If caring in a paid capacity, these time boundaries may include set times with certain individuals, set durations of time working with one individual (guidelines recommend a maximum of two hours) and not engaging with an individual outside of working hours. When caring for a family member, this may include set one-to-one time or boundaries on spaces in the home. What is important is that these boundaries are clearly created, communicated and maintained. If predictability helps people feel safe, then shifting the boundaries either way can be detrimental.

CASE STUDY 27.3 MY SPACE

Miranda is a foster carer who has fostered children for over six years. She has an important rule in her house: 'When I am in my room with the door closed, you do not disturb me unless it is urgent.'

She has often cared for children who have struggled with this rule and have made up stories to excuse the knock on her door, especially when they are first developing attachments and feeling anxious.

Iesha is a foster child who has been with Miranda for three months.

Knock knock. 'Miranda, you need to come quick, the toilet is blocked and it's going to flood the house,' called Iesha.

Miranda left her room to check. The toilet *was* blocked, and Miranda was 99% sure that Iesha was the one who did it, as she was the only one in the house.

Miranda responded, 'Wow, okay it looks like someone has put lots of toilet paper down here, so we need to get this sorted. Iesha, can you get me the bucket, mop and rubber gloves and we can get this sorted.' Miranda and Iesha got the toilet unblocked and cleaned up together, with Miranda encouraging Iesha to help as much as she could.

Afterwards, Miranda spoke to Iesha very calmly and gently. 'Iesha, I'm wondering if someone blocked the toilet to get my attention because I was in my room with the door shut. How do you feel when I'm in my room with my door shut?'

'It wasn't me!' shouted Iesha defensively.

Staying completely calm, Miranda responded, 'I never said it was, I was just wondering how you felt when my door is closed?'

'I don't like it,' said Iesha tentatively.

'Do you know what you don't like about it, Iesha?'

'I know you are writing your notes about me and I don't like it,' explained Iesha.

Miranda responded empathically, 'That must feel really hard, thinking I'm writing stuff about you. You are probably worried and feeling slightly anxious about what I'm writing. Well, just so you know, I'm not always writing stuff about you when I'm in my room. I do other things too and sometimes I just need some time to myself, just like you do sometimes. That doesn't mean anything bad is happening behind the door or that I'm not still caring about you.

'If you ever want to see what I write about you in my notes, you can always ask me, after I come out of my room, and I will show you.

'But the rule is when the door is closed you give me some time, okay? Now I need to go and take my time now. I need 30 minutes. Tell you what – if you can give me my 30 minutes, we can watch something on TV together when I come out, if you like.'

Commentary: Iesha is learning about boundaries and therefore she shouldn't be punished. She needed understanding, a plan put in place and an appropriate response. Miranda maintained her boundaries in a clear but empathic way. Miranda used a technique called *empathic commentary*, which will be covered in Chapter 34, page 328. As Iesha is learning and building trust, Miranda may need to introduce a natural consequence for being disturbed in her room; for example, 'taking time back'. ('Because I had to come out of my room for this, I need to catch up on what I was doing. That means I'm not going to have time to do "X" with you now Iesha, but if I can get my time now maybe we can do "Y" later instead.')

The problem with technology – access to email, text, message apps and telephones – is that it has become harder and harder to set boundaries around engagement. It is important to include these media within our boundaries; for example, 'I do not answer my phone after 8pm. If you need me urgently, you can message me and I will get back to you, if I need to.'

Boundaries on Behaviour

These may include:

- boundaries on physical contact and touch
- use of language, tone and volume
- limits on tangibles like food and electronic equipment
- the rules of the setting.

All settings will have rules that are applied to all. Society has laws that sometimes dictate these; at other times they are for health and safety reasons; sometimes they are based on the values of the setting, whether that be a commercial setting or a caregiver's own home.

However, as much as is reasonably practicable, boundaries should be person-centred. Whatever boundaries are set, consistency in maintaining them is important.

CASE STUDY 27.4 THE KIND CAREGIVER

Jason has limited capacity and diabetes. In his care plan, to manage his sugar levels, he is limited to how much of certain foods he is allowed to have (although this is being reviewed). One example of a limit for Jason is that he is allowed only two biscuits with his morning cup of tea. Jason always tries to persuade the staff to let him have more biscuits. Recently, a new member of staff has started, and she lets Jason have extra biscuits, her claim being that 'I was just being nice, and I want him to like me as I'm new'.

The problem is that Jason is now using this event with other staff, saying he prefers the new member of staff and he won't let others work with him. He is also starting to become aggressive when other staff refuse his request for more.

This one member of staff 'just being nice' has caused an escalation in new behavioural challenges.

Note: A second new member of staff has already raised the biscuit issue, feeling that the boundary in place for Jason is not person-centred. Jason likes biscuits, and other individuals in the home are not limited as Jason is. A suggestion has been made to buy low-fat/low-sugar alternative biscuits. This is a less restrictive measure to meet the same medical goals (which is one of the principles required in the Mental Capacity Act 2005). This staff member has raised it through management to prompt a review of Jason's care plan, and a dietician has been called in to create a more person-centred diet plan for Jason.

Commentary: The behaviour of the first caregiver created an inconsistency in the approach, which impacted on multiple relationships within the setting.

Caregivers should not just undermine behavioural plans, especially based on the desire to be liked. You don't buy trust, you earn it.

The second staff member was motivated to change the boundary based on the best interests of the individual, and they went through appropriate professional channels.

We could use a similar example of two parents creating confusing boundaries with a child. This results in either the child feeling anxious due to the uncertainty of the expectations or the child using it for their own advantage by playing the parents against each other.

Boundaries on Personal Disclosure

If we are caring for someone else, they do not benefit from listening to our woes and problems, depending on the relationship and risk factors.

CASE STUDY 27.5 THREE PRIVATE CONVERSATIONS

1. Paul often behaves in ways to trigger emotional reactions from staff. Staff reacting make Paul feel empowered and validated. If he can upset a staff member or intimidate them, it helps Paul to cope with his own emotional distress. However, he does not recognise the detrimental effect it actually has on his own self-esteem and ability to build relationships.

   A member of staff has come in and is already upset. Unfortunately, her father passed away just before the weekend. She is talking to one of her colleagues, in front of Paul, about how she is feeling.

   Later on, the bereaved caregiver is working with Paul and tells Paul he can't do something he wants to do. This triggers Paul into a rage, and he starts making extremely nasty comments to the caregiver that include comments about her deceased dad. The staff member is understandably upset.
2. It is Monday morning at a children's home, and one of the staff is talking about their weekend to a colleague, while one of the children is eating breakfast nearby.

   'I had a mental Saturday night. I went out with a couple of mates on the lash – we were necking Jägerbombs all night. Matty ended up passed out in the pub by midnight and we had to stick him in a taxi and pay the driver double in case he puked. The rest of us ended up getting some quality gear, and once I got a line of that up my nose, I was good to go for the next few hours. Until this doorman prick tried to tell us to calm down! We were only dancing on the tables... ha ha. Judd ended up planting one on this doorman and he went down like a sack of s**t, but we ended up having to leg it from the club.'
3. Two members of staff are in the dining room serving breakfast to the residents of the home. They are chatting about a colleague.

'You can tell who was working... or not working as the case may be... last night.'

'I know, look at the state of it in here. I reckon Pauline walks round with her eyes closed.'

'She's useless but she reckons she is all that, she right sucks up to management.'

'Aww don't worry. Ruth knows that Pauline is two-faced and useless, I bet she'll be gone soon.'

Commentary: These indirect disclosures carry potential consequences... especially within a professional context. The first resulted in the staff member making themselves emotionally vulnerable. The second is an example of setting a poor example. The third could have two problems – the undermining of a colleague in front of service users and, for an individual who overhears the conversation, the question arises, 'What are they saying about me if the staff talk about person "X" like that?'

The general tone of the professional relationship and principles of confidentiality can vary considerably depending on the setting and the professional role. Teachers, therapists and support workers are all different, but the boundaries may also vary depending on an individual's age, gender, disabilities, cognitive abilities and history. The following is a list of questions we could ask ourselves about the care we offer and the way we behave.

Professional Boundary Assessment

- Is this in the individual's best interests?
- Whose needs are being served?
- Will this have an impact on the service I am delivering?
- Should I make a note of my concerns or consult with a colleague?
- How would this be viewed by the individual's family or significant other?
- How would I feel telling a colleague about this?
- Am I treating this individual differently (e.g., appointment length, time of appointments, extent of personal disclosures)?
- Does this individual mean something special to me?
- Am I taking advantage of the individual?
- Does this action benefit me rather than the individual?
- Am I comfortable in documenting this decision or behaviour in the individual's file?
- Does this go against any policy or code of practice?

Boundaries on Prejudices

We all have prejudices, which are ideas based not on evidence but on assumptions about a person or group. These are most often subconscious, as we have explored within the book on numerous occasions. However, ideally, we should be aware of our prejudices to prevent them from impacting on the care of and choices we make for others.

The Equality Act 2010 outlines the professional requirement that no person should receive unfair treatment based on any one of eight protected characteristics, including age, disability, gender reassignment, marriage and civil partnership, pregnancy and maternity, race, religion or belief, or sex.

Let's look at a few stereotype statements:

- 'Autistic people all have learning disabilities or are like Rain Man.'
- 'People with dementia forget everything and are violent.'
- 'Looked-after kids are just bad kids that no one else wants.'

It may seem obvious that these are all false statements, but these are all genuine prejudices that individuals in these groups have experienced. They may be towards the extreme end of views, but even less negative assumptions like 'Autistic people don't make eye contact' can lead to misunderstanding, as some people on the autistic spectrum do engage in eye contact.

Stereotypes like those in the examples above lead to false beliefs, and these false beliefs can lead to discrimination. Discrimination can lead to abuse at worst and damage to relationships at best.

Whether building positive relationships or creating a behavioural plan, we must avoid assumptions and ensure a person-centred approach. We must also explore our own values and beliefs. This book does not go into the full details of performing mental capacity assessments or the Mental Capacity Act (2005). It is recommended that anyone who makes decisions on behalf of anyone else should be familiar with the laws and guidance that govern what decisions can and can't be made on behalf of someone else.

RISK AVERSION AND POSITIVE RISK TAKING

CASE STUDY 27.6 HE COULD DROWN

Eight-year-old Josh and his parents were going for a walk in the park, just along the river. The river was only a foot deep at this point, and Josh was just going towards the bank to see if he could see some fish.

One of Josh's mums started to panic. 'Josh, don't get so close, come away, you don't need to get so close.' Josh seemed panicked by his mum's reaction.

Josh's other mum was confused... 'He is fine. He's had swimming lessons, the water is only a foot deep and we are right here to help. If he falls, he falls – we'll take him home, get him dry and he'll learn a very valuable lesson.'

There is no such thing as no risk. Life would be very dull without any risk at all. It is easy, however, to fall into a trap of becoming excessively cautious as soon as you have responsibility for another person's wellbeing.

- It is important to recognise that it is impossible to eliminate risk entirely and that it is essential that people are given the freedom of choice and the right to make their own decisions on everything – from how they want to be cared for to how they want to spend their free time.

Don't get me wrong, caregivers are the most important people in the world but you can have caregivers and keepers. The latter try and assume total responsibility for your life prematurely, and there are many of them around.

QUOTE FROM A LADY LIVING WITH DEMENTIA

CASE STUDY 27.7 THE MAN AND THE MOUNTAIN

Sion Jair, 68, who was diagnosed with Alzheimer's in 2012, has climbed the Old Man of Coniston, a 2634-foot hill known for its steep ascent, at least 5000 times, despite many family members and professionals advising against it. The emerging science backs him up – regular, vigorous exercise is beneficial for those with the disease. He also takes great pride and joy in maintaining his independence and activity and continually repeating an opportunity for looking at one of his favourite views in the world.

The balance of risk and benefit will be unique to each individual and each situation. There is no one-size-fits-all solution, and a balanced approach will only be achieved through discussing and exploring an individual's priorities and expectations.

Care providers need a clear understanding of the difference between being defensive – which in this context means being risk-averse and taking an overly cautious approach to risk management – and taking a balanced approach to risk. Many professional caregivers become concerned about their accountability if something goes wrong, which causes them to be overly risk-averse.

A defensible decision is one where:

- all reasonable steps have been taken to avoid harm
- a person's mental capacity has been taken into consideration

- reliable assessment methods have been used and information has been thoroughly evaluated
- decisions are recorded and appropriately shared
- caregivers and their managers adopt an approach that is proactive, investigative and holistic
- all appropriate services are arranged to reduce identified risk and meet the needs of the individual concerned (as far as that person is prepared and able to accept such services)
- any occurrence of a risk event will lead to a review of the plan in relation to that risk
- policies and procedures have been followed and due adherence to legal and professional guidance is maintained – such as health and safety law/human rights.

CHAPTER 28

SELF-AWARENESS AND SELF-MANAGEMENT

CAREGIVERS MUST KNOW THEMSELVES

Caregivers are the people who will make or break the success of the plan.

Caregivers are individuals, with their own motivations, personalities and so on.

It is vital that caregivers are aware of any possible conflicts between their own view of the world and that of the individual and/or the proactive plan for the individual.

Specific points to watch for are as follows:

- Be careful to react positively even if behaviours or remedies conflict with your views. Any other response could reinforce the individual's undesired behaviour.
- Constantly monitor your own emotions. You may be having a bad day (it happens) and be like the Coke bottle that's about to explode. Strive to not let the bottle explode because of an individual's actions.
- Be aware of your own attachment style and how that reacts with individuals in care. Do you want to be liked? Do you like to be in control? Do such feelings conflict with the plan for the individual?
- Beware of the risks of meeting your own needs at the expense of the individual's.
- Know your limits, and don't be concerned about calling for help when needed; e.g., in a high-risk situation or where an individual is so distressed that you need help (perhaps from someone more experienced) to defuse the situation.
- Maintain a state of personal growth and development. Don't get stuck in antiquated views and habits just because of previous success, comfort or peer pressure.

BE A GOOD MANAGER

Try this exercise.

- Take a few moments and think of a good boss, manager, senior, supervisor or any authority figure you've had in your life. Write a list of what qualities made them a good manager and why you liked working for them. What attributes, habits or behaviours did they display that you valued?
- Now do the same thing but for a bad boss or other authority figure. Write a list of qualities and habits that you didn't appreciate and what made them a bad boss.

The examples below include a number of key words and phrases gathered on training courses run by the author over the years.

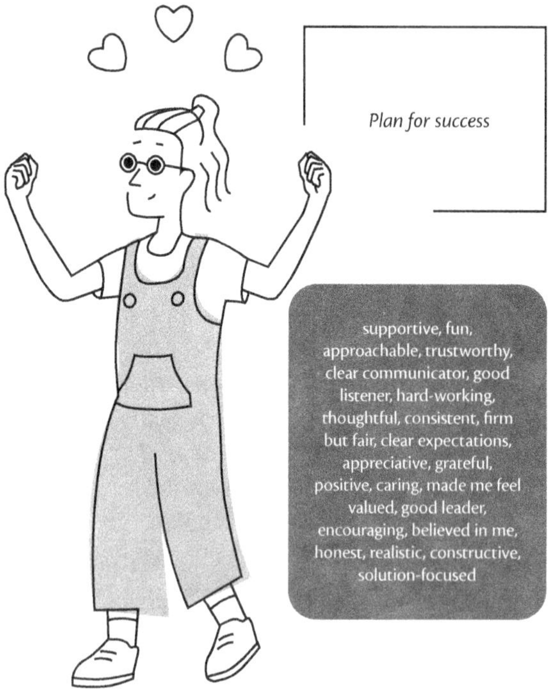
Plan for success
supportive, fun, approachable, trustworthy, clear communicator, good listener, hard-working, thoughtful, consistent, firm but fair, clear expectations, appreciative, grateful, positive, caring, made me feel valued, good leader, encouraging, believed in me, honest, realistic, constructive, solution-focused

Figure 28.1 Characteristics of a Good Boss

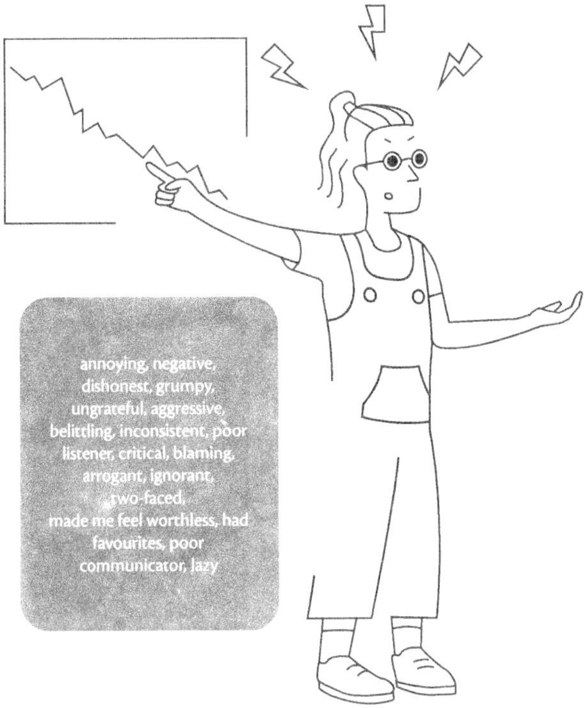
annoying, negative,
dishonest, grumpy,
ungrateful, aggressive,
belittling, inconsistent, poor
listener, critical, blaming,
arrogant, ignorant,
two-faced,
made me feel worthless, had
favourites, poor
communicator, lazy

Figure 28.2 Characteristics of a Bad Boss

We can see the fundamental differences between a good and bad manager.

Which of those two sets of behavioural traits would you prefer to work for, which would you work hardest for and which would develop your respect and trust? The obvious answer is the good manager.

In the above diagrams, if we changed 'boss' to 'caregiver/parent/support worker/teacher/social worker', would the lists of words still apply? Which list would be most likely to develop respect and trust? We could again answer with ease, 'The good.'

CASE STUDY 28.1 CHOOSE YOUR OWN ADVENTURE

You are in a meeting with your colleagues. Your manager comes in and stands over you.

'Right, we need to chat about Monday. I wasn't happy with the work you did; it wasn't to my expectations, and it needs sorting. I know you are having problems at home at the moment but that is no excuse for being lazy.'

Which of these responses should you use?

- **A – Aggressive**: Stand up, get in their face and tell them to shove their job where the sun doesn't shine, as you won't be spoken to like that.

- **B – Passive**: Freeze on the spot, keep your head down for the rest of the day, and then when you get home, snap at your kids, cry to your partner and then never go back.
- **C – Passive/aggressive**: Hold the emotions in, criticise the manager to other colleagues and then purposely be passive aggressive by stating you are too busy to help with an urgent job.
- **D – Assertive**: Have a private chat with the manager. Explain that you apologise if the work you did was substandard in their view. Explain that the way they reprimanded you, however, made you feel embarrassed and humiliated and also breached confidentiality. Ask (as this is not normal behaviour for them) if they are under some stress at the moment and if there is anything you can do to help, although, at the same time, explain that it was not an acceptable way to discuss the issue.
- **E – Avoidant/Assertive**: Raise the incident with HR.

Commentary: Hopefully you chose either D or E, but it will depend on circumstances. The point of the above is that the manager behaved inappropriately and triggered anger, shame and humiliation.

A good management rule is you should 'praise in public but criticise in private'.

However, it is common for caregivers to get caught in bad management traps at times and reprimand, criticise or disclose personal aspects about an individual in front of other individuals in the setting and/or other caregivers. And it's more than likely that many individuals would react with either A, B or C.

Sometimes a manager may have to reprimand in the moment due to a level of safety and urgency – a 'Don't do that!' reaction – but a good manager would afterwards calmly explain, in private, why they had to do that.

Also, even the best manager isn't perfect and may sometimes lose their temper and handle a situation inappropriately. But afterwards, a good manager would then accept their mistake, explain why they were upset and explain the reprimand calmly.

Being willing to recognise a mistake, accept responsibility and make amends demonstrates humility and understanding, and presents a role model of appropriate responses when inevitable mistakes happen.

A good manager is not a good manager because they are perfect; they are good because they aim to improve. It's how we respond to a mistake that's important, rather than the mistake itself.

So, if we are in a position of management, whether managing a setting or managing a person's care, wellbeing, health, education and behaviour, we must:

- be aware of our own triggers
- be present, available and open

- remove the audience where appropriate
- be consistent with responses
- learn from mistakes
- be assertive.

ASSERTION

In 'Case Study 28.1 Choose Your Own Adventure', the five ways to respond to the manager include the four main styles of interaction: aggressive, passive, avoidant and assertive.

An aggressive interaction involves the communicator thinking and acting with only their rights and feelings in mind.

Passive interactions involve the communicator putting the other person first and thinking only of that person's rights and feelings and potentially not meeting their own rights and feelings.

An avoidant style involves avoiding the interaction completely.

Each of these styles can have pros and cons; within certain situations they are not always wrong. Here are some examples:

- If someone is taking advantage of me or it's a matter of safety, it may be appropriate for us to win and get our way despite that meaning that they lose; e.g., a child refusing to wear a seat belt.
- If something matters to the other person more than it does to us, or if we need to let them learn from their own mistakes, it may mean we should let them win; e.g., an individual wants to watch a different film on a cinema visit.
- Avoidant is useful if a situation is risky to us or not important enough to pick a battle.

However, the aim of being assertive during an interaction is to allow a good balance of boundaries and connection, as we have explored through this chapter.

Assertion takes into consideration our rights and feelings and those of the other person.

CASE STUDY 28.2 CHOOSE YOUR OWN ADVENTURE – CONTINUED

In each scenario, choose the response that you feel is most appropriate.

1. You are the teacher of a class. It's the start of the day. George has arrived late to class.
   a. In a raised voice in front of the full class, 'Good afternoon George, what time do you call this? See me after please!'

   b. Don't say anything.
   c. To the full class, 'Can I just remind everyone that class starts at 9am and you are expected to be sitting at your desk at 9am.' Then quietly to George, 'Hey George, I noticed you were late this morning. Can you stay and have a chat with me at the end of class, as I want to check everything is okay?'
2. You are in the car with your partner. They reach across and change the channel on the radio, even though you were listening to the song.
   a. Snarl at them, 'Who made you king of the radio?'
   b. Don't say anything and then, as revenge, make a point of taking your time getting ready later to make them late.
   c. Say, 'When you change the radio without asking me, it makes me feel like you don't consider my feelings. I don't mind you changing the music, but I'd really appreciate being asked.'
3. A person is angry and swearing at you.
   a. 'Don't you swear at me.'
   b. Just ignore them and do what they ask.
   c. State, 'I can see you are upset and I want to help you but I can't help you while you are swearing at me.'

Commentary: In each of the above, option C is assertion. It is being used to manage an interaction in a way that is least likely to trigger escalation. We will explore these skills further in Chapter 32, page 311.

Assertion skills require a rational response rather than an emotional reaction. The next few sections will explore factors that can impact on the ability to stay rational and why we may react in certain ways.

SELF-AWARENESS OF YOUR TRIGGERS

Triggers can come from scripts, core beliefs about ourselves, attachment issues, values, prejudices and beliefs about the world. As described in Chapter 14, the possible causes of emotional/cognitive stressors for individuals are the same for everyone (page 125). Just because we feel something doesn't mean we are right!

Here are some examples to watch out for:

- Needing to be right.
- Needing to please others/be accepted/be liked, which may lead to an erosion of boundaries.
- Needing to be in control, to dictate to others (leads to a power struggle).
- Needing to solve the problem, which can detract from understanding the individual.

- Burnout – the caregiver must first and foremost take care of themselves. This is discussed more later in this chapter.
- Entitlement issues.
- It can be the case that the individual for whom the caregiver has responsibility is getting treats above the level that the caregiver feels is appropriate. This can create a conflict for the caregiver, especially if the individual seems to take the treats for granted.
- Personalising, which means taking things personally and then competing: 'I need to win; you need to lose.' The attitude should not be 'in it to win it', but to promote positive outcomes.
- Tendency to compete (leads to a power struggle).
- Tendency to blame.
- Being thin-skinned in response to criticism.
- Your reputation – you may be concerned that such a relationship could, e.g., undermine the opinion that you're always in control.

SELF-AWARENESS OF EMOTIONAL REACTIONS

We are all human, and at times we can be pushed to and beyond our limits. Our *own* alarm bells may sound.

When that happens, how do we manage our own behaviour within the relationship?

Do we withdraw and just move away and avoid?

Do we go into boundary enforcement, where it's a case of 'I'm not budging' or 'Rules are rules'?

Do we slip into 'consequence overdrive', such as 'Right, that's it – you're not going on the Xbox for the rest of the week'? And does the punishment even fit the crime?

Do we give up on structure completely, going 'Oh, do what you want'?

Do we go into lecture mode?

All of these are emotional reactions rather than rational states.

If we find ourselves caught up in these questions, we should reflect a little and ask ourselves, 'Why did I react like that? What could I have done differently?'

In fact, we should use the 6STM on ourselves!

BARRIERS TO POSITIVE RESPONSES

- **Cultural differences:** One of the participants may perceive the other's behaviour as rude or inappropriate, based on cultural differences (e.g., eye contact, as mentioned in Chapter 4).
- **Poor listening skills:** Often when we are listening there are external

and internal barriers that mean we don't genuinely listen to the other person. This can affect our ability to see things from their point of view.

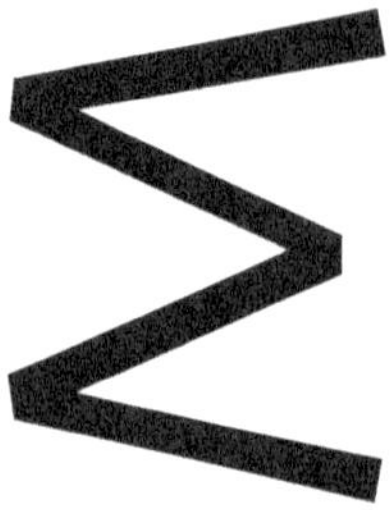

Is the letter above an M or a W? It depends on our point of view.

- **Making assumptions:** We can all be guilty of this. We can make assumptions about a person within milliseconds. We base that on such things as body language, dress, demeanour and so on.
- **Being judgemental or having prejudice.**
- **Being preoccupied or in a hurry.**
- **Emotional reactions:** As discussed in the previous section.
- **Defensiveness:** This can in turn lead to blaming the other person.
- **Blaming.**
- **Our hot buttons:** These can lead to an emotional response.
- **Language differences:** Words and phrases that can easily be misinterpreted or not even understood.
- **Wanting to win.**

Dale Carnegie, in the book *How to Win Friends and Influence People*, says:

> Nine times out of ten, an argument ends with each of the contestants more firmly convinced than ever that he is absolutely right. You can't win an argument. You can't because if you lose it, you lose it; and if you win it, you lose it. Why? Well, suppose you triumph over the other man and shoot his argument full of holes and prove that he is non compos mentis. Then what? You will feel fine. But what about him? You have made him feel inferior. You have hurt his pride. He will resent your triumph. And – A man convinced against his will... Is of the same opinion still.[68]

If our true aim is to develop positive relationships, trust and connection, then our aim should never be to win.

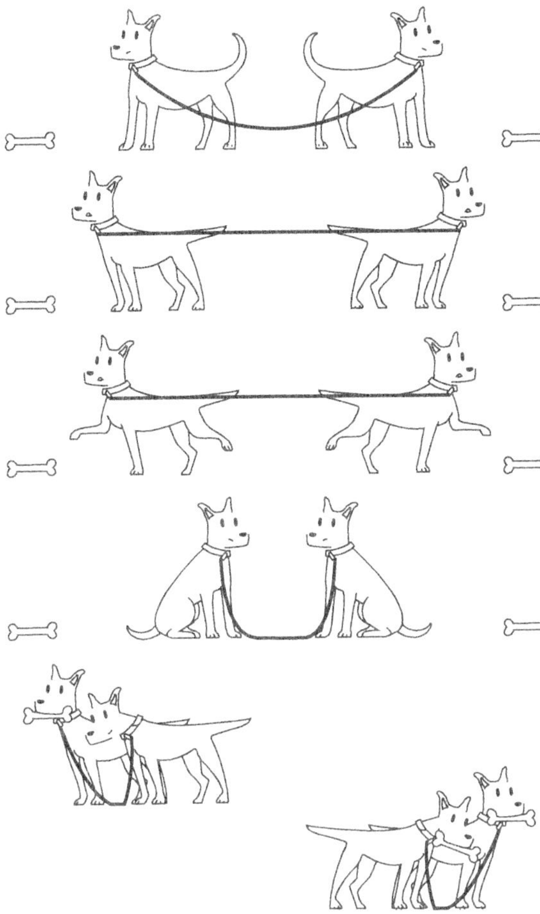

Figure 28.3 Cooperation

SELF-CARE AND RESILIENCE

Working with emotionally dysregulated people causes emotional dysregulation. Working with people who have experienced trauma can cause trauma. A significant indicator of increased likelihood of developing dementia is home-caring for a relative with dementia (not for hereditary reasons but due to high unmanaged stress).

It is absolutely vital that we pay attention to our own wellbeing.

We cannot care for others if we do not care for ourselves.

CASE STUDY 28.3 THE AEROPLANE ANALOGY

When the masks drop down from overhead on an aeroplane due to a drop in cabin air pressure, who should we help first – ourselves or the child next to us?

The answer should always be: 'Us.' Why?

The drop in pressure will reduce the oxygen levels in the cabin (hence the mask supplying oxygen). A reduction in oxygen by just a small amount can reduce the efficiency of your brain function and reduce your ability for fine motor function. If you try to help the child first, the reduced oxygen may limit your ability to successfully get the mask on the child at the same time as your brain is experiencing an ever-decreasing oxygen supply, ultimately resulting in unconsciousness for you and the potential deaths of you and the child.

However, by effectively getting the mask on to your own face, your fully oxygenated brain is more likely to successfully help and save the child.

Commentary: The aeroplane analogy is synonymous with being a caregiver, parent, etc.

To be selfless, we must first be selfish.

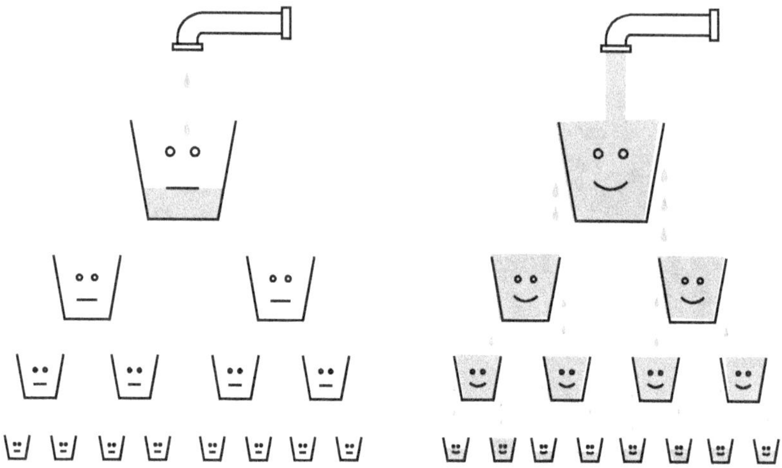

Figure 28.4 The Life Bucket

Gary Vaynerchuk,[69] entrepreneur and author, uses a great analogy for self-care:

> I always return to the concept of a life bucket. You need to fill it with happiness. I think the right way to do it, is just to spend all of your time to fill up that bucket, and then once you're totally full, you can then go on the offense and fill other people's buckets as well. I think most people don't have their bucket full, thus, they're always in the process of trying to fill their bucket as well as everyone else's and they always fall short.
>
> They are never really focused on either and it never works. You can't give unless you have something to give. You need to mix passion with practicality. You need to be selfish in order to be selfless.[70]

The only addition that could be made to this quote is that when you are a caregiver, the ideal is that you fill your bucket enough: to last your shift; to visit; to support. And then you can go for a refill.

CASE STUDY 28.4 I CAN'T COPE WITH MUM

Kate's mum lived alone and had been diagnosed with Alzheimer's. Kate would go down to her mum's every morning and evening and usually popped in at lunch when she could. She supported her mum with her meals, medication, dressing and hygiene, and bedtime routine.

Kate also had regular phone calls from her mum in the early hours of the morning, as Kate's mum would panic about 'the children being missing', a common delusion Kate's mum experienced.

Kate was tired and had just had some bad news. She was not in the mood for her mum's needs today. But as usual, she sucked up the stress.

Kate's mum was sitting in the chair, and Kate asked her what she wanted for lunch. Kate's mum said she had eaten. Kate knew this wasn't true. Unfortunately, although Kate would usually manage to distract her mum and get some food down her, today it escalated into a blazing row between Kate and her mum.

Kate stormed out of the house after ensuring her mum was safe but a nasty atmosphere was left behind.

On the drive home, Kate burst into tears.

Commentary: Kate was left with a feeling of guilt, maybe even shame, as she knew she had upset her mum. It's also not how Kate wanted to remember her mum.

Kate should have organised for someone else to go to see her mum if she was feeling that tired and overwhelmed, but sometimes the guilt placed on us by ourselves or by others doesn't allow us to be selfish to be selfless.

There are several risks attached to poor caregiver self-care:

- **Blocked care**: This is where a caregiver loses all compassion and empathy towards an individual as a defence mechanism to their own stress linked to burnout.
- **Burnout**: A state of emotional, mental and physical exhaustion caused by excessive and prolonged stress.
- **Compassion fatigue**: A condition characterised by a gradual lessening of empathy over time, caused by caring for other people who may not care for themselves.
- **Secondary traumatic stress disorder**: A reaction to taking on clients' trauma by experiencing ongoing stress reactions created by the client. This is similar to PTSD.

- **Becoming abusive or neglectful towards an individual:** This happens when the straw breaks the camel's back.

Yes, from time to time, caregivers will struggle. But caregivers, *and their management*, should be mindful of that happening, be aware of the possibility and prepare for it.

All the coping strategies described for individuals in care are applicable to everyone (see 'Coping Strategies', Chapter 22, page 197).

A selection of self-care and resilience strategies are given below:[71]

- Manage appropriate boundaries.
- Make time for your closest relationships: 'Trusted people that will make you take self-care.'
- Talk with others about what you are going through.
- Really prioritise exercise. (And don't wait for motivation... it's a myth. Motivation begins with action.)
- Follow a healthy diet and good sleep practices.
- Reframe a difficult experience. (It's not that you can't; it's that you find it difficult. You can't yet.)
- Turn stressful situations into learning opportunities.
- Learn from others who are role models of resilience.
- Give yourself a break from media, social media and the news. (Rarely do they contain things that directly affect your life, but the negativity can infect you like a virus.)
- Keep your life simple.
- Practice relaxation techniques.

CASE STUDY 28.5 BUT WHAT DO THE NON-SMOKERS DO?

The staff at a care home were reviewing their stress reduction strategies in line with the Target system.

A comment was made that smokers always got a break and time out, but the non-smokers missed out.

It was decided to introduce mandatory non-smokers' breaks. They had to take a minimum of four five-minute breaks per shift. They were no longer allowed to be martyrs and say, 'It's okay, I'll manage.' The management team made them log their breaks.

The non-smokers commented that they didn't know what to do or where to go in their break.

A plan was created. A square was placed on the wall outside.

4 seconds – **breathe in**
4 seconds – **hold**
4 seconds – **breathe out**
4 seconds – **hold**
Repeat.

Try it now for yourself. Even just one cycle can increase relaxation.

Figure 28.5 Square Breathing

Non-smokers were to go outside and trace their finger on the square five times. Each side should take four seconds to trace.

The non-smokers said they would feel silly, until it was pointed out that the benefit the smokers got from their break was not actually from smoking (once the initial hit of nicotine had rebalanced their nicotine-withdrawal stress). The cigarette was offering no benefit other than... time away from the job and a way to regulate their breathing. Inhale the smoke, hold the smoke, exhale the smoke, hold the breath to allow the next drag. The non-smokers were getting exactly the same benefit, without having to smoke.

- Celebrate successes or even the challenges.

CASE STUDY 28.6 THE REWARD CHART – FOR THE CAREGIVER!

Lisa had behavioural difficulties. Often her parents were at their wits' end. Phrases from their lips were along the lines of the following:

- 'She's done it again.'
- 'Why can't she get it right?'
- 'What are we doing wrong as parents?'

So, a reward chart was set up. When Lisa displayed one of the identified behaviours that challenge, rather than despair, the parents got a star put on *their* reward chart. At the end of the week, stars meant prizes that the parents picked themselves as their treats. When there were sufficient stars, the parents would treat themselves: maybe a long soak in the bath followed by a glass of wine, a night away or a new item of clothing.

Not only did this turn the negative into a positive and the despair into hope, it also helped them to change their reactions to Lisa's behaviour.

Rather than getting upset and angry and shaming Lisa (accidently) they started responding to negative behaviour with nonchalance and minimal reaction, reducing its reinforcement. It also allowed them to focus their big responses on the positive behaviours.

This chapter has further explored our individual responsibilities to manage the setting. The tools and principles referred to in this chapter can be used in all relationships. Even though this section is included in Stage 3: Proactive Planning, it also informs responses and prevention strategies too.

PART 6

THE 6-STAGE TARGET MODEL STAGE 4

Recognise Escalation

CHAPTER 29

THE STAGES OF ESCALATION

In Stage 4 of the 6STM we will explore recognising escalation. When we refer to escalation, we are referring to any state outside a person's baseline state. Thinking back to the window of tolerance described in Chapter 12, page 117, this may be hyperarousal (fight/flight) or hypoarousal (freeze/submit).

Within the context of Stage 4 of the model, caregivers should be recognising signs (what is seen or heard) or symptoms (what is felt) of both baseline states and escalation states:

- of themselves
- of the individuals they know well
- that are typical to human behaviour.

This stage will also describe the process for supporting an individual to recognise their own symptoms of escalation and emotions.

Please take advantage of the bonus chapter 'Dynamic Risk Assessments', which describes how to recognise dynamic risk factors that could impact on appropriate responses. The chapter can be downloaded at https://library.jkp.com/redeem using the code ESGBAKQ.

THE STAGES OF ESCALATION

Behaviour doesn't occur in a vacuum; there are causes and reasons that trigger behaviours. As we explored in the self-test in 'Case Study 14.2: How Angry Do You Get?', the bottle of Coke analogy and the window of tolerance container example, multiple events stack up and can result in crisis. We also explored in Chapter 10 the factors that keep the lid on the bottle, factors that inhibit escalation.

In the bottle of Coke analogy, the idea is that we may not know a bottle has been shaken until we try to open it. This is also true with people.

Sometimes we get no indicators, and the person explodes. However, as this chapter will explore, there are usually 'signs or symptoms' of escalation. We need to learn to recognise those in ourselves and the general population and to recognise any signs that are specific to an individual. We will also explore why sometimes these are missed.

But why is recognition of state important?

CASE STUDY 29.1 WHERE *IS* HE?

Imagine you're waiting for a friend at the cinema. You'd arranged to meet at 7.45pm, the film started at 8pm and it's now 8.05pm.

You may feel frustrated because you haven't heard anything from your friend and you're worried about him. So there are emotions in play:

- There is the concern about your friend's wellbeing.
- Your friend hasn't met expectations and therefore you feel slightly annoyed about that.

But your rational brain says, 'It's okay. I'm sure he's struggling to find somewhere to park, and he hasn't messaged me because he's still driving. I'm sure he'll be here soon.'

So your rational and emotional brain can balance with each other (you are still inside your window of tolerance).

Another ten minutes go by – it's 8.15pm and he's 30 minutes late. The emotional brain starts to take over, where everything becomes much more black and white: 'I'm right, he's wrong.' All the excuses you allowed for in your first stage of frustration are no longer good enough. 'He should have found somewhere to park by now. If he was going to be this late, he should have found some way of letting me know.' At this stage, you feel angry at the situation (anger is indirect).

If your friend then turns up and doesn't offer an apology, you might find this is another trigger to push you further into an aggressive state (aggression is a directed emotion towards person/s, objects or concepts you disagree with, such as a political viewpoint). At this point you might shout, '*Where* have you *been*? I've been worried sick about you.' Or you might hold your emotions in but struggle to engage with your friend or enjoy your film.

You are unlikely to act with violence due to multiple inhibitors and your ability to self-control.

Because the situation and your expectations were not met, you progressed further up the escalation stages. So, at the point of your friend's arrival, even if your friend had offered a valid excuse for their lateness, your ability to empathise, see their point of view and forgive them has been inhibited by your emotional hijacking. It may also take you a while to fully 'calm' down from your heightened state.

The escalation is shown in Figure 29.1.

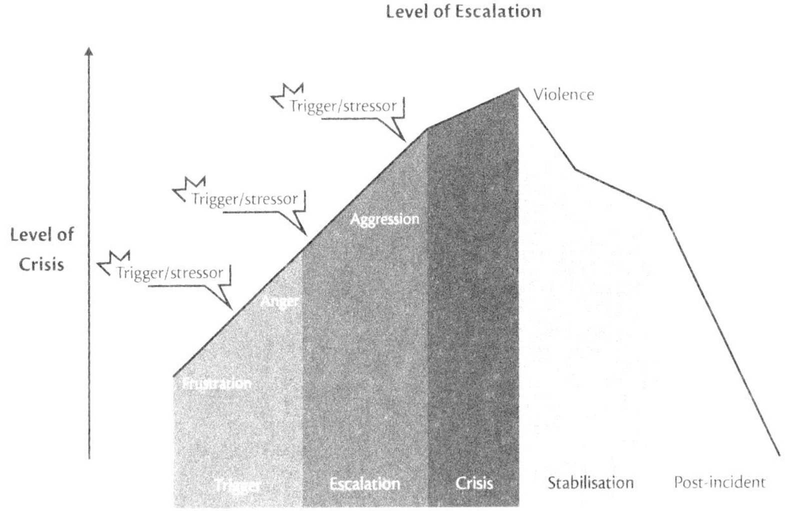

Figure 29.1 Emotional Hijacking Escalation

Commentary: In this example, if your friend had sent you a text message when you were still at the frustrated stage, he'd probably have a better chance of meeting a nicer 'you' when he arrived, even if he didn't turn up until 8.15pm. A small intervention (of information) offered earlier in the escalation cycle may help to manage expectations and prevent further triggering into the higher stages.

The point being: the earlier an intervention occurs (when a person still has some rational control), the better chance we have of meeting a person's needs and preventing escalation.

The escalation model shown above is a simple model to understand the stages of escalation. Let's explore a more detailed model.

THE ESCALATION ROLLER COASTER

The following diagram uses the analogy of a roller coaster to depict the cycle of escalation – from a 'baseline' (normality) state to crisis state and then de-escalating down to baseline. It is helpful if we can identify where an individual may be within that cycle, how much their sympathetic – emotional – nervous system has taken control, as that knowledge will help us to find the appropriate response.

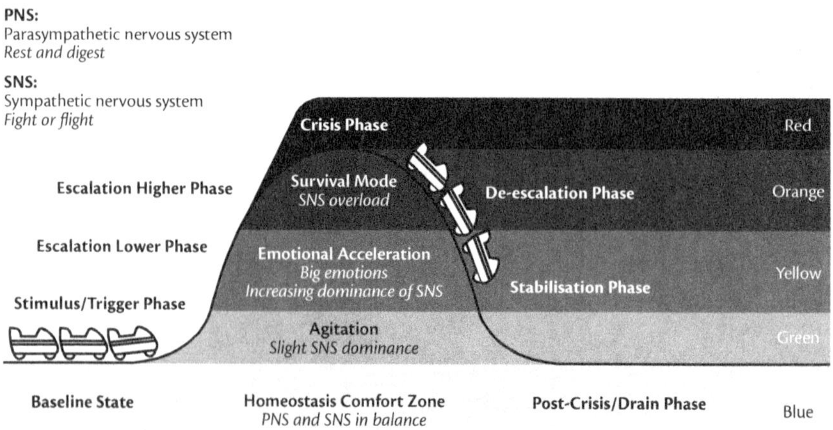

Figure 29.2 The Escalation Roller Coaster

The Diagram Explained

The Colours

BLUE

At the base is the 'blue' zone. This is the baseline state or 'comfort zone'.

The individual is in a state of homeostasis – the rational and emotional brain or the PNS and the SNS are nicely in balance with each other. The individual feels engaged, they have positive relationships, they're feeling safe, content and happy.

The individual is not yet on the roller coaster. (They are inside their window of tolerance.) One of our aims when supporting a person is to maintain this state. This is especially important when someone is in the stabilisation period of trauma/transition recovery.

However, as discussed earlier in the book, there is huge benefit to expanding our window, as it allows us to develop our resilience and develop connections with others more effectively. Also, although comfort zones feel good and safe, they are like balloons – if you are not expanding them, they tend to shrink; and we are like goldfish – the smaller our tank, the less we grow.

CASE STUDY 29.2 MATERNITY LEAVE

Shanti is on maternity leave; she worked for a big cosmetic company in their marketing department. She had been with the company for two years but had only moved to the marketing department seven months prior to going on leave.

Shanti has spent the last ten months with her newborn baby. She only sees a few key people during the week; her only outings have been to the local shop and an occasional trip into town. She has not made it to the gym or the other clubs she used to attend since she found out she was pregnant.

Shanti is supposed to be going back to work next month. She is feeling anxious. She is even thinking of handing in her notice. She just feels she won't fit in anymore. Shanti is aware that there have been some staff and process changes. She feels out of the loop and overwhelmed by the prospect of returning.

Commentary: Shanti's comfort zone has shrunk to such an extent that stepping out of it feels too much. Shanti's company could have managed this return/transition better by allowing her to come in occasionally, keeping her in the loop about personnel and process changes and including her in conversations if she was willing. They could also manage a staged return to work (just like the priming and staged desensitisation in Stage 3: Proactive Planning).

GREEN

This is the click, click, click phase at the beginning of a roller coaster. A stimulus and trigger phase. The individual gets a little shake of the Coke bottle. This is not necessarily a bad place. Managed levels of stress can be extremely positive. If we examine the stress continuum model below,[72] we can see that stress, which triggers our SNS slightly, can actually improve our focus, our reaction speed and our ability to multitask. That is why some people claim to 'work well under pressure'.

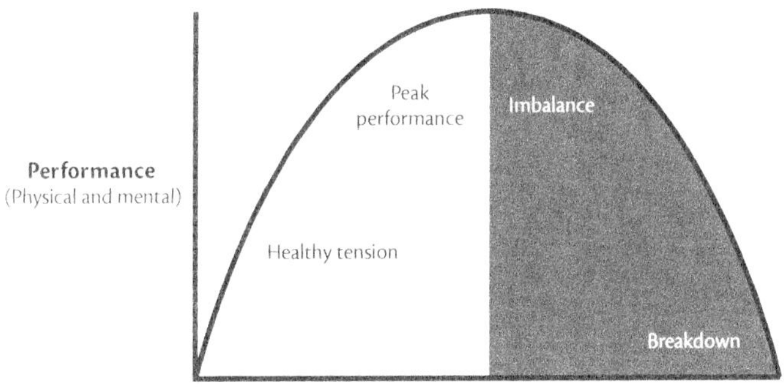

Figure 29.3 The Stress Continuum Model

USED WITH PERMISSION FROM CORNELL HEALTH, 2024

We can experience this effect when starting a new job, going on a first date, expanding our horizons with a new hobby or even learning a new skill – like a child walking along a wall unaided.

So, individuals should be encouraged to enter the green zone – provided they have the support, strategies and resilience to come back down before they enter the yellow to red phase.

If too much stress is stacked on a person, or their usual coping strategies are impaired, unavailable or fail them, or they haven't developed effective coping strategies, they will continue up the roller coaster.

CASE STUDY 29.3 THE LIGHT AT THE END OF THE TUNNEL

The following similes are examples of those given by numerous people who struggle with emotional dysregulation.

> Sometimes it feels like I'm walking down a tunnel. The tunnel is full of my stress, negative feelings, anger, it's overwhelming. The only way to get out of the tunnel is to keep going. There is a light at the end of the tunnel, but to get out, to feel relief, I have to hit someone or hurt myself, to explode in a rage. It's the only way out.

> When I'm struggling with my bad thoughts, the voice in my head tells me I'm useless, ugly, that everyone hates me, that I will always fail. It can feel like I'm drowning. I can't get air into my lungs, it feels like I'm dying. I need to cut like I need to breathe. Cutting myself feels like taking a breath at the surface. It's a release.

Commentary: In both narratives, the individuals don't seem to have alternative strategies to allow themselves to re-regulate, calm down or feel okay; they only recognise a maladaptive way to meet their need and manage their stress. To re-enter their blue zone, as discussed in Stage 3: Proactive Planning, caregivers should work with the individual to develop a plan.

YELLOW

The emotional brain is beginning to take over, and emotions may start to spill out. The person may now struggle to think logically and rationally and can easily be escalated. This is the same as the 'angry' phase in 'Case Study 29.1 Where *Is* He?', and they may still be able to maintain control, depending on their resilience.

ORANGE, RED

The individual experiences levels of stress beyond their abilities to inhibit; the usual healthy coping mechanisms are failing, and the emotional brain starts to take over. Put simply: the SNS (the emotional system) begins to take control.

The click, click, click ratchets on and on until the crisis phase is reached. The individual is now very high up on the roller coaster; fight/flight is now in control. Aggression, violence and emotional crisis follow.

The individual has left their window of tolerance.

After the crisis phase, there is usually a natural de-escalation. The emotional charge that has built up to reach the crisis point is released, and the person often begins to calm naturally. And so the roller coaster descends, but the individual can easily be retriggered, as they are still in a heightened emotional state.

Once stability – the blue zone – has been regained, the individual may feel very tired or distressed. Often, once the rational brain has re-engaged, they may reflect and feel they've messed things up, or they may become worried about the consequences.

Everybody's Roller Coaster is Different

The diagram below shows a number of different examples of roller coasters.

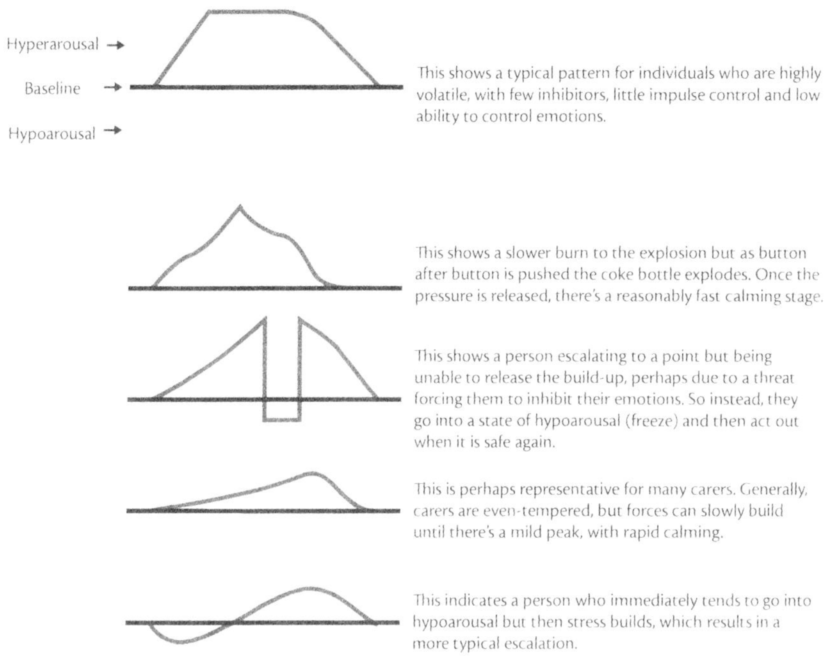

Figure 29.4 Different Roller Coasters

The flat horizontal line represents the baseline.

It's quite possible that the shape of the escalation line varies according to circumstances. A person's home life may have fewer inhibitors because their partner loves them unconditionally and may forgive and empathise with their mood. A person may be more controlled at work because there's a greater chance of consequences. Inhibitors are often internal as well as external. As explored in Chapter 10, consequences change depending on who is involved, and when and where the event occurs. All of these can change the ebb and flow of escalation.

CASE STUDY 29.4 JOHN'S ESCALATION

Stage A: John, who usually goes into town on a Thursday, is told that because the home is short-staffed, they will not be able to take him into town but will try

to find someone to take him later. John argues with the staff member but ends up walking out before anything is resolved, and he takes himself off to his room.
Stage B: John comes out of his room and goes to the lounge, where other individuals are involved in an activity. The staff member involved is busy with these people, so John stands for a moment, staring at the staff member, and after a few huffs and puffs leaves the room and heads to the Senior's office door.
Stage C: Outside the office, John barges past Jim, another individual, and bangs on the door. Staff member Jane is inside on the phone; she doesn't turn around on hearing the bang. John bangs again. Jane continues with the phone call. John kicks at the door and shouts through it at Jane. Jane activates her alarm and other staff come running. Jane comes to the door and opens it saying, 'John, calm down. I am not going to talk to you until you have calmed down.' John begins to speak, but Jim says, 'I was here first, wait your bloody turn.' John pushes Jim, who falls over. Staff grab John and there is a struggle.
Stage D: John is physically supported to his room. Staff ask him to calm down, as they cannot understand what he is saying because he is so aroused. PRN medication is offered, but he refuses. Eventually he can talk to Sylvia, a staff member he trusts, who says she will do her best to arrange to get him to town tomorrow if not today.
Stage E: Sylvia comes to John's room, where he is calming. They have managed to arrange a staff member to take him into town this afternoon. Sylvia tells him Jim is annoyed but unhurt. She suggests they talk to Jim when both he and John are ready. Sylvia asks John if he would like his music on. John says yes, and then she gives John some time to calm alone.

You might like to think about the following questions for a moment:

- When should de-escalation have been used?
- What should have been done and said differently by the staff in this incident at each stage?
- What was done to promote de-escalation?

Commentary: De-escalation should have occurred as early as possible for John. Someone could have checked on him. In B, John is in the green and yet is ignored. In C, John goes into crisis before de-escalation begins.

It is quite imaginable that in discussions with Jane later on, she might report: 'John kicked off for no reason!'

John's bottle of Coke had been shaken numerous times, and despite the warning signs, no one responded appropriately, leading to the staff reacting to John's behaviour. John's escalation cycle is most like the second example in the different roller coaster images.

CASE STUDY 29.5 JOHN'S ESCALATION USING THE TARGET SYSTEM AND THE 6STM

Prevention of incident: Effective staffing levels to meet client needs and contingency plans for staff absence; staff training in the Target system; positive values and proactive mentality from staff.
Proactive management: Knowledge of John.

Identify Behaviour

Agitation from John (we know from past incidents that John gets upset when his routine is changed).

Understand/Empathise

John finds change stressful, and he struggles with disappointment. He looks forward to going into town. John prefers to know what he is doing and when.

John likes staff members Sylvia and Toby.

John likes going into town, watching sci-fi films and listening to music.

Proactive Plan

If a change in John's routine is occurring, he should be given as much warning as possible; he should be presented with a clear alternative of when he will be going into town. He should also be supported emotionally and given alternative things he can do in the interim.

Response Plan

John is rarely aggressive, but if something has upset him, saying 'I'm sorry' and showing understanding works well for John at all stages of escalation. John needs connection when upset and will actively seek it.

Recognise Escalation and Recommended Responses

Blue: John is talkative and friendly; he has good eye contact and clear communication.
Green: John doesn't like confrontation and will often walk away from you when he is upset. He then tends to get more upset and will come out looking for help or attention. He responds well when calmly offered it.
Orange: John will often go to tell management when he is angry, and he can be aggressive at this point with banging and shouting. Prompting John into a quiet space and listening to his complaints settles John well. Then redirect him to a preferred activity.
Red: We have not witnessed John in crisis.

Commentary: If changing John's routine is a known trigger for John, then staff should create a proactive plan before they tell him and not wait till the horse has bolted. Even if the strategy they use fails, there should be a plan.

Let's refer back to the fire analogy in 'Case Study 2.1 Similarity to Fire', page 22.

If you identify an activity that you know carries a risk of starting a fire, you don't wait for the fire to start before you act. You plan.

- You ensure you take precautions before you start the task.
- You try to make the area safe before you begin the task.
- You perform the task in the safest way possible.
- If, despite the planning, a fire starts, you try to put it out immediately – you don't let it spread before you act.
- You also follow appropriate procedures and plans to ensure you and others are safe in the event of a fire.

CHAPTER 30

SIGNS OF ESCALATION

In John's escalation example ('Case Study 29.4 John's Escalation' in the preceding chapter), we (in hindsight) can see the warning signs from John as a sequence of escalation, but Jane didn't see the build-up. The 6STM version of the event may have allowed Jane to be aware that John coming to the office is a red flag. However, there are still factors that can impair this awareness beyond knowledge.

Can you find the
the mistake in here?

A B C D E F G H I J
K L M N O P Q R S T
U V W X Y Z

Figure 30.1 Can You Find the Mistake? (1)

If you haven't seen the picture above before, it may have taken you a couple of moments to spot the mistake. You may have started by reading the alphabet to see if anything was out of order or missing. But did you spot the second 'the' in 'Can you find the the mistake in here?'? This simple example can be related to real life. What we perceive and pay attention to are not the same. Sometimes we focus on one thing, like a particular person or task, and then we miss other information within the environment.

It's easy to focus on the job we're doing and forget what else is going on around us.

Can you find the mitsake in here?

1111 2222 3333 4444 5555
6666 7777 8888 9999

Figure 30.2 Can You Find the Mistake? (2)

In this second example, it is likely you found the error immediately, as you now know what to look for. Knowing what to look for allows us to better notice. So if we are pre-informed of an individual's signs of escalation, we are more likely to notice them.

CASE STUDY 30.1 THE CONSULTANT

A school has hired Kiara as a consultant to help support Daniel, a child who has behavioural issues. The teacher who has Daniel in her class has said that he is really changeable in his moods, that he seems to start disrupting the class and behaving badly at random and that his mood shifts are sudden.

Kiara sits at the back of one of the classes to monitor Daniel.

About 20 minutes into the class, Kiara notices that Daniel's behaviour has changed. The teacher doesn't seem to have noticed, but Daniel has dropped his pencil on the floor three or four times. He is looking around the class more and fidgeting. Daniel gets up and goes over to the bookshelf and gets a book, then returns to his seat. He gets up again and takes it back. He starts to slightly pester the child sitting next to him. This continues for a while with no recognition from the teacher, who is busy teaching and supporting other students. Fifteen minutes go by, and Daniel is now running around the class knocking books off tables and going up to the front of the class and taking the marker pens that the teacher is using... now the teacher notices.

A proactive plan will include ensuring that information on how to recognise escalation is in an individual's care plan; this can be taken from incident reports, interactions and monitoring of an individual.

Table 30.1 Daniel's Signs of Escalation

State	Signs for Daniel
Blue – baseline	Daniel can sit and engage in learning. He can be quiet and attentive.
Green – trigger	Daniel will begin to fidget and tends to drop and pick up things from the floor
Yellow	Daniel will tend to find reasons to stand and move around.
Orange	Daniel will begin to pester other children.
Red	Daniel will become disruptive; he will be unable to sit still and will try to get the teacher's attention.

This information would ideally be paired with guidance on how to respond appropriately for each stage of escalation; this will be explored in the next section.

PRE-COMMUNICATION

In Stage 3: Proactive Planning, we also referred to pre-communicators – specific signs that a person may give leading up to a behaviour. It is useful for staff to have access to a communication chart, especially for individuals who do not have typical communication abilities.

Here is an example of a simple communication chart.

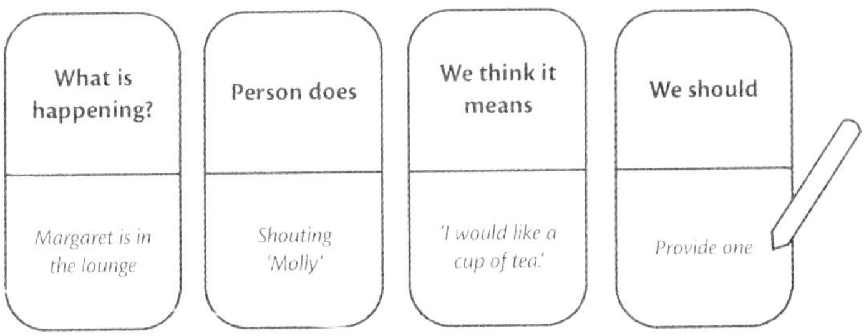

Figure 30.3 Simple Communication Chart

Examples

When Margaret is in the lounge and starts shouting 'Molly', we think it means 'I would like a cup of tea' and we should provide one.

When James stands up and repeats the phrase 'Get your coat' with increasing pace, we think it means he wants to go to the shop. We should show him his schedule, so he knows when he is going to the shop next.

GENERAL SIGNS OF ESCALATION

There are also general indicators of escalation that apply to the majority of people as they move towards aggression and violence, specifically.

Some signs are general signs of arousal caused by increased adrenaline and fight-or-flight mechanisms being activated. These can be seen in any individual who is experiencing stress or frustration.

Other signs indicate anger, moving to aggression. They include evidence of the individual using strategies to intimidate or evidence of an internal struggle to self-regulate or control reflex behaviour.

Green to Yellow Signs

- Change in mood and level of anxiety
- Pacing, movement (toward you or away); restlessness, fidgeting, stimming
- Changes in what they are saying, tone, pace and volume
- Changes in baseline behaviours (e.g., are they frowning when normally they're content?)
- Changes in communication – increase or decrease in words
- Eyes – watchful, scanning, assessing
- Concentration problems
- Disorganised behaviours – trying to distract themselves
- Gestures – jerky/uncontrolled
- Attempting to use learned self-calming techniques – humming, singing, biting nails – but they're not working
- They tell you that they are getting angry, upset

Yellow to Orange Signs[73]

- Huffing and puffing
- Facial indicators – staring, frowning, rubbing forehead, reddened complexion
- Posturing – facing up to another, a show of strength
- Raised voice
- Aggressive body language/actions – pointing, clenched fists, hitting things, throwing objects down in frustration
- Words expressing threats – including swearing
- Argumentative and belligerent – won't follow requests
- The acronym STAMP can be used to describe some behaviours exhibited by a person who is moving into bigger emotions:

S – Staring: Prolonged glaring at people
T – Tone: Sharp, sarcastic, loud, argumentative
A – Anxiety: Flushed face, heavy breathing, rapid speech, reaction to pain
M – Muttering: Talking under breath, criticising people to self or others, mimicking others
P – Pacing: Walking around in a confined space, walking into areas that are off limits

Orange to Red Signs[74]

Here is a list of things to watch for that could closely precede an attack:

Face

- Pale, flushed, lips tighten over teeth
- Eyebrows drop to cover/protect eyes
- Break stare, then look at intended target
- Chin drops to protect neck

General

- Breathing rapid and deep
- Clenched fists
- Stance goes from square to bladed
- Body movement may stop, or rocking from heel to toe
- Lowering of entire body to lunge

These are all potential signs of escalation. Let's just review or describe some indicators of hypoarousal:

- Silence
- Staring into space
- No response
- Low energy, lethargy
- Can't say no
- Difficulty concentrating
- Decreased reactions
- No emotions

There are also longer-term indicators that someone is struggling emotionally and escalating; these are more typical signs of chronic rather than acute stress:

- Aches and pains
- Chest pain or a feeling that their heart is racing
- Loss of appetite or excess eating
- Exhaustion or trouble sleeping
- Headaches, dizziness or shaking
- Poor concentration, memory challenges
- Loss of enjoyment in things previously enjoyed
- Muscle tension or jaw clenching
- Stomach or digestive problems
- They report an increase in negative thoughts or hallucinations/delusions
- Self-reporting

The list of indicators is non-exhaustive. It is important to remember that some individuals will have specific indicators that do not follow this list.

CASE STUDY 30.2 PAYING ATTENTION

Joan, a new care worker at a mental health unit, was working in the communal area and meeting some of the individuals while under the supervision of an experienced staff member.

Joan noticed a man enter the room, look at her and then leave the room. He had done this three times so far. The fourth time he entered the room, he walked past everyone, stood by the TV and just started staring at Joan. Joan noticed and mentioned it to the supervising staff.

The staff informed her, 'That is Arjan. He struggles with new people and will take some time to get used to you. He's lovely once you get to know him but don't engage with him yet. He will need to see you here a few times to accept you. He loves colouring so we will help you to build a relationship with him by doing some with him in a few days.

'He is okay at the moment; he's just watching. But if he stares and starts grinning at you, that can mean he is going to hit out. So keep your distance a little for now and make sure you are not blocking his way out – if he can just leave the room, he tends to, rather than hit.

'I will stay with you until he's settled, but that's why you did the breakaway training in induction. Okay?'

Commentary: Because Joan is new, she is naturally situation aware and spotted Arjan. Awareness is an important tool in behaviour management.

SITUATION EVALUATION

The following diagram shows various stages of awareness.

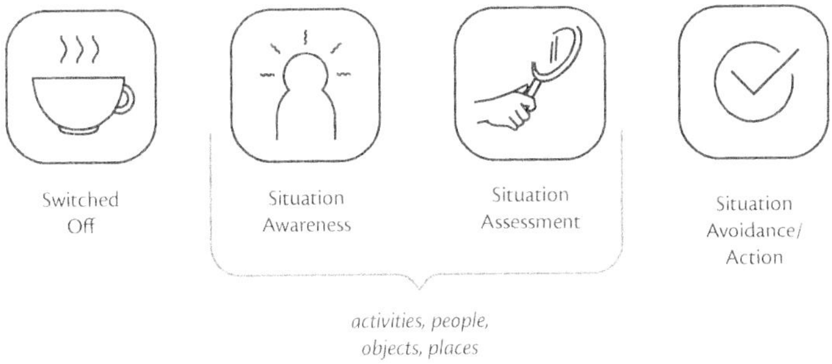

Figure 30.4 The Awareness System

Most people are generally 'switched off' from the situation, thinking of the next cup of tea, jobs they must do and so on. This is a common state when we are in our comfort zone; it is comfortable and familiar. It is easy to become complacent. We often actively seek this state despite the environment or situation we are in, especially as we become habituated to it.

In this state it is highly likely that we will miss escalation signals.

A situation-awareness state allows us to better notice escalation, evaluate the risks and then act or avoid as appropriate.

CASE STUDY 30.3 HIGHWAY HYPNOSIS

Have you ever driven home from work and then realised you couldn't really remember the journey? You were on autopilot.

People are most likely to get a speeding ticket from a speed camera they knew was there within a 25-mile radius of their own home.

This is a switched-off state. You are more likely to have an accident in this state.

Good drivers stay in a situation-awareness state, as the best drivers don't rely on themselves being a good driver or not; they work on the assumption that everything else is unpredictable.

If they were driving down a road and there were children playing with a ball at the side of the road...

- a switched-off driver wouldn't notice the kids
- a paranoid driver would slam on the brakes and panic about the children running out (this is not a state we want)
- a situation-awareness driver would notice the children and assess; e.g., 'What if they run out? Could I stop? Can I safely swerve out of the way? Should I slow down?'

CHAPTER 31

INTROSPECTION

We will explore possible responses in Stage 5: Respond Appropriately, but having an informed approach that includes dynamic as well as planned assessment can increase safety for everyone.

SELF-MONITORING: BE AWARE OF OUR OWN STATE

We are human; it can be easy to forget this. In Chapter 28, page 267, we explored potential personal triggers and the importance of self-awareness, self-management and self-care. It is important that we are aware of the symptoms of escalation, as that is the sensation we will experience when we are stressed or emotional. There could be things in the HELP acronym that are shaking up your bottle of Coke. If you are then going into a situation where another person may be distressed, the human stressor can be significant. Thinking back to our explanation of amygdala hijacking in Chapter 11 (page 105), if something causes that alarm bell to go off loudly enough, the rational brain will be overruled, no matter how good our inhibitors.

Watch for your own warning symptoms, which might include the following:

- Increased heart rate
- Dry mouth
- Legs like jelly
- Freezing
- Shiver down spine
- Muscular tension
- Nausea
- Speechlessness, struggling to find the words
- Needing the toilet
- Increased body temperature
- Sweaty palms

Although the symptoms cannot be seen, we often make the incorrect assumption that people can 'smell your fear'. But you can't see a knotted stomach.

You may feel the next few examples, but they may also be recognised by others:

- Shaking
- Flushed face
- Increase in volume and intonation of speech
- Nervous laughter
- Clenched fists

If these are noticed by others, they may draw conclusions, possibly incorrectly. A flushed face can indicate being frightened or being aggressive. We can't control our face going red, but we can use techniques to hide some visible signs.

If we become aware of such symptoms, what can we do?

Duck Syndrome

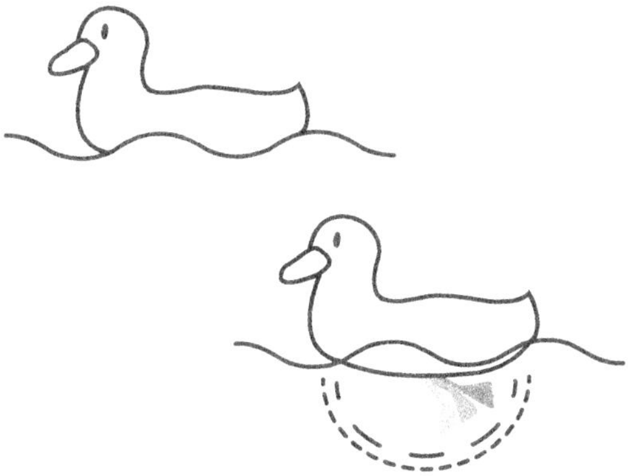

Figure 31.1 What's Happening Under the Surface?

Somehow a duck always seems serene and calm, even though under the water its legs might be paddling frantically.

And we all know the expression, 'Like water off a duck's back.'

To retain that cool demeanour, to maintain our self-control, to project an image of calm, to keep our rational brain in control – here are a few tips:

- Control your breathing. Consciously slow it down.
- Relax your muscles. Consciously think about relaxing your shoulders.
- Think positive thoughts, maybe even recite a mantra internally, such as: 'I can handle it, I can handle it.' Even if an individual becomes aggressive, 'I can handle it.' If they cut themselves, 'I can handle it.'
- Stay in the present. Don't think, 'What if this happens and then that happens...?' or 'Last time this happened and then that happened...' Pay

attention to current feelings. Try to find one sensory input to label – the feel of the floor on your feet, the colour of that door. Focus on the individual's body language and be curious.

- If all else fails, and it's appropriate and possible to do so safely, withdraw and take some time to regain composure.

INDIVIDUAL'S INTROSPECTION

Part of Stage 3: Proactive Planning included reference to introspection work. This is done by helping an individual to recognise their own feelings, mood and escalation and working with them to explore what they could do, and what we may be able to do, to help them re-regulate. A form based on the following example could be a useful tool to use with them. This regulation scale was created as a resource by the Government of South Australia Department for Education.[75]

Table 31.1 Sample Mood Monitoring Form

Regulation zone		Why do I feel like this?	What signals am I getting from my body (interoception)?	What can I (or someone else) do to help?
Red: Panic Zone	Red: SNS overload			
	Orange: SNS dominant			
Green: Learning Zone	Green: Slight SNS dominance			
Homeostasis: Emotional and physiological balance				
Blue: Comfort Zone	Blue: PNS dominant			

The principle is for the individual to become more aware of their emotions by connecting emotions with feedback they are getting from their bodies. As mentioned in other areas of the book, mood monitoring is an ongoing process that both the caregiver and the individual will continually work on. It will be informed over time by incidents, emotional awareness and reflection work.

By better understanding and monitoring their emotions, individuals can become aware of changes in feelings that could lead to unhelpful behaviours. They can also begin to adjust self-strategies to better manage their emotions. This requires learning.

CASE STUDY 31.1 POTTY TRAINING

When potty training a young child, first we need to get the timing right. There is no point in trying to teach a child how to use a toilet before: 1) they can recognise the feelings in their own body; 2) they have the communication skills to follow instructions; or 3) they have the physical skills to undress and use the toilet/potty. Signs that the time is right can vary from child to child, but some basic indicators may include the following:

- You're changing fewer wet nappies.
- Your child's bowel movements are more predictable.
- They broadcast bodily functions.
- They dislike dirty nappies.
- They can perform simple undressing.
- They understand bathroom language.

Not all of these are needed; most are useful. However, the child being willing to participate and motivated to try will allow much quicker success. It is nice to get them involved and let them say goodbye to nappies for the last time.

To start with, the child may not recognise 100% when they need the toilet. So, to begin with, the parent must monitor and notice the signs. If the child starts jiggling, we direct them to the toilet and then reward their success. Some kids respond to praise, others to stickers (it's always best to find their favourite motivator to reinforce the success).

We may also set a routine – perhaps every 20 minutes we may encourage the child to try. This increases the opportunities to reinforce a success. We could even include good handwashing as part of the routine to promote multiple good habits.

CASE STUDY 31.2 EMOTIONAL TRAINING

When emotionally training, first we need to get the timing right. There is no point in trying to teach a person how to emotionally regulate before: 1) they can recognise the feelings in their own body; 2) they have the communication skills to follow instructions; or 3) they have the physical abilities to take alternative actions. Signs that the time is right can vary from person to person, but some basic indicators may include the following:

- We are experiencing fewer episodes of the behaviour.
- The behaviours are more predictable.
- They may communicate some feelings.
- They dislike the consequences.

- They can perform alternative strategies.
- They understand emotional language.

Not all of these are needed; most are useful. However, the person being willing to participate and motivated to try will allow much quicker success. It is nice to get them involved and let them say goodbye to their inner demons.

To start with, the person may not recognise 100% when they are experiencing emotions. So, to begin with, the caregiver must monitor and notice the signs. If the individual starts fidgeting, getting louder, repeating questions (or whatever their signs may be), we encourage them to choose a calming activity or an incompatible pleasurable activity (that they have chosen or we recognise for them) and then reward their success. Some people respond to praise, others to tangibles (it's always best to find their favourite motivator to reinforce the success).

We may also create a schedule of calming or pleasurable activities for the person to do on a set routine throughout the day. This increases opportunities to reinforce a success and helps to lower stress. We could even include other positive behaviours, like exercise, as part of the routine to promote multiple good habits.

CASE STUDY 31.3 BEHAVIOUR THAT CHALLENGES... MALADAPTIVE OR NOT? (PAGE 20) – REVISITED

Scene-setting: This revisits the case study about Liam. Some time has passed, and Liam's caregivers decide that he is ready for a different approach.

Liam loved to jump. When he went to bed he would jump on his bed. His foster parents bought him a trampoline for outside and one for his room too.

Liam struggled with sensory overload and would often have meltdowns when he couldn't cope with too much stimulation.

His foster parents noticed Liam would do a little jumpy movement and stimming behaviour for a while before meltdowns.

They spoke to Liam and asked him how he had felt just before a particular meltdown had occurred.

'I feel sick' was his reply.

It was explained that this was anxiety, and he was asked if his little jumps and movements helped.

'Sometimes' was his response.

It was agreed with Liam that when he felt that way he should go to his room or trampoline and jump for ten minutes. His foster parents would help him.

Initially, the parents would spot Liam's stimming and redirect him. Over the course of a year, Liam would do it himself. His 30-minute meltdowns sometimes became just a two-minute jumping session.

Commentary: The above case studies are similar in essence and are designed to show the use of common-sense approaches to manage our expectations of what should and shouldn't be a known skill (like emotional intelligence) and to use our recognition skills to aid teaching and improve outcomes.

The Mood Monitoring Form breaks the plan into different symptoms and responses to the different levels of escalation. The foot of the form is the homeostasis area – for recording feelings when the individual feels comfortable, content and warm; this is where the PNS (the rational brain) is in control.

Moving up the form, there is the stressor/trigger phase, where the SNS is starting to activate. This is the 'Learning Zone', where the individual has some abilities to make choices about what they do next. As the SNS takes over, those choices disappear; the emotional brain is hijacking the rational brain and crisis is coming.

For each level, the individual can record the following.

- 'Why do I feel like this?'
  E.g., 'There's too much noise, nobody's listening to me.'
- 'What signals am I getting from my body?' (This is known as 'interoception'.)
  E.g., 'My heart is pounding, I feel queasy, my shoulders feel tight, I can't concentrate, I feel hot,' and so on. This could include such apparently minor sensations as: 'There's a label in my shirt that's irritating my back.'
- 'What can I (or someone else) do to help?'
  E.g., 'Speak calmly to me; take me to my room so I can listen to music; give me a sensory toy to play with.' This is where caregivers can work with the individual to identify possible strategies. Then, if that stage is reached again, the individual has some control – they have contributed to the options and can be given the chance to choose the preferred strategy at that time.

The idea is for the individual to learn ways of getting off the roller coaster – to recognise the signals that 'something is going to happen soon unless I do something to avoid it'.

The following is an example of how a completed form might look:

Table 31.2 Sample De-escalation Form for an Individual

Regulation zone	Why do I feel like this?	What signals am I getting from my body (interoception)?	What can I (or someone else) do to help?	Regulation zone
Red: Panic Zone	Red: SNS overload	I'm in crisis, I'm scared, so shout and hit to feel safe.	I feel like someone else and so can't focus.	I need you to give me space, but don't be angry.
	Orange: SNS dominant	I'm getting overwhelmed and scared.	I feel hot and can't focus.	Prompt me to my calm space.
Green: Learning Zone	Green: Slight SNS dominance	I'm getting anxious as I feel unsafe.	I feel sick in my stomach and I feel hot.	Calm breathing.
Homeostasis: Emotional and physiological balance				
Blue: Comfort Zone	PNS dominant	I'm happy and content. I like the people around me.	I feel calm. I'm aware of the world around me and I can listen.	Talk calmly to me, be friendly and don't rush me.

Metaphors

Metaphors can be a useful way to explain feelings to some individuals. Examples include 'the bottle of Coke' and 'the marbles in a container' that have been used within this book.

CASE STUDY 31.4 USING THE ROLLER COASTER

Roger was doing some introspection work with Bradley in post-incident reflection after Bradley had assaulted one of the other children in the home. Roger used the roller coaster metaphor.

'Bradley, I want you to imagine your emotions are like a roller coaster. You know at the beginning of a roller coaster, you often have that bit that goes... click... click... click as you start going up to the first big drop? Well, I want you to imagine that all the things that upset you, that wind you up, are like another click on the roller coaster pushing you closer and closer to the big drop. And when you reach the top, that's it – all your feelings and anger come flying out, and yesterday that resulted in you hitting Anthony. Unfortunately, that meant it wasn't safe to go to football as we were supposed to. I'm so sorry you missed out, so I was wondering if we could work together to look at other things you might be able to do when you are getting wound up.

'Cause Bradley, when you're at the top of the roller coaster, I understand you had nothing else you could do. But when you're at the bottom of the roller coaster you can get off.

'Can you remember yesterday when you had just started feeling like you were on the roller coaster? How did you feel?

'So rather than keep going up the track, what do you think we could do instead?'

Roger and Bradley end up creating a plan of three things that Bradley could do when he is feeling agitated. This was shared with other staff at the home and Bradley was prompted to use one of these if any staff recognised he was getting agitated. Bradley received reinforcement for choosing these options.

In Stage 6: Learn from Incident, we will look at 'mood monitoring' as part of reflective practice that can be used to help an individual look at how they were feeling at the different stages of their escalation and, from that, how work can be done to build their own self-awareness and self-management.

PART 7

THE 6-STAGE TARGET MODEL STAGE 5

Respond Appropriately

CHAPTER 32

RESPOND APPROPRIATELY

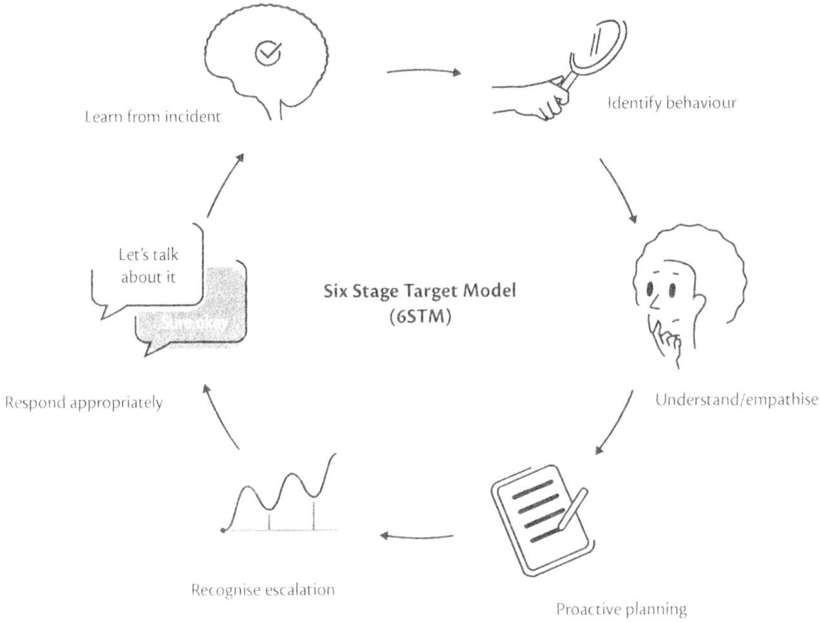

Figure 32.1 Six Stage Target Model

So far in this book, we have covered:

- how to identify both positive behaviours and behaviours that challenge that are maladaptive
- understanding why a person may be using a maladaptive behaviour
- creating a plan to develop positive skills, promote positive behaviour and reduce escalation
- methods to recognise escalation in ourselves and others.

In Stage 5: Respond Appropriately, we will explore appropriate responses and positive engagement.

Stage 5 will be split into three sections.

The first (Chapters 32–34) will look at general principles of positive engagement and de-escalation to develop understanding, and techniques to better interact or calm situations.

The second (Chapters 35–37) will look at the specific process of responding to an unexpected event of agitation, anxiety or aggression and how to use all the skills explored so far to bring about successful de-escalation.

The final section (Chapter 38) will focus on responding appropriately to individuals based on pre-planned behavioural management strategies for behaviours that challenge.

POSITIVE ENGAGEMENT

In Chapter 22, page 193, we explored the importance of positive relationships and development of trust to be able to better support a person with learning new skills and developing more beneficial behaviours. We also discussed, in Chapter 2 about prevention, the importance of having a positive attitude and culture to reduce the risks of behaviours that challenge from occurring (page 22).

THE ATTITUDE AND BEHAVIOUR CYCLE

We have already seen this diagram in Chapter 3 (page 27), but it's worth repeating here.

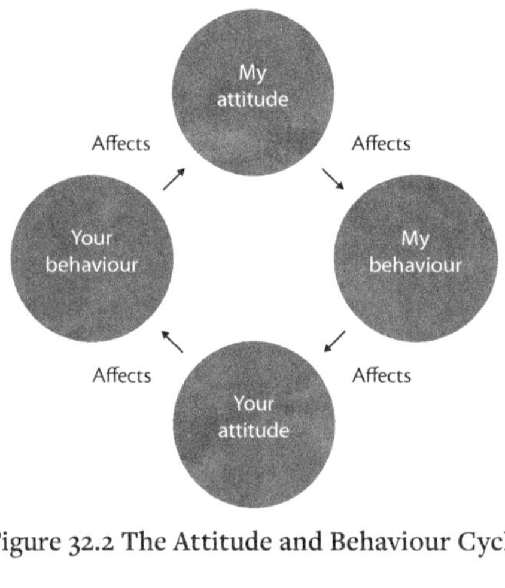

Figure 32.2 The Attitude and Behaviour Cycle

The diagram puts in a nutshell how human interactions can spiral. The spiral can twist in a negative or positive direction. The importance is the connection between how *our* attitude (made up of our thoughts and feelings) affects *our* behaviour. And then, how our behaviour affects the attitude (thoughts and feelings) of others.

It must primarily be the responsibility of the caregivers to be aware of their attitudes and how they are affecting their behaviours.

As caregivers, our prime responsibility is to be aware of our attitudes and how they affect our behaviour. We must ensure that the spiral twists in a positive direction.

CASE STUDY 32.1 THE GAS BILL

Brian is an unemployed man who lost his job due to starting to drink. He became an alcoholic after his wife passed away and has struggled to get work since. He has two children, and both are now teenagers; he worries that he can't give them what they deserve. Brian is calling a gas company, as he thinks he is being overcharged for his gas. He is very short on money at the moment and was hoping he was due a rebate on his gas, as that is what happened at a similar time last year. Brian has just spent 15 minutes trying to get through to talk to a person.

Sharon has worked in the customer services department at the gas company for the last five years. She is coming to the end of her shift, she is tired and her back is starting to hurt. Sharon has had to deal with so many customers who think the gas company owes them something and complain when their bills come in, who are surprised that prices go up... like they do every year. Sharon takes her last call of the day from Brian.

Sharon: Good evening, Sharon speaking. How can I help?

Brian: Finally, it's taken me ages to get through to anyone; your system is s**t. I just need to talk to someone about my bill. You lot are trying to rob me and I can't afford it.

Sharon: You need to speak to the accounts department about that sir; they are in at 9am tomorrow.

Brian: I'm not calling back again and waiting in that f***ing queue system. Put me through to your manager.

Sharon: Sir, if you continue to swear at me, I am going to have to terminate the call. It's not my fault that you're not happy with your bill.

Brian: Don't you dare hang up on me, it's your f***ing company's fault and you think we little people don't matter. You're all stuck up little...

Sharon hangs up the phone. She turns to her colleague and says, 'Why do I always get the angry wasters who think we can just magic up money for them, right at the end of my shifts?'

Commentary: In the above example, both Brian's and Sharon's feelings and thoughts that make up their attitudes have a direct impact on their behaviour and communication.

The outcome is the fault of both. However, who had the greater responsibility? Brian, because he wanted his need met and questions answered? Or Sharon, because she had professional responsibility, is providing a service and is the one with the power and authority?

If we put Sharon in the position of primary responsibility, not only did she need to manage her own attitude, but she also needed to be aware of how Brian's behaviour was having an impact on the interaction and her attitude. Let's imagine that Sharon is a caregiver... the same applies.

It may seem unfair that we have to put in the most effort, but as discussed in previous chapters, we cannot control other people's behaviour; we can only control our own. Also, we may be the ones with the professional or moral responsibilities due to our role as a caregiver/support provider. We could also assume that our emotional maturity or our abilities to regulate our emotions and behaviours may be better and so we must become the teachers through role modelling control.

To be able to control any situation, you must be able to control yourself first.

CASE STUDY 32.2 THE RUDE STUDENT

A teacher is delivering a course to a new group of adult students. About an hour into the delivery of the session, one of the students gets out a newspaper, places it on the table and starts reading it while the teacher is talking.

The teacher can't believe what he is seeing. The teacher is enraged, marches over to the student, slams his hand down on the newspaper in irritation and says, 'What do you think you are doing? That is so rude. If you don't want to be here, there is the door.'

The student packs up his stuff and walks from the room, calling the teacher an arsehole. The other students are left in shock; some can't believe their fellow student's behaviour. Others think that the way the teacher handled the situation was unprofessional.

Student's behaviour: Ignoring the teacher, reading the newspaper.
Teacher's attitude: Thinking – rude, ignorant. Feeling – angry and defensive.
Teacher's behaviour: Aggressive, dismissive.

The attitude of that student and the other students was affected.

We will revisit this example in Chapter 34 to look at how things could have gone differently.

One of the biggest causes of escalation and behaviour that challenges is miscommunication.

Effective communication can prevent escalation, improve relationships, reduce frustration and allow successful de-escalation.

Please take advantage of the bonus chapters 'Communication' and 'Tips for Improving Communication'. These chapters expand on the 'Means, Reasons and Opportunities Model' shown on page 181 and include the following topics:

- How people interpret things differently
- Body language and paralinguistics
- Barriers to communication
- Special notes about communication in relation to autism and dementia
- Avoiding character attacks
- The XYZ formula for assertive communication and feedback
- Using positive language
- The 'five-step appeal' strategy

These chapters can be downloaded at https://library.jkp.com/redeem using the code ESGBAKQ.

CHAPTER 33

DE-ESCALATION THROUGH POSITIVE ATTITUDE AND EMPATHY

First let's explore three definitions of de-escalation.

- The art of resolving conflict through communication rather than force. (Some people are naturally gifted but everyone can learn additional skills, and even the greatest artist never stops learning.)
- To build rapid rapport and a sense of connectedness with an agitated person to reduce the likelihood of escalation to physical violence. This sense of connectedness is established using specific verbal, psychological and non-verbal techniques that emphasise controlling one's own emotional response to threat while guiding communication. (This definition will underpin many of the strategies explored throughout the remainder of Stage 5: Respond Appropriately.)
- The principle of just not making things worse. (This definition may seem simple, but it summarises an understanding of human nature and human interaction. People get angry – that is life, but the way we respond can either escalate or de-escalate the situation.)

CASE STUDY 33.1 THE CAT'S TAIL

If you pull a cat's tail, what will it do? It will either scratch you or run away; the cat doesn't think about why you pulled its tail, what might have caused you to pull its tail and what the consequences of its actions will be – it just responds with fight or flight. So, for animals, it's a case of stimulus leading to a reaction.

Whereas humans have the ability to think, and the way we choose to 'respond' to any given stimulus could either escalate (negative) or de-escalate (positive) the situation.

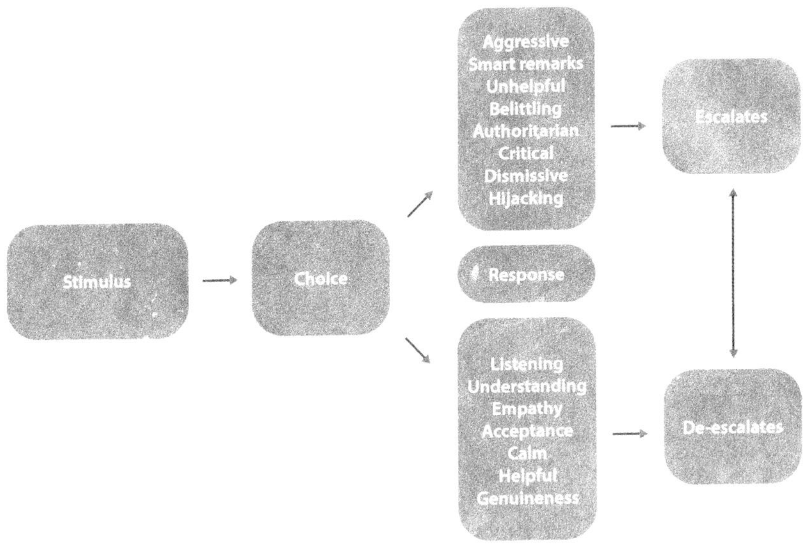

Figure 33.1 Escalate/De-escalate Choices

> Note: do not confuse 'hijacking' with 'amygdala' or 'adrenal' hijacking. What we mean here is hijacking the conversation with remarks such as, 'Do you know, the same thing happened to me, and...'

The rest of this chapter will explore the appropriate responses that increase the likelihood of de-escalating a person in any sort of emotional distress.

The act of de-escalating a person using these methods can build trust and connection between people.

ACTIVE LISTENING

People want to be understood – understood in what we are saying and how we feel, and understood about our intentions and our challenges. Such understanding can help us feel connected and valued, which can build self esteem and a sense of trust and safety.

To understand a person, we need to be able to listen to them. Listening is not just hearing what they say. It refers to the mechanism of exploring what a person is saying with their words, what they may not be saying with their body language or actions and what the thoughts and feelings behind this communication are. This is not a passive action; you must actively listen.

If an individual comes to us with a complaint, or says something is wrong in their world, then clearly, they want to be heard. They may not be looking for a yes/no answer; they just want to be listened to.

Or maybe we can sense through a person's behaviour that they have something to say, that 'something's up', and we can open communication.

We may do this using verbal attending.

Verbal Attending

Verbal attending is acknowledging what we see in the individual's behaviour that is making us curious. We can use this to make a non-judgemental approach. We can acknowledge the behaviour and then see if we can help.

Use expressions such as the following:

- 'I'm aware you are staring at me; is everything okay?'
- 'You seem to be wringing your hands; I'm wondering if you're feeling anxious.'
- 'I've noticed that you are pacing up and down; I'm wondering if you need some help.'
- 'I can see that you have clenched your fists; are you feeling angry about something?'
- 'You are gritting your teeth and I know you do that when you are getting upset; can I help?'
- 'You seem restless; would you like to talk to me about it?'
- 'You seem to be a bit quiet today; is there anything worrying you?'

Some people just want to vent. Inviting them to talk so you can understand them allows you to be emotionally in control of any criticism (it's nothing personal), as you asked for it, but it allows them to get their feelings out.

'I can see you are angry... why don't you tell me everything that's bothering you?'

SOME HINTS FOR ACTIVE LISTENING

Listening is 'seen', not 'heard' – you need to show you are listening.

- Stop anything else you are doing and give the person your full attention.
- Use non-verbal cues to show you're listening, such as occasional nods of the head, or 'uh-huh' or 'I see'.
- Paraphrase – in your own words, repeat what the individual has said, asking if you've understood correctly. This has two benefits: it shows the individual that you have been listening, and it ensures you have correctly understood the situation.
- Use open questions to encourage the person to open up – 'who, what, why, where, when, how?' – instead of questions that invite a 'yes/no' answer, which cut off the opportunity for expansion; e.g., 'Tell me what happened...' or 'Where were you when this happened?'

- Use closed questions only if you want to clarify a piece of information; e.g., 'Michael said you hit him. Is that correct?' or 'Were you in the dining room?'
- Answer questions as required, and only ask questions that are relevant.
- Silence is golden. If you are silent, it is common for the other person to fill the silence.
- The 'SOLER' Model, developed by Gerald Egan,[76] gives us some useful techniques for demonstrating active listening:
  - **S – Sit**: This is not always possible but it demonstrates you are giving your time and it signals non-aggression.
  - **O – Open posture**: Even if it's cold, resist arm folding, which can be perceived as defensive or judgemental whether intended or not.
  - **L – Lean**: Lean slightly towards the individual; this shows interest.
  - **E – Eye contact**: Use soft eye contact rather than staring.
  - **R – Relaxed posture**: This indicates calmness.

Selective Response[77]

- Do not be defensive, even if comments or insults are directed at you. They are not about you. Do not defend yourself or anyone else from insults, curses or misconceptions about their roles or behaviours.
- Do not try to argue or convince.
- Answer only informational questions, no matter how rudely they are asked (e.g., 'Why do I have to fill out these f***ing forms?' – this is a real information-seeking question).
- Do not react to language you may find offensive (e.g., 'Don't swear at me'), as this response can easily create a barrier. The chances are that it's not directed at you; it's just the individual's frustration bubbling over.
- Do not answer abusive questions (e.g., 'Why are you all such a*******s?'). This sort of question requires no response; it isn't asking for information. Just deflect and restart *communication*.

BARRIERS TO ACTIVE LISTENING

CASE STUDY 33.2 THE PILOT'S TROUSERS

Try this activity with someone else – a small group works really well. Tell them you are going to read them a story and at the end they must answer a question to see how good a listener they are. Let them know they can make notes if it helps.

'You are the pilot of a plane travelling from England to Australia via Singapore. In London, 142 passengers are on-board. At Singapore, 37 get off and 41 new passengers get back on. The flight continues to Australia.'

'That is the end of the story – are you ready for the question? What is the colour of the pilot's trousers?'

A typical response from the group is: 'You didn't tell us.'

But look (listen!) carefully... '*You* are the pilot...' So the answer should be whatever colour trousers they are wearing or: 'I'm not wearing trousers.'

Commentary: Most people don't start listening straight away, which is why 'alerters' (as described in the bonus chapter 'Tips for Improving Communication', which can be downloaded at https://library.jkp.com/redeem using the code ESGBAKQ) are useful; and most people make assumptions about what the important part of the information is. In the example above, people tend to focus on the passengers in the story rather than the pilot.

CASE STUDY 33.3 AN UPSET TUMMY... OR IS IT?

Finley keeps complaining of tummy ache every morning before college.

Finley's keyworker, Keith, thinks something is going on and decides to talk to him about it, as Finley used to enjoy college and was doing really well on his courses.

Finley says he hates college, the work is really hard and he just doesn't like going any more.

Option 1: Keith says he is happy to help Finley with his work and is happy to talk to teachers to see if more help can be given.

Option 2: Keith picks up on Finley's reluctance to explain what he is finding hard and decides to focus additional questions on his classmates, the teacher and what else Finley does when he is at college. Finley gets visibly upset when talking about his other classmates and doesn't seem to indicate a connection with any of them. Finley also seems to be spending non class time alone and he is not eating properly at college. Keith decides to try to talk to the college about Finley and see if they know of anything that is happening and if Finley can get some additional support around the social side of college life.

Commentary: It is easy to take what a person says at face value... especially if you are busy or have a pre-conceived idea of what they are going to say.

Active listening takes effort. It can be quite hard work. We typically don't listen for long continuous periods of time before our brain may switch to another thought or we start thinking about what a person is saying rather than continuing to listen.

This is just one of a number of internal barriers to active listening.

Internal Barriers

- **Other thoughts**: As described above, it's difficult to keep focused.
- **Pre-judgement**: Our mind is made up, no matter what the individual may say.
- **Preparing our argument**: While we're listening, we're mentally composing our response ('That's wrong, I'll tell them so-and-so when they shut up'), thereby diminishing our power of listening.
- **Boredom**: You may find some people boring. It takes an effort to stay with them.
- **Too deep**: If the individual gets into detail, we can lose focus.
- **Fact listening**: Focusing on the facts and disregarding emotions and side clues. E.g., hearing 'the hamster was four years old' without taking note of the tears in the speaker's eyes.
- **Tiredness**: It's easy for the brain to switch off when we're tired.
- **Uncomfortable subject matter**: We can easily stop listening because we just don't want to hear more.

External Barriers

- **Noise**: There may be noise in the room or outside.
- **Discomfort**: E.g., uncomfortable chairs, facing the light or you or the individual has a pain such as a headache.
- **Other people**: There may be others passing by.
- **Distractions**: E.g., the TV being on, things going on through the window.

Genuine listening that is focused on trying to understand the person and see their point of view about a subject allows us to develop a connection with the person. If our aim is to build trust, and we genuinely care about creating positive outcomes for the individual, listening is a key first step.

A phrase to bear in mind throughout de-escalation is:

> Connection before correction.

The next chapter looks at one of the most important principles in the book – empathy.

CHAPTER 34

EMPATHY

CASE STUDY 34.1 THE DEAD HAMSTER (PART 1)

Peter, who is 40 years old, comes and tells you that he is upset because his pet hamster has just died. How could you respond?

Would you be flippant or belittle Peter? 'It's only a hamster,' or 'Hamster sandwiches tonight?'

Would you offer practical solutions or clichés? 'Can't you get a new one?' or 'Oh well, everything dies in the end.'

Would you ask questions that focused on the information you wanted to know, so you could decide whether the feelings were justified? 'How old was it? What did it die of?' or 'Why are you upset?'

Would you hijack the story or the emotions? 'I had a hamster die on me two years ago – you'll get over it, I went out and bought a new one.' Or burst into tears because you are reminded of the loss of your own pet?

Would you try to point out the lessons or the positives? 'If you'd looked after it like I told you...' or 'At least he's not suffering anymore, he's gone to a better place.'

Would you be dismissive or ignore him altogether? 'That's sad, but look, we have a lot to do today, let's get to it.'

Would you try to find a solution and move them on through the grieving process? 'Let's have a funeral.'

All of these responses could lead to disconnection, whether you thought they would help or not. Many people may be more sympathetic – 'Aww, bless' – but most people aren't looking for pity and this can still cause disconnection.

CASE STUDY 34.2 THE DEAD HAMSTER (PART 2)

Five-year-old Mira comes and tells you she is upset because her hamster has just died. How could you respond to a child in that type of situation?

Would you recognise their feelings and apologise? 'I am so sorry to hear that.'

Would you acknowledge their feelings and be accepting? 'You seem really sad, you must be finding this really hard.'

Would you actively listen in a non-judgemental and non-directive way (you let them dictate what they say)? 'Please talk to me and tell me all about it.'

Would you remain calm, control your own emotions and only relate for their benefit? 'I've never had a hamster, but I lost my dog last year and I found that really hard... so I know it can feel hard to lose something you care about.'

Would you offer your compassion, availability and support? 'There is nothing I can say to make it better, but I'm here for you, and if there is anything I can do to help, I will.'

These are all examples of showing empathy and building connection. In the example of a dead hamster, it may feel more natural to demonstrate these positive responses to the five-year-old child than a 40-year-old man.

We are more likely to feel more empathy towards the child's loss due to our values, beliefs, attitudes and prejudices. We may still move on to practical solutions with the child, like buying a new hamster or having a memorial, but it is more likely the child would be allowed to grieve and be allowed to just experience their emotions with a caregiver available to share the feelings before the next step is taken.

Commentary: Empathy is the ability to understand and share the feelings of another. We can relate to the child more than Peter.

- Some people are born leaders; some aren't.
- Some people can run fast; some can't.
- Some people are great at arithmetic; some aren't.

But with all of these examples, even those who aren't naturally gifted in the subject can improve their skills by training and learning from others.

- Some people are naturally empathic; some aren't.

So what makes an empathic person? What can we learn from them?

There are three factors that make up genuine empathy:

1. The ability to recognise an individual's emotional state – happy, sad, angry, overwhelmed, anxious.
2. The ability to modify one's own behaviour to accommodate and *accept* the individual's feelings, not to try to *correct* them.
3. The ability to *share* the individual's emotional state. To be *willing* to feel the feelings of the individual.[78]

Number 3 can be challenging when the person we are empathising with is in pain. Sharing in an individual's emotional state and feeling what they feel can be draining and carries the risk of triggering our own internal turmoil. This can carry the risk for us of not knowing how to overcome these feelings; this may lead to burnout or compassion fatigue described in 'Self-Care and Resilience', Chapter 28, page 275. This is another reason for self-care.

CASE STUDY 34.3 THE PERSON IN THE HOLE

(Adapted from the analogy of Brené Brown.)

Imagine there's a person in a deep, dark, cold, damp hole in the ground. Why they're down there – it could have been life that sent them down there, it may have been their own choices that sent them down there – is irrelevant; they are down there none the less. The hole may represent depression, grief, loneliness, failure or any state a person may be in that reduces wellbeing.

Some people will walk past the top of the hole and won't even care to glance down to the person below. This will never allow connection to occur.

Some people will look down the hole and show sympathy: 'Aww bless, that looks rubbish... well I'm going to have to go but good luck.'

Some people do try harder and encourage solutions – 'Have you tried climbing out?' – or offer comfort through clichés or pointing out silver linings: 'We've all been in a hole at some stage in our life,' or 'On the bright side... it could be deeper.'

These examples all exhibit *sympathy*. Sympathy drives disconnection. Most people don't want to be pitied. The person will still feel alone and may even feel worse.

Sympathy is feeling *for* someone.

Empathy is feeling *with* someone.

So, what is empathy?

Empathy is being willing to climb into the hole with the person.* We need to experience what the person is experiencing. We need to see their situation from the bottom of the hole. 'I can see why you didn't climb out; it's so much deeper from the bottom,' or 'I'm so sorry, I didn't realise your foot was chained to the floor.'

Climbing down the hole is hard; we have to be willing to feel the feeling that they are feeling. It takes time, which isn't always available; it can be uncomfortable; we may have even been in a similar hole in our past. Some people don't feel they know what to say because their urge is still to make it better, but even being in the hole is better than doing nothing; we could say, 'To be honest, I don't know what I can say, but I'm here, and I will help in any way I can.'

Being willing to join the person and connect gives us the best chance of helping the person out of the hole when they feel ready.

---

* It is important that we have our own ladder so we can climb out of the hole as needed. We also need the self-awareness to know if we shouldn't go into the hole in case we get stuck, because then how could we ever hope to help the other person out? (See the information on self-care and self-awareness, Chapter 28, page 275.)

CASE STUDY 34.4 THE DEAD HAMSTER (PART 3)

1. Five-year-old Mira tells you her hamster has just died. Your reaction is likely to be to empathise (connection) and then move on to overcoming the grief: 'Let's go and get a new one' (correction).
2. Forty-year-old Peter tells you his pet hamster has just died. This tends to evoke a slightly humorous picture – a grown man upset over a hamster?

   But imagine Peter going on to say, 'I'm upset because my wife left me two years ago, and she took my two daughters to the other side of the country. They moved into a flat where no pets are allowed, so I agreed to look after their hamster. I only get to see my daughters once every six months now, but I get a text message from my daughters every week asking how the hamster is.'

   Does this change our understanding? Peter isn't upset about the hamster – it's the connection to his daughters that feels lost.

   The story behind the hamster may help us to relate to and accept Peter's feeling, as it feels more age-appropriate or in alignment with whatever our prejudices are.

   We needed to go into the hole with Peter and listen to his story before we judged, dismissed or tried to solve Peter's problem.

   So we need to empathise (connection) to find out what's really going on before looking for solutions (correction).

Commentary: The story changed everything... and it's important to understand that there is always a story (whether the individual knows it or not).

To connect with an individual, we must have the ability to:

- listen to their story or be curious about it
- see things from their point of view
- put ourselves in their shoes and see the world through their eyes
- acknowledge their feelings
- step alongside them.

It's about saying 'I can imagine myself in your shoes, looking with your perspective of the world, having experienced all the other things that have happened to you and your history. And I understand why you feel this way.'

Typical statements from an empathic person would be:

- 'I think I would feel like that too in that situation.'**

** Note that 'I would feel like that too' is not the same as 'I know how you feel'. It is highly unlikely that we can actually know what the person is feeling.

- 'You're right.'
- 'I'm sorry you've had to deal with this.'
- 'This seems like such a tough situation; I'm here with you.'

The goal is to *connect*. But when we care about someone, we often want to remove their pain straight away, make it better or solve their problem for them. This puts a lot of pressure on the other person to try to be better, to have a problem that you can solve, to have a reason to feel the way they do that you can change. This can often make the experience worse for them.

CASE STUDY 34.5 I'M DOWN BECAUSE I'M DOWN

Ronnie is a grown man who lives with depression; he knows that his parents and friends will always be there for him. He knows he can always call them if he's down because of something bad happening – loss of a job, a broken relationship, whatever. They'll be there to support Ronnie and be a shoulder for him to cry on.

The problem is that sometimes Ronnie is down because he's down. Life can be going well but Ronnie still feels low. There's no problem to fix. When Ronnie feels like this, he finds it hard to connect to people.

His parents want to find the reason – to find something that can be fixed because they want to make it better. This makes Ronnie feel guilty that he feels as he does.

Ronnie's friends try to help by encouraging him to go to the pub, have a good night out; that'll cheer him up. Often Ronnie will put on a mask to keep his friends happy so they don't feel down or pity him.

Ronnie's parents and friends are diving into *correction* before *connection*.

There isn't a quick fix for Ronnie. He won't feel like this forever, but Ronnie cannot imagine how he can feel better when he is low. He needs someone to just join him in the hole, even if just for a bit. To let him know that it's okay, that he has a friend who knows it's hard and feels tough. He needs to be accepted for who he is in that moment. It's okay to remind him that things will get better, but it's okay if he is not ready yet. Once Ronnie feels accepted for who he is – is allowed to connect with someone else despite his pain – there is a better chance that Ronnie may ask for help to climb out.

Earlier, in 'Case Study 5.4 Kev's Story', page 39, we looked at how Kev was badly treated. His story has an interesting follow-up, showing how a different response could have made a huge difference in Kev's life. You may like to review the original case study before continuing here with the follow-up.

CASE STUDY 34.6 KEV'S STORY – THE SEQUEL

This is a paraphrasing of Kev's words from an interview about his childhood. Kev was raised in care.

Many of the kids I knew in children's homes are now either in prison or unfortunately some of them are dead. I feel I was one of the lucky ones – I got out. I was eventually fostered by one of my teachers and her partner, and they helped me turn my life around.

Not all the staff at the homes were bad.

I remember one time I got angry about something and a good staff member told me to 'go outside and breathe off. Stay away from everyone that's making you angry.' But when I went out, I kicked a plastic sandpit so hard that it just completely smashed. And I panicked, thinking I would definitely get restrained and punished. But luckily that same staff member just said, 'Don't worry about it, it can be replaced, we all lose our temper sometimes and make mistakes.'

I mean, if you make a mistake, what's the last thing you want?

It's so easy for someone to cause escalation – saying the wrong thing, being aggressive, even standing in a threatening way. Kids pick up on those signals. And restraint – whether eight or nine, or in your 30s – if you take away someone's freedom, they're going to lash out and become angrier with life, with people and with yourself.

Instead, you want help – to be able to blow off steam or be talked down: 'You're not bad, you're not in trouble, it's not your fault, we're on your side, I get you're angry, we want to help you.' If the majority rather than the minority of staff had used that approach, maybe things would have been better for everyone.

In the examples above it can be challenging to overcome our beliefs and habits to demonstrate empathy. The double empathy problem below helps to explain.

The Double Empathy Problem[79]

This occurs when there is a reciprocal misalignment of emotions between two people. Emotions can be shaped by culture, by an individual's history and so on. Where these background factors differ, two individuals may find it very difficult to empathise.

CASE STUDY 34.7 WHY AREN'T YOU WEEPING?

Kathy comes from a culture where the death of a close relative is a time of sorrow, of mourning. The funeral of the deceased is a sad affair, as people comfort each other about their loss.

Kathy's friend B-J asks Kathy if she would like to attend the funeral of one of B-J's close relatives. Kathy agrees.

At the funeral, Kathy is shocked, bewildered and totally confused, because there is music, laughter and gaiety as those attending rejoice in celebration of the deceased's life.

Kathy just cannot understand this point of view. Equally, B-J cannot understand why Kathy wants to be sad at the event.

How difficult is it for these two people to step into the other's world?

CASE STUDY 34.8 THE DOG FARM

Diana is a dog lover. One day she sees a programme about dog farms, where dogs are reared and slaughtered for human consumption. Just like in Diana's country, where cattle are reared and slaughtered for the table.

Diana cannot grasp how such cruel and abhorrent behaviour towards dogs can happen.

Equally, a person from a country where dogs are eaten will find it hard to understand why Diana treats her dog as a companion – having it in the house, caring for it.

How difficult is it for these two people to step into the other's world?

This double empathy problem can also be seen when caring for people with autism. The brains of autistic people work in a slightly different way to the neurotypical person. They experience the world in a different way. They feel emotions in a different way. So it can be difficult for a neurotypical person and a person on the autistic spectrum to see the world from the other's point of view.

Difficult but, with effort, not impossible.

Again, let's refer back to the 40-year-old man and the dead hamster. Until we can understand his background – that he's not as upset by the death of the hamster as he is by the connection with his young daughters – we find it hard to empathise.

NON-JUDGEMENTAL CURIOSITY – EMPATHIC COMMENTARY[80]

Building on the discussion about empathy, we can now apply certain empathic techniques for gaining connection when we're conversing with an individual who is experiencing some distress. Empathic commentary can be used as a responsive strategy to build connection and manage a situation; it can also be used within post-incident reflection to empathically explore behaviours and their causes. Empathic commentary is a principle that naturally occurs between attuned caregivers and younger children.

It is a process where we put aside our own feelings and allow ourselves to be completely open to the feelings of the child. We then mirror their emotions using our body language and vocal pace and express what we see and feel.

Imagine an infant's mother saying the following:

- 'Who's a happy little boy right now; you're loving that ice cream aren't you?'
- 'Someone is looking very cross right now; you didn't like your sister taking your toy did you?'

- 'So many tears; your knee must really hurt.'

These are all examples of empathic commentary that provide a demonstration of empathy, as well as helping the child to understand and recognise their own feelings and experiences.

When using empathic commentary responsively, we are communicating and allowing the person to understand that we are trying to make sense of their feelings – to accept them and empathise with them. Having information on a person's history and what they've come from can sometimes allow us to access that empathy more easily, as well as relate (out loud) to the things from a person's past that may be the reason why an individual is feeling this way in this moment.

Having someone demonstrate that they understand a person's emotions (or at least are trying really hard to understand them) and why they might be feeling them helps the person to make better sense of their own feelings and reactions, and can allow the person to better understand themselves. It also helps the two people to develop connection and trust, thus increasing the likelihood of successful de-escalation.

This strategy is incredibly useful for individuals who are dysregulated, especially children and young people who have experienced trauma. It can be used with adults too (particularly if we want to build emotional intelligence); just be careful not to become patronising or infantilising by using any childish tones or language. Dr Amber Elliott in her book *Why Can't My Child Behave?* (p. 85) gives numerous great examples and explanations of this tool. She outlines a number of simple rules. These are intended for use with children but only need some simple adaptations for use with adults.

Some Rules for Empathic Commentary[81]

Work hard to be empathic. Despite what the child's behaviour might make carers feel, it is important to concentrate on the child's emotions and how their experience makes sense of the emotions and behaviours.

- It is important for carers to try to mirror their child's facial expression and the emotion that makes sense of their behaviour, if these are different, and the child's energy levels, in a calm, contained way.
- Carers should endeavour to demonstrate their empathy with words but, more importantly, with their tone of voice and body language.
- It is useful for carers to be tentative about how they convey their understanding of the child's emotions and behaviour.
- Be brief and don't overcomplicate what is said in the commentary.
- There is no need for carers to ask their child questions; if what the carer says is tentative then their child will have an opportunity to correct them.

- If the emotion is ambiguous or contradictory then carers should commentate on this ambiguity rather than trying to force one single interpretation of the child's emotional state.
- Avoid using comments that either praise or chastise. Try to be judgement-neutral.
- *Responsive empathic commentary*, i.e. commentary for use *during* the child's difficulty, should be brief, clear and concise.
- *Preventative empathic commentary*, i.e. commentary for non-problematic times, can be slightly wordier and contain more explanation. It should still only be one or two sentences.

An example of the commentary *during* an incident would be: 'You seem angry. I'm wondering if you are upset because we had run out of your cereal this morning, but you don't know how to feel happy again. Can I help?'

An example of reflection *following* an incident might be: 'So earlier you got really angry at Bob, but I'm wondering if you were still feeling angry about running out of your cereal in the morning, but you didn't know how to feel better so you ended up getting angry at Bob. Maybe we could try and figure out other ways of expressing anger or coping with being upset.'

The following examples are given to demonstrate the type of response we should aim for in any given incident – always aiming to understand the individual's emotions and building *connection* before *correction*:

- An individual is ranting, 'You hate me, you're angry with me, you don't want me here, everybody here hates me...'

  The instinctive response might be: 'No, I want you to be here. I'm not angry.'

  Whereas the empathic commentary would be: 'I'm so sorry that you find that so hard. It must be really difficult to feel the people around you don't like you.' And further comments can continue to build a connection:
  - 'I can see that it feels like I'm angry with you, and it must be a really difficult feeling to have. It's no wonder it feels horrible, and you feel like you'd be better off elsewhere. And, although it doesn't feel like it, I do really want you here.'
  - 'I'm thinking maybe you're feeling a bit sad today because you and Jess fell out yesterday.'
  - 'Sometimes it's hard for you to stop the excitement turning into getting overwhelmed, isn't it?'
  - 'You're really enjoying your breakfast this morning. It's nice to see.'
  - 'You look so happy when you jump on the trampoline!'

And here are a few examples of what to say to an individual who is upset about losing control of a situation:

- 'I reckon it feels so much better when you get to make the decisions for yourself. I can get it.'
- 'It seems that I annoyed you when I asked you to change the channel, because you wanted to keep watching your programme. I understand that must feel frustrating.'
- 'If you're not in control, then you feel really bad! So it's no wonder that you want to tell your sister what to do!'
- 'I'm so sorry that I find it hard to understand why it feels so bad when you're not in control, but I'm working on it to try and make it feel better.'

Exercise

Take a moment to compose an empathic response to the following situations. One possible example is included for each below.

- An individual is chatting non-stop at you while you are cooking food.
- An individual has shut down and disengaged after being asked to do a task.
- An individual says they hate you and they want to leave after you asked them to stop an activity.
- An individual is very hyperactive before they go out for the day. You realise you are getting impatient in your interactions with them.
- An individual comes home and walks straight to their room, slamming their door without interacting with anyone after being out for the day.

Example responses:

1. 'You seem to really want my attention right now. You seem to find it hard when I'm busy with other jobs.'
2. 'Something about me asking you to do (task name) has really stressed you out, hasn't it? It seems that you need to shut down for a little bit.'
3. 'Me asking you to stop doing (activity) seems to have made you really angry with me. I am trying to understand why it feels so tough when you are asked to stop something.'
4. 'You've got so much energy this morning and I can't keep up. I end up getting frustrated with you, don't I? I'm sorry.'
5. (Maybe through the closed door) 'Hey, I'm wondering if you've had a

tough day and need some time to be on your own, but I want you to know I'm here, and if you want to talk to me, I always want to listen.'

Empathic commentary takes practice to develop as a habit but can be an excellent tool.

The fundamental principles are acceptance, validation and empathy put into a non-judgemental narrative about the individual's feeling *that is not asking them to change their feelings or behaviour* but just helping them to understand their own feelings and feel like someone else understands them too.

There are a number of other empathic skills that can build connection, as follows.

ACCEPTANCE

Acceptance is not the same as resignation; it's not the reaction of: 'Oh do what you want.' It also isn't allowing a person to cross personal/professional boundaries or just mistreat other people. Acceptance recognises that every person thinks and feels differently about everything that happens in life. How a person thinks and feels depends on their individual values and beliefs, which are further shaped by experiences and relationships. If we all thought the same, life would be dull.

Acceptance of those who may have had very different experiences of life and people is really important in allowing them to feel validated.

CASE STUDY 34.9 LEGACY OF ABUSE

A child who has experienced authority figures as abusive may perceive any authority figure as bullying and dangerous and so may react defensively and excessively to what we may perceive as a low-level request. (The request becomes the 'green room', the trauma from page 108.) The feelings of danger are real for the child, so the reaction is valid based on the past despite it being inappropriate to the present. We must accept the feelings so that the child can see we are different from the people of their past – we are not a threat. We understand that they feel they needed to react like that, and that's okay. Then, once they feel calm, we can introduce the idea that maybe they didn't need to react like that.

CASE STUDY 34.10 NOBODY'S LISTENING TO ME

An individual feels frustrated because no one is listening to him, despite staff feeling that they do. His view or feeling is that he is not being listened to, or at least not feeling valued. Maybe the staff hear him but don't act on his words. Acceptance of the feelings and acknowledging how frustrating that must feel will help the individual to feel listened to and that his feelings are valued.

CASE STUDY 34.11 'HELP THAT LITTLE BOY!'

An individual living with dementia is becoming distressed because they are hallucinating, and they see an unattended young child under a table. The individual is genuinely feeling distress that this child needs help and no one is helping. 'Someone needs to help that little boy. Someone needs to get him out – he could get hurt.' Accepting the feelings without validating or denying the hallucination is the best way to calm a person. We can accept the feeling: 'I can see how upset you are, and we need to get this sorted, don't we? A young child shouldn't be left unattended, and we don't want anyone to get hurt. *We will make sure everyone is safe*. Let's go this way and I will get someone to make sure everyone is safe.'

Acceptance means that:

- although we may not like, approve of or agree with a *behaviour*, we *accept* the person
- we accept their *feelings* and *don't try to change them*
- we value that they see the world differently
- we want to *understand* the person and explore their point of view
- we can even look for the positive in their viewpoints, which may help *us* to grow.

Once an individual realises that they are being accepted, they can experience relief in being able to spontaneously drop pretences and be ready to convey innermost feelings. They can do that because they no longer fear loss of esteem or being judged.

The individual feels safe in saying 'I hate so-and-so' without getting a reply of: 'No, you don't hate so-and-so.' Such invalidation of feelings can cause the individual to suppress their true feelings, thereby presenting to the world an untrue image of themselves. In turn, this can cause distress and shame: 'I'm not the person I should be. I'm bad.'

For example, an 'acceptance' response to 'I hate so-and-so' would be: 'It must feel really hard if you hate that person, and I know they used to be your friend. So you must feel really challenged by what's happened.'

REFLECTION OF EMOTIONS AND CONTEXT

Reflection is the principle of holding up a metaphorical mirror to a person's behaviour, actions, feelings or words. It can demonstrate active listening and understanding, and ensure clarification in our understanding.

Reflection can be *content-only*, which is sometimes called paraphrasing – this involves the process of repeating back to the other person, in our own words, what they have said to us.

For example:

> Person A: I want to go to the shops later to get some flour and eggs.
> Person B: You need to get some items from the shops.

Or:

> Person A: My family don't care about me. They are always doing things without me and constantly going out together without inviting me.
> Person B: You feel that your family don't care because they exclude you.

Or:

> Person A: I told Gary that I didn't like that flavour of yogurt but he keeps buying it. I don't want it in my fridge, as it just gets wasted.
> Person B: You are saying that Gary keeps buying a yogurt you don't like.

The following examples are *context-only* reflection. This can also be done by almost directly repeating the person's words but changing the tone of the reply to convey an inquiry.

For example:

> Person A: I hate that caregiver.
> Person B: (using an enquiring tone) You hate them?
> Person A: Yeah, they always ignore me.
> Person B: You feel they ignore you?
> Person A: Yeah, the other day I asked them for a drink, and they didn't get me one.

Within this exchange, we are using reflection just to prompt further explanation without judgement or a request for justification of their feelings.

We can also reflect *feelings* rather than context.

For example:

> Person A: My family don't care about me. They are always doing things without me and constantly going out together without inviting me.
> Person B: You sound upset.
> Person A: I am. It hurts my feelings and makes me sad.

Or:

> Person A: I told Gary that I didn't like that flavour of yogurt but he keeps buying it. I don't want it in my fridge, as it just gets wasted.
> Person B: You sound frustrated.
> Person A: I am. It feels like he is doing it on purpose to annoy me.

We can also use a combination of both variations to reflect feelings and context.

For example:

> Person A: I don't get to spend time with my parents often. Mum is always working at the school and Dad is often away a lot travelling for work.
> Person B: It sounds like your parents aren't around much and that makes you sad?

Or:

> Person A: Why can't I go to the shops? I want to get some food and I don't want to wait until 3pm so someone can go with me. I want to go now.
> Person B: You seem angry that you can't go to the shops when you want to.

Reflection is a method of *connection*, not correction or solution.

APOLOGISE

In the right circumstances, a well-delivered, sincere apology can create positive feelings, create a perspective of shared values and offer resolution after a disagreement or a mistreatment.

Some people find that giving an apology can trigger shame and be extremely difficult, as it may feel like an admission that they are inadequate – that, rather than having made a mistake, there is something inherently wrong with them. Others believe that offering the first apology after a disagreement is an admission of guilt and responsibility for the entirety of an event that involved wrongs on the part of both parties; they think an apology from them may allow the other person to take no responsibility for their own part in the issue.

When It's a Good Idea

- If something we've done has caused pain for another person, even if it was unintentional. It opens up the doors to communication, which allows us to reconnect with the person who was hurt.
  'I'm sorry I didn't listen to you earlier.'
- Apologising can allow expression of regret that they have been hurt, whether by us or not, which lets them know you really care about their feelings. This can help them feel safer with you.
  'I'm so sorry that happened to you.' 'I am sorry that you feel upset.' 'I am sorry you are feeling ignored.'
- Apologising for a wrong we did also allows us to discuss what the 'rules' should be in the future, especially if a new one needs to be made, which is often the case when we didn't hurt the other person intentionally.
  'I am sorry I made you angry by being late and not letting you know. Now I know how important that is to you, I will always try to let you know if I am ever going to be late again.'

This doesn't mean that we need to take responsibility for things that were not our fault. We can express regret at unintentionally hurting someone's feelings, but we don't have to say we did wrong.

Taking responsibility may mean specifying what we did that we believe was wrong, but we may also mention what we believe was not wrong on our part, thereby protecting ourselves from taking responsibility for the whole issue.

An apology can also include a simple statement such as: 'I am sorry that you felt that way.' It does not necessarily have to state that we did something wrong. Instead, it is an acknowledgement that the other person was hurt but without apportioning blame.

Finally, there is a disarming honesty in explaining our genuine intent behind our actions that may be affecting a person's feelings – as long as it is said in a non-defensive or non-confrontational tone: 'I'm sorry, I was only trying to help.'

CASE STUDY 34.12 THE BUZZER 1

Aneta is busy supporting an individual with some personal care. It has been a tough morning, they are short-staffed and Aneta has been rushing around but is still behind. Deidre's buzzer is going off, and this is the fourth time in the last hour. Aneta finishes what she is doing and knocks on Deidre's door before entering.

'Where have you been? I have been waiting ages. You're lazy you lot, swanning around. I need the toilet,' snaps Deidre.

'You are not the only resident here, Deidre. We are very busy, and we can't just jump because you want some attention. If you are not going to be grateful, why should I help you?' retorts Aneta.

Aneta then spends a very uncomfortable ten minutes with a sullen, grumpy and withdrawn Deidre.

CASE STUDY 34.13 THE BUZZER 2

Aneta is busy supporting an individual with some personal care. It has been a tough morning, they are short-staffed and Aneta has been rushing around but is still behind. Deidre's buzzer is going off, and this is the fourth time in the last hour. Aneta finishes what she is doing and knocks on Deidre's door before entering.

'Where have you been? I have been waiting ages. You're lazy you lot, swanning around. I need the toilet,' snaps Deidre.

'I'm so sorry if you feel like you've been left waiting, Deidre. It's a busy morning and we are bit behind unfortunately, but I'm here now, how can I help?' replies Aneta with an apologetic tone that finishes with a sympathetic smile.

'I need the toilet, please,' says Deidre.

CASE STUDY 34.14 BETTY (CHOOSE YOUR OWN ADVENTURE)

Betty is 86 years old and has been poorly for a number of years. She has cancer and some signs of vascular dementia. Betty approaches a caregiver.

'Am I dying?' says Betty to the caregiver, visibly distressed.

Choose a response:

- **A**: 'Oh Betty, don't worry – you're fine. Come on, let's get a cup of tea.' You lead Betty to the lounge.
- **B**: 'Well Betty. Aren't we all going to die in the end? Come on, don't be silly.' You walk away.
- **C**: 'You look really upset.'

  'I am,' says Betty.

  'Would you like to talk to me about things for a bit?' you ask.

  'Yes please,' says Betty.

  You sit down with Betty. 'What's upsetting you, Betty?' you ask with genuine interest.

  'I am just feeling scared. I don't want to be in pain when I die.'

  'This is really worrying you isn't it? It sounds like you are unsure about what is going to happen. Betty, if I'm honest, I'm happy to talk to you for as long as you like, but I may not be the best person to give you the answers. Would you like me to arrange a chat with one of the nurses who may be able to answer any questions you might have?'

  Betty says she would.

Commentary: In this example, response C uses reflection, active listening and acceptance to develop trust. It also expresses a good use of boundaries, recognition of potential limitations and being willing to help to find corrections/solutions.

ALIGNMENT

In everything a person ever says, there will be at least 2% of truth. We often tend to focus on the untruth and create a confrontation. If we focus on the truth first, it can be very disarming.

Many people, when behaving in a certain way, are expecting a negative reaction; they are almost anticipating the 'No, I disagree'. It can immediately disarm a situation if first they hear a 'Yes, you are right'.

> **CASE STUDY 34.15** CAN'T I GET A DRINK ROUND HERE?
>
> Bibi is raging: 'I'm fed up with it here. None of you lot listen to me. I have been waiting for half an hour. I must have asked five members of staff for a drink and every single one of you just wanders past me and ignores me completely. Nobody will help me. Nobody will do what I want them to do. I hate it here.'

Commentary: Bibi may be exaggerating. He hasn't asked five members of staff; there are only three on duty. It hasn't been half an hour. People don't ignore him.

What is the truth? First, Bibi wants a drink. He also *feels* he has been waiting too long.

It would be easy to point out the untruths. 'We do listen to you. You haven't been waiting 30 minutes...' We have created a confrontation, potentially escalating the situation.

How much better to focus on the truth? For example: 'You're right, you shouldn't have to wait for a drink... let's go together and get you one.'

Or: 'Are you saying you'd like a drink?'

We've aligned with Bibi; he has nothing left to argue about. We're on his side in regard to the truths, and we didn't react to the untruths.

Sometimes we can align with a person's feelings but then recognise how the facts of a situation may mean a situation cannot be changed.

'You seem really frustrated and I think I would feel the same if I was in your situation. Unfortunately we need to get this authorised by the right people to get this changed.'

We may even align with a person against a principle, system or rule, distancing ourselves from an authority. (This does not mean we need to disagree with the authority.) 'Yes, you're right, this isn't fair, and I understand that this makes things difficult for you. However, this is the rule, and it's not personal.' Again, we have aligned with the individual, leaving no room for further aggravation.

Note that the response begins with 'yes'. This simple word can be very disarming.

This technique is especially effective if accompanied by physical alignment; for example, sitting next to the individual rather than opposite or standing.

In general terms, we're looking for a point of agreement – the 'yes' point. We're showing we're an ally.

CASE STUDY 34.16 ALIGNMENT – THE DOG WALKER IN THE PARK

Clarice is walking through a local park with her dog off the lead, despite signs clearly stating that it is mandatory for all dogs to be kept on leads. A park warden approaches Clarice to address this issue.

Terry: Excuse me madam, I don't mean to disturb your walk today. My name is Terry, I'm a park warden here, I hope you are enjoying the park. Please could I ask you to put your dog on its lead?

Clarice: Why?

Terry: It's a park rule, I'm afraid.

Clarice: Well, my dogs are trained and aren't affecting anyone. They don't exercise properly on the lead. My dogs are fine.

Terry: I completely understand, and your dogs do seem very well trained; unfortunately it's just the park rules.

Clarice: Well that's not right. Why should my dogs be punished just because other people can't control their dogs properly?

Terry: You're right – it would be great if everyone trained their dogs properly so we could let dogs just run around, but the park has to set rules to ensure everyone is safe, and if other people see your dogs off the lead they'll think that they can do the same. I'm sure you wouldn't want any person or dog to get hurt because people aren't following the rule.

Clarice: Okay, but I'm not happy.

Terry: I understand, but thank you.

CASE STUDY 34.17 ALIGNMENT: THE DELAYED CONTRACT

Jamie runs an electrical contracting firm and has been called to the office of the site manager who is unhappy about a delay in completion.

Jamie has encountered this site manager on numerous occasions and knows him as quite a confrontational and critical individual who will often rant and rage about things not going as he expects.

As Jamie enters the site manager's office, the site manager is sitting at his desk facing the door. There is a chair opposite for Jamie to face his opponent. Instead, Jamie immediately says, 'Good morning.' He then proceeds to grab the chair facing the site manager and moves it around to the same side of the desk as the site manager. He sits down and says, 'So, I believe things aren't as far along as you were expecting, so shall we take a look at the situation and see what we can sort out together?'

The site manager is initially slightly taken aback but then proceeds to move the appropriate schedule documents over in front of Jamie so that they can both explore the options and solutions.

Commentary: In the second example, physical positioning is used to demonstrate and create alignment to allow connection and de-escalation to occur before moving forwards with a solution.

SELF-CONTROL AND CALMNESS

Remember: Self-control and calmness are as contagious as fear and panic.

As described earlier, we need to appear like the duck – serene, even though under the surface there is a lot going on.

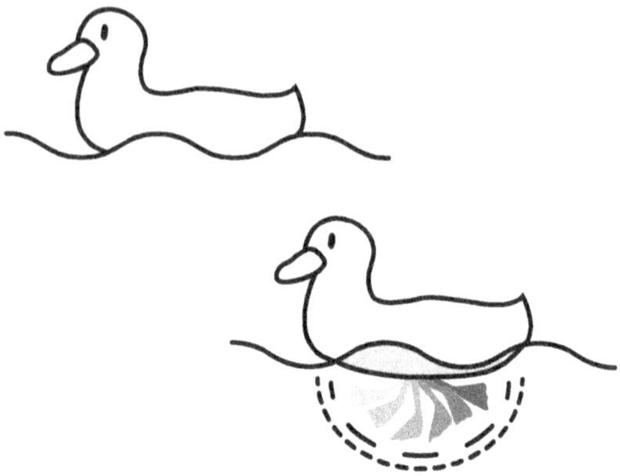

Figure 34.1 What's Happening Under the Surface?

Tips to Bring Calmness to the Incident

Voice

- Use a modulated, low, monotonous tone of voice (our normal tendency is to have a high-pitched, tight voice when agitated).
- Do not get loud or try to yell over a screaming person. Wait until they take a breath and then talk.
- Speak calmly at an average volume, although positive mirroring (carefully mirroring the individual's emotions) may be more appropriate at times.
- Be respectful, even when firmly setting limits or calling for assistance. The agitated individual is very sensitive to feeling shamed and disrespected. We want them to know that it is not necessary to show us that they should be respected. We automatically treat everyone with dignity and respect.

Positive Mirroring

Staying calm should not be confused with being nonchalant or not caring. If we act too unaffectedly, we can come across as disingenuous.

CASE STUDY 34.18 I'M IN A RUSH...

You're in a massive rush, and you have a complaint about something. You go to the shop, up to the counter, saying, 'Look, I really need this to be sorted out, it's not right and I'm in a rush.'

If the assistant responds with an excessively slow-paced, low-volume 'Okay... let's just stay calm, let's see what we can do,' you may consider the assistant to be non-empathic – they're not taking you seriously.

Whereas if they say, quickly, 'Right, let's get this sorted, I'm on the case,' you'll see that the assistant realises it's important; they are mirroring your emotion in a controlled way.

Mirroring is an act in which one person unconsciously imitates the body language, actions, speech style or attitude of another person. Mirroring often occurs naturally in social situations, particularly in the company of close friends or family. For example, friends sitting having a drink together may use similar language and gestures, pace of speech and laughter and may even all take a sip of their drinks at the same time. We tend to like people who are like ourselves, and so mirroring those around us is an innate quality.

We also use mirroring as a way of understanding other people; one way we empathise with another person is when we subconsciously mirror their facial expressions, which then informs our brain what emotion is being felt.

Mirroring can be used as a way of improving connection and trust with a person.

CASE STUDY 34.19 THE COLD-CALLER

Salespeople use mirroring as a way of improving rapport (positive connection), as we are more likely to buy from someone whom we like.

If a cold-caller rings our phone when we are in a sombre mood and they are high energy and enthusiastic, we are likely to find them annoying and want to hang up.

If a cold-caller rings when we are feeling energised and happy and they are slow and melancholic, we may feel disconnected and want to avoid them.

If a salesperson matches our mood, pace and language, we are far more likely to listen for longer.

CASE STUDY 34.20 THE CAR SALESPERSON

I'm sitting opposite the car salesman, feeling defensive and prepared for the overbearing sales pitch. I'm leaning back with my arms folded, waiting for the pushiness to begin.

However, instead of an excessively chirpy, enthusiastic car pusher leaning forwards to draw me into a sales routine, the salesman seems relaxed, also leaning back in his chair, his arms casually folded. He just starts to ask me questions.

What is it I'm looking for? What is most important to me? What cars have I driven before and what did I like about them?

He seems genuinely interested and hasn't mentioned a deal or an offer at all yet. I begin to relax. We end up chatting for a while about family and how important the car is to the family for everything we do. At this point, we are still facing each other, fairly upright in our chairs. My arms are no longer crossed; his aren't either. He asks if he can show me something, and he gets a brochure from a drawer and places it on the table between us. He turns it upside down and I have to lean forwards to see what he is pointing at. I feel genuinely interested in the car he is showing me.

Commentary: In the second case study, mirroring was used to relax the customer, and then, once rapport was developed and the customer was relaxed, the salesperson was able to get the customer to lean forwards. When we are interested in something, we naturally lean towards it... when we lean towards something, our brain is slightly tricked into feeling more interested in it.

This slightly manipulative tactic can be used for positive outcomes during de-escalation and can be used with individuals who are verbal or non-verbal, including those with dementia or on the autistic spectrum.

CASE STUDY 34.21 MIRRORING TO CALM SOMEONE WHO IS NON-VERBAL

Drew is distressed; he is getting overwhelmed by the busy environment and, despite being relocated to a calmer space, is struggling to regulate.

Drew is non-verbal autistic. He is stimming by rocking back and forth quite quickly, and he is breathing quickly and making a noise. Danny, his keyworker, has seen this many times and is there to help bring Drew down.

Danny starts by tapping at a fairly rapid pace on his leg. Each time Drew rocks, Danny taps. Tap, tap, tap. After a little while, Danny starts to slow his tapping down, step by step. Drew seems to be slowing his movements and breathing alongside Danny. Very soon, Drew is calmer. (This technique is sometimes called cross-over mirroring.)

Positive mirroring is the process of mirroring an individual's mood and behaviour when they are in an escalated state but in a controlled way so that they do not perceive that we are becoming aggressive or confrontational.

By positive mirroring to build rapport, we can then role model calming behaviour to draw the individual to a calm state.

We will also use this tactic alongside other tactics, including redirection/distraction.

Let's return to a previous case study to see how some of the strategies mentioned can be applied.

CASE STUDY 34.22 THE RUDE STUDENT – DIRECTOR'S CUT WITH ALTERNATIVE ENDING

A teacher was delivering a course to a new group of adult students. About an hour into the delivery of the session, one of the students got out a newspaper, placed it on the table and started reading it while the teacher was talking.

The teacher couldn't believe what he was seeing. The teacher remembered a few golden rules:

- **Respond rather than react**.
- **Identify behaviour**: Is this maladaptive?
- **Understand/empathise**: Be a better detective rather than a judge – be curious.
- **Proactive plan**: Be a good manager – praise in public, criticise in private.
- **Recognise escalation**: Remember to manage the risk as well as your own emotions.
- **Respond appropriately**.

The teacher felt he needed to address the behaviour, as other learners were noticing it and were being distracted by it. Although this behaviour wasn't hazardous, it was affecting the wellbeing of the environment. However, the teacher recognised that this was unusual behaviour from a learner – the blatant display of disinterest and perceived sign of disrespect was communicating that something was going on for this learner; something was affecting his attitude, which was, in turn, affecting his behaviour. The teacher became interested, not irritated; fascinated rather than frustrated.

The teacher wanted to find out 'What is wrong for you, how are you feeling or what has happened to you?' that has triggered this behaviour in the student.

He recognised that this would be better achieved in a position of privacy rather than publicly shaming or questioning the student, but he also recognised that he needed to be mindful of potential escalation (the student was a stranger and therefore had the potential for unpredictability).

The teacher set a quick activity for the rest of the class to engage in and got them all started. The student continued to ignore the session and his peers, preferring the newspaper. The teacher approached the student and quietly invited him to have a quick chat.

The student and teacher stepped into the empty corridor. The teacher ensured he left the classroom door open and positioned himself where the class would still see them, thus managing the risk if escalation occurred.

The teacher positioned himself in alignment with the student and said, 'Sorry to pull you out of the class, but I am finding it really hard to engage with you. I've noticed you seem disinterested in the session. Have I done something to upset you or is there something going on that I'm not aware of, because I'm finding this really difficult?'

The student looked caught off guard and responded, 'I'm sorry – it's nothing to do with you. My mum is in hospital and she is really poorly. I wanted to go and be there with her but work have told me I have to come into work and do this stupid f***ing course otherwise I won't get any shifts.'

The teacher empathised completely and now understood the student's behaviour. He continued to align and connect with the student before requesting a solution.

'I am so sorry to hear about your mum. I hope she is okay and I completely understand why you don't want to be here. Are work aware of the situation?'

The student replied that they were.

'I would love to let you just go home, but unfortunately it sounds like both of us could be in trouble if I did that. Look, I get that you aren't going to be a model student today, your mind is elsewhere, so I'm not going to ask you to overly engage or force you to enjoy the session. I do need you to put the newspaper away though, as that looks really bad for both of us. All I can promise is that I will crack on and try to get you finished and away as soon as possible. Is that okay?'

The student begrudgingly came back to the classroom, put away his newspaper and seemed to visibly make a bit more of an effort at engaging. He did keep checking his phone and was the first out the door at the end... but now the teacher could excuse the behaviour because he understood the emotions.

A number of months later, the teacher and the student crossed paths again. The student made a point of approaching the teacher.

'Hey, I just wanted to apologise about last time. I didn't behave well.'

The teacher replied, 'Don't worry about it. How's your mum doing?'

'She is doing good – all clear,' replied the student.

Commentary: Through the example given, we can clearly see the improved outcomes for both parties. There is no escalation, and the situation stays calm. A positive relationship is maintained between the teacher and the student, which should improve future interactions.

To summarise how many of these tactics differ to old-logic principles, let's revisit a case study from earlier in the book.

CASE STUDY 34.23 'PLEASE SIR, I WANT ANOTHER BISCUIT' (PAGE 58) – REVISITED WITH NEW-LOGIC EYES

A child asks if they can have another biscuit. The answer is 'no', and the child's response is to explode.

They go into a meltdown, full fight response.

Knowing the child's history, the caregiver responds with a genuine, calm and empathic tone, 'Wow, this has really upset you. I'm sorry I couldn't let you have another biscuit. It's so hard not getting something you wanted. I see you are maybe needing a bit of time to cope, so I'm just going to wait with you until you feel ready.'

The child is confused: *the caregiver is not shouting at me or ignoring me. They just seem to be understanding and calm but they are not giving in and letting me have a biscuit. This is different??*

The child feels overwhelmed and tries something new: 'You don't care about me, you hate me.'

The caregiver responds, still calm. 'That must feel horrible thinking I don't care. I'm wondering if in the past you only felt noticed when you got angry or upset so it's hard to be calm. When you feel ready and calmer we can go and sit and watch telly together for a while if you like.'

The caregiver stays with the child until they are calm, and the caregiver's calmness helps the child regulate. The fact that the caregiver didn't shout or walk away but accepted the child at their worst and still wanted to engage starts to affect the child's perspective of the world and how adults behave. This time in approach begins to build trust between the caregiver and child and also teaches that anger doesn't work as a way to get what you want.

DAPPER – A USEFUL ACRONYM

DAPPER summarises a useful and positive but prepared approach with an individual. We want to ensure we signal non-aggression and a non-confrontational position at the same time as being prepared in case escalation cannot be prevented.

It promotes a balance between connection and personal safety.

D – Distance
A – Attitude
P – Position
P – Posture
E – Empathise
R – Read the situation

Distance

Proxemics, or the distance between sender and receiver, can change the way communication is interpreted. An aggressive person will often invade personal space. 'Getting in someone's face' is a common idiom for someone being aggressive, so maintaining appropriate space from an individual may be an important way to demonstrate a lack of threat. It can also help to keep us safe if an individual suddenly lashes out or strikes us. It is also important to recognise that what we perceive as a comfortable distance depends on the setting and relationship.

The more we trust people, the closer we allow them to be. Our perception of 'too close' for someone we don't know varies according to the number of people around; for example, an open park, a packed concert, a full train, an empty café.

Therefore, we should be aware of the distance we maintain between ourselves and the individual; for example, relative heights play a part, or someone with dementia may see a caregiver as a friend or stranger from one minute to the next.

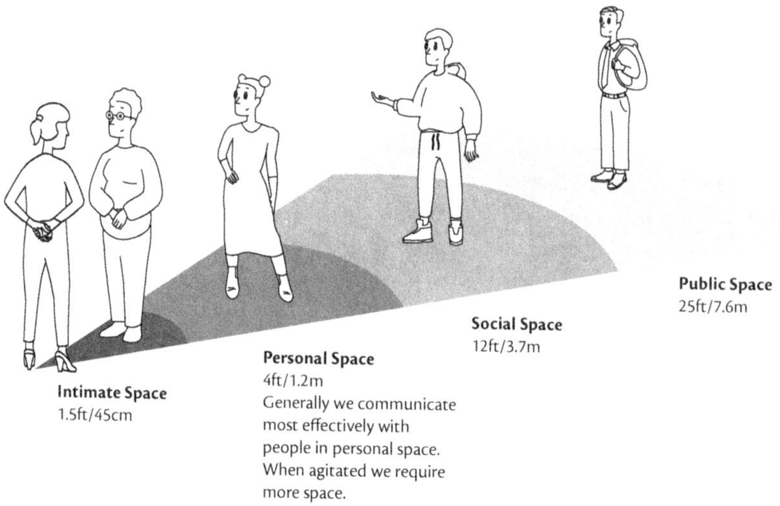

Figure 34.2 Proxemics

Attitude

Our whole attitude should indicate: 'We're here to help; we're here to support; we're not *against*, we're *with*.' We should show positive body language and unconditional positive regard for the individual using all of the communication skills described previously.

Position

As well as distance, there are other positions that should be avoided and considered when looking to de-escalate. We should avoid the following:

- **Blocking exits/doorways**: Making a person feel trapped.
- **Standing square on**: We should stand at an angle to demonstrate alignment.
- **Standing over someone**: We should try to come down to a person's eye level, by either sitting with them or kneeling down. If we need to stand, we should try to ensure that the angle between them and us is not too steep (we don't want them to have to look up to allow eye contact).

- **Allowing other people to invade or intimidate**: Crowd control and team management is important to avoid escalation by others.

Posture

Our posture should be open and relaxed but prepared. We should always have our hands in an available position to defend our space or protect from any attack in worst-case situations.

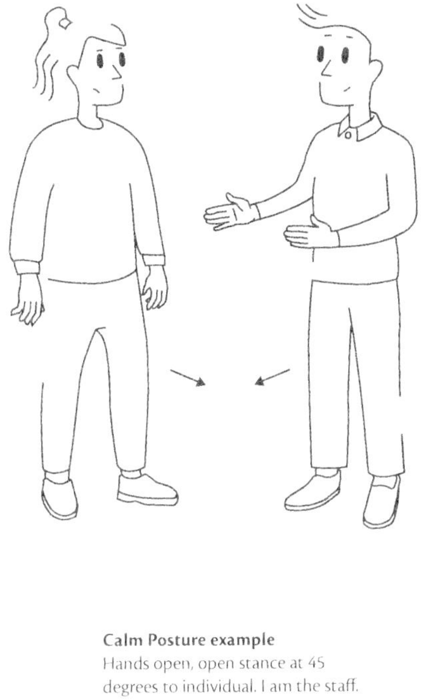

Figure 34.3 Calm Posture

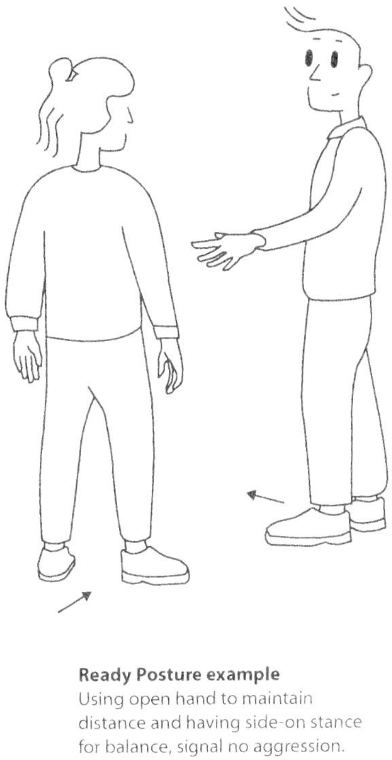

Figure 34.4 Ready Posture

Empathise

As already described, we should try to see the world as the individual sees it – to recognise the emotions and their causes. Use all the skills described in the previous content, especially Chapters 33 and 34, to show alignment and understanding. It is much harder to be aggressive to someone who is desperately trying to understand you.

Read the Situation

Read the situation for our own safety: Carry out your own dynamic risk assessment. See the bonus chapter 'Dynamic Risk Assessments' for more information. This can be downloaded at https://library.jkp.com/redeem using the code ESGBAKQ.

Read the situation of the individual: Where is the individual on the escalation roller coaster?

Be aware that any inadvertent mistake on our part, such as crowding, touching, blocking exits and so on, could be a trigger to further escalation.

Special Note about Proxemics when Working with an Individual with Dementia

We may be working with a person who sees us as a stranger, even if we have engaged with them a thousand times. For them, it might seem like they are meeting us for the very first time. If we behave with familiarity, that could trigger an unhelpful emotional response.

REORIENTATION IN CONFUSED STATE

When interacting with an individual who is experiencing a different sense of reality to us – whether that is caused by psychosis, delirium or dementia – we can use any of the strategies that have been explored in the situations in this book. Whether what the individual is saying is true or not, the person's feelings are true. We should still focus on the connection first.

This doesn't mean we don't explore potential causes. Are there shapes, noises or circumstances that the individual's brain may be misinterpreting and can the environment be adapted to reduce these? For example, a person claims that someone keeps knocking on their window and they won't stop, and you realise that a tree branch may be tapping on the window in the wind... can this be removed?

> **CASE STUDY 34.24** THE TV IS TALKING TO ME
>
> A distressed-looking individual approaches their caregiver. 'The TV is talking to me. It's saying that bad things are going to happen.'
>
> The caregiver responds. 'You seem really upset and scared. I think I'd feel the same if that happened to me. Let's move away from the TV room and go and find somewhere where you can feel safer.'

So far, we have looked at the importance of understanding communication, listening skills and a variety of empathic tactics. These all combine to try and develop a connection with an individual not only to reduce escalation and distress, but also to prevent further escalation if a person is distressed, unhappy or angry about something.

In the next chapter we will look at correction, solution and other potential tactics to draw escalation to a close.

CHAPTER 35

BRINGING ESCALATION TO A CLOSE THROUGH SOLUTION OR RESOLUTION

We could use the term 'rapport' to summarise the last chapter, which explored de-escalation through positive attitude and empathy.

Rapport means a close and harmonious relationship in which the people or groups concerned understand each other's feelings or ideas and communicate well.

As we have seen throughout this book, when you build rapport with someone, you're better placed to influence, learn and teach, particularly as the trust that you've built means other people are more likely to accept your ideas, to share information and to create opportunities together.

By using the skills of communication, listening, empathy and acceptance, we have hopefully ascertained the individual's position, their concerns, their emotions. This can allow us to look to manage or even resolve the situation.

Rather than stay in an indeterminate loop, it may become necessary to move on to some sort of resolution or look to alter the individual's behaviour or outcomes. This may be done through a variety of methods that will depend on the behaviour and its cause or function, and on where the person is on their emotional roller coaster. Are they on the way up or on the way down? We need to respond in the right way at the right time.

In this chapter, we will look at the correction/solution opportunities we can offer once connection is made and also which strategies tend to be most appropriate at what stage of escalation.

First, let's look at 'correction' or 'solution'.

BRINGING ESCALATION TO A SOLUTION OR RESOLUTION

The goal of de-escalation is to build rapid rapport and a sense of connectedness with an agitated person in order to reduce the likelihood of escalation to crisis. The collaborative view then allows us to work with the individual to achieve the outcome that is hopefully best for them or as close as we can get.

In the last chapter, we looked at Brené Brown's analogy of the person in a hole in the ground to represent empathy.

If we have rapport and connection, a point can often be reached where we present options or opportunities for the person to leave the hole. This may be to resolve the issue and get them out of the hole permanently, or a temporary solution to be able to achieve outcomes and they can return to the hole later if they need to; or we might need to redirect focus from being in the hole to addressing other needs.

ESTABLISHING WHAT THE PERSON WANTS

As described in Chapters 29 and 30 on recognising escalation, if a person is in a heightened state, they may not be able to clearly articulate or even contemplate what they need. They may need a trusted helper to guide them to appropriate outcomes or support them to use appropriate strategies to meet their own needs.

To respond appropriately in the moment, we can use the 6STM dynamically.

We have recognised escalation, and so we carry out the following stages.

We identify: Is this a behaviour for which we have a pre-existing plan? Is this something that needs my immediate attention, or should I ignore the behaviour (but not the person)? If we don't have a plan but we feel the person needs our support and it's safe and appropriate, we can engage.
We try to understand and empathise: Why this? Why now? What is wrong for them, what's happened to them or how are they feeling?

We can use the motivation triangle again here as a reminder to explore the cause or purpose of the behaviour.

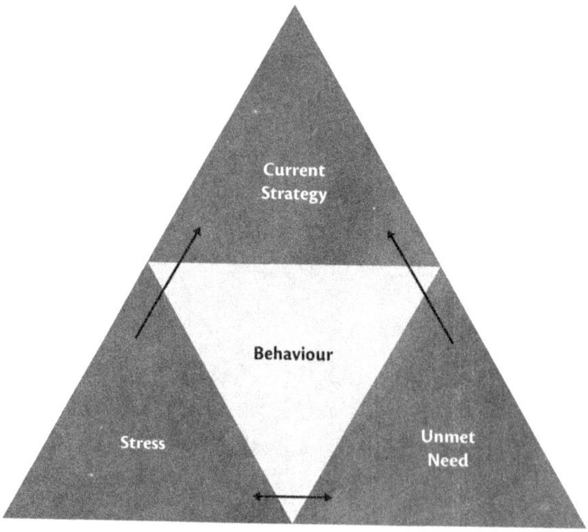

Figure 35.1 The Motivational Triangle

'In this moment can I understand the need or what's causing the stress and why they are using this strategy rather than any other?'

Once we establish our hypothesis, we can begin to create a **plan** either with the individual or for the individual if they are unable to collaborate.

Can I meet the need or help them to meet their own? Can I eliminate the stress or help the person to cope with it?

Only then can we **respond appropriately.**

The remainder of this chapter includes practical steps that can be taken to help meet the individual's needs. The following chapter includes practical steps to help eliminate the individual's stress.

MEETING THE NEED

If the individual is trying to gain/get or avoid/escape:

- a person
- an activity
- a tangible, sensory stimulus
- help or control

then is this appropriate, safe and available, and therefore can we facilitate this or do we need the person to act a certain way before this need should be met?

CASE STUDY 35.1 MY DVDS HAVE BEEN STOLEN!

Simone is angry and alleging that another individual in the home has been into her room and taken a number of her DVDs. The caregiver present is aware that this is correct.

The person who took the DVDs has actually gone out for the day and taken the DVDs with him. The caregiver has listened to Simone and acknowledged her feelings and validated that it isn't appropriate for someone to take her property without asking. The caregiver realises that although they have managed Simone's escalation through connection, a solution needs to be found to allow Simone to calm and move forwards.

The caregiver could use one of the following.

- 'Simone, I can see you are very angry, but I need you to sit down with me, so we can talk about this calmly.'
- 'Simone, I know you are angry, and I think I would feel angry too if someone had taken my stuff without asking. What would you like to happen now?'
- 'Simone, I understand you are angry about this, and we need to find a way to stop this from happening in the future, and I want to get this

sorted for you, but I can't get this sorted when you are so angry. Why don't we go out for a walk to calm down and when we get back we will get this sorted?'

- 'Okay Simone, I cannot get the DVDs back right now but I'll make sure they are returned to you tonight when they come back. Were you wanting to watch one of those films today? Okay, then I will see if we can either get another copy or find it on Netflix. Or, for today, we may have to choose another film instead and then you could watch that other one tomorrow.'
- 'Simone, I'm sorry you are so upset and I wish that I could just sort it. Unfortunately, the person who took your DVDs has gone out for the day and taken them with him, so there is nothing I can do right now. I am happy to log your complaint and we will get it sorted later. Let's sit down and get it written down, and maybe we can move on for now as I don't want this to ruin your whole day.'
- 'Okay Simone, I completely understand why you are upset and I want to get this sorted for you but there is nothing that I can do right now, so either we can move on for now, and we can sit and have a drink and I can help you to get this sorted later when we can do something about it – or I can give you some space to get calm and then we can have a drink together in a bit. What would you prefer?' ... 'I understand, but they are the only two choices we have right now, so which is it?'

Commentary: When looking for a solution, be honest. Lying to a person to calm them down may lead to future escalation if they become aware of the dishonesty. However, do not volunteer information that may further upset the person.

There is not one response that is correct; they all contain strategies that may work to bring the situation to a close. Some set clear boundaries, others give the control to the individual themselves and some are looking to redirect from the problem to the solution.

They include some of the following strategies.

REQUEST A SPECIFIC BEHAVIOUR

In Chapter 37, we will refer to 'Prompt' as a stage of de-escalation; the bonus chapter 'Tips for Improving Communication' (which can be downloaded at https://library.jkp.com/redeem using the code ESGBAKQ) describes the use of positive language and the five-step appeal. We are looking to request a preferred behaviour and ideally one that is incompatible with the unwanted behaviour or has a calming effect.

Taking a deep breath, sitting down, slowing down what they are saying or eating and drinking are all incompatible with stress and so may work to de-escalate.

Having pre-prepared plans of what positive actions we could choose from can improve the likelihood that we can respond rather than react. We should always request and suggest rather than command and demand. And we should never use threats such as:

- if you do this, then I'll do that
- if you don't do this, then I will do that.

These ultimatums are likely to cause escalation or at least damage and lose trust, rapport and connection, as this is now a power struggle that even if we win... if our aim is improved outcomes for all... we lose.

See the discussion on feedback in section 'Explain the Choices and Their Outcomes', later in this chapter, where we'll look at pointing out consequences as a choice.

FUTURE-ORIENTATED QUESTIONS

Encouraging the individual to rationalise what they would like to happen can be a good starting point to explore options and begin to discuss how a need can be met. If we find that the answers are overly emotive and unreasonable, we may need to provide boundaries on what the possible options are, or decide to wait until the person is calmer, before we explore this question further.

SUPPORT TO FIND A WIN-WIN SOLUTION (COLLABORATE/COMPROMISE)

Collaboration can take time, as it's about finding what the person needs and exploring what they see as a win but at the same time ensuring that the overall outcome is a win.

Their win may not necessarily mean getting exactly what they want, but it's about managing the gap between expectations and reality.

CASE STUDY 35.2 MISSED TRAIN

Briony's taxi was late to pick her up, and she knows she is cutting it fine to get the last train home. She's not had a good night, she has work tomorrow and she is feeling incredibly stressed. She makes it to the station and runs to the platform to see a train disappearing from the station. She has a sense of dread that it was her train but hopes she is actually in time. Briony sees a platform assistant, Jenny, just walking down the platform. She runs over to Jenny, who is in uniform.

'Excuse me, that wasn't the train to Manchester, was it?'

'Fraid so, reckon you're gonna have a long walk, haha,' Jenny replies flippantly.

'That's not funny. That can't be the last train – I need to get home.'

> 'Are you telling me I don't know my own job? That was the last train love,' snaps Jenny.
>
> 'F*** you, you stuck up bitch. Thanks for nothing.'

Commentary: In the above scenario, we need to look at all the expectations that Briony may have had in this situation and then look at how many of them were met and what could have been improved.

Expectations may have included the following:

- Another train
- To be listened to and be shown empathy
- Professionalism
- Respect and manners
- Signposting to other options
- Help or support to find another solution

Briony received none of these.

We could criticise Jenny here for her reactions, but what if Jenny is ill, that was the last train so it's now the end of her shift, and she has had this situation 100 times before where 'customers just expect you to magic up a train'?

It doesn't make Jenny's behaviour right but maybe we could relate to it. However, Jenny did have a responsibility, especially as the professional, to manage the gap between expectations and reality. Of course she couldn't magic up a train, but the other expectations are reasonable and could have been met.

Win-win is the ideal outcome that may include the following:

- **For them**: Having their needs met, i.e., getting what they want, being treated with respect and dignity, receiving a helpful explanation of why they can't have their needs met, being listened to and understood.
- **For us**: Managing the situation professionally, de-escalating the situation, maintaining positive relationships, having a stress-free day, maintaining boundaries and others being satisfied that we did our best.

It is not always possible to accommodate all of these, and sometimes no matter what we try we cannot find a solution where all parties are 100% happy, which is where compromise may be the best we can hope for. But the last point on the win for us is that our overall goal should always be that we and others are satisfied that we tried our best.

OFFERING PRACTICAL SOLUTIONS

Being knowledgeable or at least being willing to find out more is a demonstration of collaboration. Practical solutions are not always desired.

We have all had a situation that has made us emotional. We have gone to someone looking for understanding and support and received nothing but advice, solutions or silver linings and felt dissatisfied or even patronised by the response. But sometimes we genuinely need some help to meet our needs and may value that type of support.

When responding to an emotional situation, it isn't wrong to ask that very question: 'I know you're upset. Do you want me to help you find a solution or do you just need me to listen?'

There may also be a point in the interaction where this changes: 'I know you needed me to just be understanding, but I'm worried that we are a little stuck, so I'm wondering if we should look at things we could do to make this better or move forwards.'

POINT OUT THE FACTS

A bit like finding a solution, at times we may need to direct emotion towards a rational outcome and point out the facts. This is a bit like in Simone's case study earlier in the chapter, where her preferred outcome may well be to have her DVDs back immediately, but that's not practical in that moment and so it may need to be pointed out carefully.

Don't forget, the individual may be very aware of the facts and pointing them out may be perceived as patronising or belittling, but sometimes they need to be drawn into focusing on the realities of the situation and to be aware that their behaviour is not going to change the facts.

This can sometimes be a useful strategy when mediating a situation between two people, especially if one appears to be trying to dominate the situation: 'I can see that you are both upset about this, but until I have heard both sides of the story, I cannot help you both to resolve this.'

Pointing out the fact that you need to hear both sides informs the aggressor that shouting louder or being more aggressive is not going to change the situation.

We should also be willing to calmly explain any limits and rules. This may need to be done in an authoritative and firm but respectful tone to emphasise that they are fixed and serious. If rules have not been created by you (they are the setting's rules or laws), you can explain that: 'I understand you feel this is unfair, but these are the rules that we have to follow here.'

If you are the person who set the rules, it may be fair to explain why the rule is in place: 'I know you think I'm being unreasonable and you don't understand this rule, but it's something that is important to me and I must enforce it.'

If it is a rule that you negotiated with the individual themselves (e.g., behavioural plans, care plans), you can refer to that: 'We agreed to this rule together and so we need to stick by it for now. If when everything is calm you want to talk about it, we can; but that is not happening now, while you are upset.'

Just like when giving feedback, which will be covered shortly, we can list consequences of inappropriate behaviour without threats or anger. Use expressions such as: 'Look, these are the rules. I want you to understand that if you make this choice, this will be the outcome; if you make this choice, this is the outcome. I know what I would prefer for you. The consequences are fixed – the choice is yours.'

Note: If a person makes what you feel is the wrong choice, or if they seem to regret and become upset about the choice once the consequence is initiated, we should never shame: 'I warned you/it's your own fault/you made your choice!!'

We all make mistakes, but mistakes are stepping stones in learning. If we are trying to build a person's self-esteem and self-worth to improve their behaviour, then shaming, blaming or communicating an 'I win/you lose' narrative post-incident will have the opposite effect and will not develop trust.

Narrating empathically to show understanding and relating to 'choices being tough sometimes' is far more appropriate: 'I can see you might be regretting your choice and that must be hard. But it's okay to regret a choice; we will try again tomorrow, and we will get there.'

EXPLAIN THE CHOICES AND THEIR OUTCOMES

Like pointing out the facts, we may try and draw a situation to a resolution by outlining what choices are available and allowing the person to make the choice themselves.

One example of this is feedback.

Feedback involves identifying or pointing out the potential outcomes of a person's behaviour without demanding a change. If carried out by a trusted person in a non-judgemental manner, it can support de-escalation.

We begin by listing potential consequences of inappropriate behaviour, without threats or anger.

Model:

Behaviour = Effect
versus
Alternative = Effect

Feedback may help prevent someone who is beginning to escalate from escalating further or prevent future escalations.

'Look, I know you are finding this hard, but if you continue to get angry and we can't get calm then we will not be able to go out later as it won't be safe. If we can sit down and talk calmly, I'm sure we can get this sorted and we can enjoy the rest of the day.'

This is often not a useful tactic when someone is highly agitated, as they may perceive it as a threat or command.

CHALLENGING

'Challenging' is the skill of highlighting incongruence and conflicts in an individual's thoughts, words and actions. Gently confronting or challenging an individual can open an opportunity for exploration of feelings and outcomes. Challenging should always be offered thoughtfully and not in a way that is likely to be perceived as judgemental or reprimanding. It should have a clear person-centred purpose – and not be challenging for the sake of it. It is important that we are aware of how the individual might respond to challenge. Challenging should only be used if you have first developed trust and rapport with the individual.

Challenge must be offered in an encouraging and non-judgemental way, and we must continue to be empathic, acknowledging that seeking change is likely to be difficult for the individual.

Challenging may be most appropriate during a debrief rather than during an emotional episode but can be a tool worth being aware of.

Below are some examples of situations where challenging may be relevant, with some examples of its use.

Challenging Negative Thoughts: 'What Are the Facts?' or Offering Alternative Views

'You say that you hate Sally because she was rude to you; can you give me an example of when she made you feel that way?'

'Okay, so you felt she was rude because she didn't say hello to you when she came in the room, and I understand you finding that rude. Do you think Sally meant to be rude?'

'Could there have been any other reason why Sally didn't say hello? Was she doing anything else at the time? Okay I'm not saying this is true, but maybe Sally just had other things on her mind and wasn't ignoring you – she was just distracted. Now, that doesn't make it okay, but I have definitely accidently ignored people before without realising it. It seems like we can't be sure of why Sally didn't say hello, can we? I'm not sure whether getting upset will help us. Maybe we could talk to Sally when you are calm and see if everything is okay?'

The last example shows the tone, pace and relationship between the caregiver and the individual. The individual's escalation must be at an appropriate level before this type of challenging can result in de-escalation.

Challenging Inconsistencies: What They Are Saying and Their Actions Are Incongruent

'I have noticed that even though you said you are feeling okay, you don't look happy. Would you like to talk about it?'

'You have said to me that you want to find better ways to cope with your feelings, but you haven't done any of the strategies that we agreed to. Can I do anything to help you right now?'

Challenging Their Behaviour Towards You

'I am feeling that you are getting very angry with me, but I promise you I'm only trying to help and understand what is upsetting you.'

'I know you are upset right now but I am feeling like you are making me the enemy and I'm not trying to be.'

'You keep calling me stupid, and I'm not stupid but it's making me feel upset. Please can we change the way we are speaking to each other?'

DELIVERING A GIFT

One way to de-escalate a situation is by delivering a gift. This does not mean giving the person a present (although it might work). The gift is an indication of positive effort to help a person, which may not really require that much effort on our part.

The gift might include giving them what they want.

Is there any reason why they shouldn't get what they want? Or is it just about us not wanting to give in? Sometimes it might be completely appropriate to let the person gain or avoid whatever it is they want in that moment. Note that it may be a short-term strategy that could lead to long-term consequences if not managed properly. However, especially in situations that could result in harm due to escalation, it may be the safest and easiest way to resolve the issue. We just need to be extremely mindful of not reinforcing a maladaptive behaviour just for convenience.

SIGNPOSTING

It may be possible to suggest additional help (as in alternative options, additional information or support that you can't offer).

CASE STUDY 35.3 CRISIS CENTRE

A well-known mental health charity has experienced a number of incidents where individuals have dropped into their office in mental health crisis looking for immediate support.

This charity does not offer this service, but its office has recently relocated, and it has taken over the site from a former crisis drop-in centre. This is what the individuals were looking for and expecting.

The charity has successfully managed each situation and de-escalated the individuals who, on each occasion, were highly distressed.

It is then pointed out to the charity that it would be worth their while to have pre-prepared information that staff have access to. This would have details about where the nearest convenient drop-in centre is located, transport options and a phone number that they could give the person or even call on their behalf to support their needs.

This would aid their ability to de-escalate, as they have a signposting option pre-prepared.

Commentary: After the first 'fire' of an individual raising this issue, the charity should have put immediate plans in place to be prepared for the next time it happened. This is the process of moving from *reaction* to proactive plans and response strategies.

PASSING THE BATON

Sometimes it is appropriate – due to our knowledge, skills or resources – to refer to someone else who has additional powers or skills to help the person. In a care setting, this could be a manager or social worker.

This is the correct thing to do when:

- you recognise that you have exhausted your resources and options
- the situation is beyond what you should be managing
- it will make the individual feel respected and important, therefore validating their issue.

It shouldn't be used as an easy get-out or every time you encounter a behaviour you don't know how to manage; this would result in your role in the relationship becoming redundant and you undermining yourself.

CHAPTER 36

ELIMINATING OR SUPPORTING TO COPE WITH THE STRESS

Meeting an individual's specific need is not always possible due to resources, circumstances, care plans or just the realities of the situation, but that doesn't mean we can't take steps to eliminate or reduce the stress for the individual.

We have mentioned the acronym HELP throughout the book, and we need it again now.

Is the stress caused by human, emotional/cognitive, location or physical circumstances?

If we recognise that the cause of agitation or distress is any of these, then can we either alter the environment or situation to reduce the stress or support the individual through the process of calming using other means?

Again, many of the strategies and principles discussed in the previous chapter and in this chapter can have a significant de-stressing benefit – as a problem shared is a problem halved – and human connection (if a person can engage) is the quickest way to de-escalate, as discussed all the way back in 'The Window of Tolerance and Polyvagal Theory', Chapter 12, page 117.

SWITCHING

CASE STUDY 36.1 SWITCHING (THE TEAMWORK TOOL!)

Darren was very agitated. One of his caregivers, Phil, had entered the room and seen Darren's distress. Jez, another caregiver, also heard the commotion and came to the room, but seeing that Phil was already involved, he maintained his distance. (Jez was trained and therefore knew that two staff could potentially overwhelm Darren or make him feel ganged up on, but he did position himself so that Phil knew he was there, without invading or blocking any exits.)

Despite Phil's every effort, Darren started to escalate further and was starting to invade Phil's personal space; he was posturing and was directing his agitation towards Phil.

Jez could see that Phil was starting to react to Darren's behaviour and so felt the time was right to switch faces.

Jez approached from Darren's side and spoke calmly but firmly as he approached.

'Darren, I can see you are getting upset. Can I help at all?'

Darren looked towards Jez. Phil took a few steps back to create some space.

'I'm fed up of waiting to go out and he's...' (pointing aggressively at Phil) 'not listening,' shouted Darren.

'I'm sorry you feel that way Darren. I think Phil is just trying to find out what's going on but let's see if I can help. Phil, would you mind seeing if you could find out what's happening with Darren's transport for us? Thanks.'

Phil, who was also trained, knew that Jez was not undermining him, and he also realised that his own bottle of Coke was beginning to get shaken up by Darren's behaviour. So he appreciated the support and the exit opportunity and left the room to find out the information.

Jez continued to talk to Darren. 'Now Darren, Phil's gone to find out what's going on for you but why don't we sit down and you tell me why this has got you so agitated today? You don't usually get so agitated about your transport – is something worrying you?'

Darren calmed and started talking to Jez about what was going on and soon de-escalated. Phil popped his head in and told Darren and Jez that the transport was all sorted and would be arriving at 2pm.

Later on, after Darren had been out and returned, Phil approached Darren. 'I am sorry if you didn't feel I was listening to you earlier Darren – is everything okay now? Did you have a good afternoon?'

'It was good. Thanks Phil.'

Commentary: This is an example of a positive team approach that used switching as a natural de-escalation tool.

Aggression is directed towards a person, but anger is indirectly focused on the situation. Sometimes, when a person becomes aggressive, removing the focus of their aggression allows the individual to de-escalate to being angry at the situation. This can allow a second person to better engage and build rapport and a solution.

Switching may need to be repeated a couple of times, but switched-out caregivers should always aim to reconnect after the incident.

CASE STUDY 36.2 'GET AWAY!'

Gladys has dementia and is meant to be going to the hospital. The transport ambulance arrives, and the driver and an escort come to help Gladys to the vehicle.

Gladys becomes extremely distressed as they are walking her down the corridor, and she backs away from the two men.

Gladys has her back to the wall and both men are trying to de-escalate her. Gladys is lashing out and shouting, 'Get away, get back, leave me alone. You're not taking me anywhere.'

Sarah is a caregiver at the home and is just grabbing Gladys's night bag to go with her to the hospital when she hears the commotion. She heads down the corridor and sees what is happening.

Sarah moves quickly down the corridor, and as she gets closer, she raises her voice. 'You two, move away from her, leave her alone.' Sarah then positions herself alongside Gladys, looking out at the two ambulance men, who, understandably, look confused.

She continues, 'It's okay Gladys, I'm here.' Turning to the two men, she says firmly, 'I need you both to move away.' She gestures for the two men to go down the corridor. Sarah mouths 'sorry' to the men as they move away.

'Oh Gladys, are you okay? You seemed so frightened.'

'They were trying to take me away.'

'That must have felt very scary, but you're okay now. You are safe. Let's go to the lounge and get a drink to settle your nerves.'

Sarah takes Gladys to the dining room and organises a cup of tea with a biscuit for her. She then goes to apologise and explain to the two men what's happened.

After a few minutes, Gladys seems settled, so Sarah feels she can try again. 'Gladys, you are going to hospital today to have some tests done. I'm coming with you and the transport has arrived. Would you like to walk down to it now?' Gladys agrees and Sarah walks Gladys down to the ambulance. As they go, Sarah keeps talking to Gladys about Gladys's favourite subject, which is her grandchildren. And they get onto the ambulance with the very two men who, just ten minutes before, Gladys had thought were trying to abduct her.

Commentary: Sarah recognised Gladys's emotional reaction as one of fear that had not been de-escalated by the two ambulance drivers. It is very likely that Gladys was disorientated about who the men were and what was happening. Rather than siding with the men and potentially increasing Gladys's distress she used alignment, positive mirroring and empathy to de-escalate the situation and redirect Gladys, allowing her to calm. Sarah then used a different approach to achieve the same desired outcome.

HUMOUR

Humour can be an amazing tool for de-escalation if used by the appropriate person in the appropriate way. It is difficult to indicate exactly what those criteria are, and some people seem to have a natural ability to diffuse situations with humour; others often get it wrong and actually cause escalation.

Humour works better when rapport is there, and the person should never feel humiliated or belittled through the humour, but laughter is almost the polar opposite to aggression, distress and anxiety.

Humour can work to distract or redirect or even put a situation into perspective if used effectively.

CASE STUDY 36.3 KNIFE AT MY THROAT

Karen had worked at the home for five years but had only met Brett five months ago when he came to live there.

One day Brett was in the kitchen and Karen came in and asked him if he could please tidy up the plates that were on the draining board. Brett glared at her as she went to leave the room. Before she knew it, Brett had come up behind her and was holding a small knife against her neck.

Karen immediately panicked but, for some unknown reason, rather than showing fear, she stated, 'If you cut my throat and we get blood on the floor… I bet you'll still expect me to clean it up for you.'

Brett moved the knife, smiled and laughed slightly. 'Probably,' he said with a smirk, and he put the knife in the washing-up bowl and then started putting the plates away.

Commentary: This is an extreme example that is based on a real event, and we would never recommend humour as an appropriate strategy in such a dangerous situation. But there are many situations just like this where calm humour has worked effectively in extreme circumstances. The lad involved was moved after the incident to a more secure setting – which may have been right or wrong – but staff should never be put in such a dangerous situation.

In Dan Hughes' PACE model mentioned in 'New-Logic Approaches', Chapter 6, page 59, the P stands for playfulness. Playfulness or a sense of fun has been proven to improve relationships and develop trust and attachment, especially in children who have never experienced much fun or play before. It should be used as an everyday attitude to deal with situations or as a way to build fun into everyday life. However, it can also be a way to redirect and can sometimes be a way of communicating, 'I know you are trying to get a reaction from me but you're not going to get it. Instead I'm going to use fun, silliness or paradoxical responses' (an opposite response to the one expected) 'to deal with this.'

Examples can involve anything from suddenly looking out of the window and claiming to have just seen a pigeon wearing dungarees fly past, to dropping down to do some press-ups and saying, 'If you're going to hit me, I'd better warm up first.' Or even claiming to be distracted by the thing on their ear that you can't identify.

CASE STUDY 36.4 THE SABOTAGE

Casey is at the computer and her foster mum, Gabby, is busy doing jobs around the house.

Gabby hears banging and comes downstairs to see Casey banging the printer and computer, shouting that she can't do her homework because the printer is broken.

When Gabby comes over, she sees that a kitchen fork has been put into the printer mechanism to stop it working.

Gabby explains, 'Look at that – there is a fork in the printer. What an amazing idea for a place to keep cutlery.' She walks off into the kitchen and grabs all of the spoons and forks from the cutlery draw and returns to the printer. She then begins to arrange the spoons and forks in the printer while narrating what she's doing. 'I think spoons on this side and forks on the other. It may make dinner taste a little funny, but they do say the first bite is with the eyes and our dinners are going to be very colourful now.'

Casey's expression changes from being very cross to confused, and now she starts to laugh. Gabby and Casey laugh together.

Gabby then says, 'Well, now we have sorted the printer, I'm wondering if you'd like some help with your homework?'

Commentary: This approach may seem counter-intuitive, as our instinct to punish the action of sabotaging the printer may seem strong. But what if Casey just doesn't know how to ask for help but needs it? So, yes, she has chosen an inappropriate strategy, and we may need to help her to learn better ones, but when she is already escalated she may not be able to accept the help, and it's hard to do homework or focus when you feel overwhelmed. Maybe she did the best she could by blaming the printer rather than feeling shame by saying, 'I'm too thick to do this work by myself.' Gabby allowed Casey to de-escalate and then helped her to meet her need for help. When everything is calm, they can talk about supporting Casey to learn better ways to meet her needs.

We first put out the fire; only after that do we try to learn from it.

PARADOXICAL RESPONSES

Doing the Unexpected

CASE STUDY 36.5 I WASN'T EXPECTING THAT!

1. Zeke is overwhelmed and is finding anything he can grab to throw in anger and distress. He even takes his shoes off and is ready to throw them.

   Tim, a caregiver, has an idea, and says to Zeke, 'Hey, tell you what – I bet you can't get that shoe into the bin.'

Zeke is distracted and takes up the challenge, and the situation is calmed.

2. Zoe is very angry; she's saying she is going to run away, and the two caregivers are feeling at a loss about what to do. Do they grab her to stop her leaving or walk away and ignore her? One of the caregivers spots a football and decides to try something different. He kicks the ball to his colleague and says, 'To you.' The caregivers start passing the ball between them, inviting Zoe to join them. Zoe yells, 'I'm not playing f***ing football.' But the caregivers are clearly having a good time, and after a few minutes, Zoe joins in; everyone ends up laughing.

REVERSE PSYCHOLOGY

Reverse psychology, also known as 'strategic self-anticonformity' if you ever want to show off your vocabulary, is a tactic that involves advocating a behaviour that is different from the desired outcome.

'I don't want you to do "A"' (but I actually do) or 'You should do "A"' (because I actually want you to do 'Z' instead).

The idea is that by pushing for the opposite of what you really want, the other individual will choose to engage in the behaviour that is truly desired.

While it can be seen as a way of managing another person's behaviour, it can also be used as a form of manipulation.

Reverse psychology has its pros and cons. It can be an effective way to alter behaviours, especially with individuals who have a tendency to not conform. However, it can make a person feel manipulated if they realise what's happening, which could damage trust. Also, it should not be used on individuals with low self-esteem, as they are more likely to conform due to their lack of confidence in their own judgement.

Reverse psychology should only be used sparingly, if at all, and we should be prepared for it to backfire.

Examples given in the article 'How Does Reverse Psychology Work?' by Kendra Cherry, MSEd are:[82]

- Discourage the desired behaviour. ('You wouldn't enjoy that.')
- Forbid the desired behaviour. ('Don't do that.')
- Suggest that the person couldn't do the desired behaviour. ('I'm not sure you can do that yourself.')
- Downtalk the desired behaviour. ('I wouldn't choose to do that.')
- Compare the desired behaviour unfavourably to something else. ('You should do this because it's so much better than that.')
- Encourage the behaviour you don't desire. ('I'm glad you are doing that.')

Always present these with acknowledgement that it's their choice. ('I wouldn't do that but it's your choice.')

> **CASE STUDY 36.6** I'LL DO WHAT I WANT
>
> Trevor was in the supermarket with Teddy. Teddy seemed to be in a difficult mood and was not coping well with shopping. Teddy said he wanted to go home now. Trevor responded that they were nearly done – just a couple more items to get.
>
> Teddy decided that this was enough, and he sat down in the aisle.
>
> Trevor knew he was in for a battle if he managed this in the wrong way.
>
> 'That's a brilliant idea Ted. If you stay down there, I'll know where you are, and you're pretty safe on the floor. I'll go and get the last few bits,' said Trevor with genuine appreciation.
>
> 'No!' Teddy shouted and stood straight up to walk with Trevor.

Commentary: You can potentially see an immediate issue with this example... what if it hadn't worked and Teddy hadn't moved, calling Trevor's bluff? Would it have been safe for Trevor to leave him there or would he have had to back-track? An alternative might have been to say, 'That's a good idea Ted. Let's take a rest – it's been a long day. I'll sit with you. Phew, it doesn't matter if we get home a bit later,' and for Trevor to sit on the floor near Teddy.

REDIRECTION/DISTRACTION

Redirection and distraction are often the most effective tactics when the need is unmeetable but we need to bring the situation to a close.

The strategy is best used if it is person specific, as what might redirect one person wouldn't redirect another.

In distraction, the focus is on trying to do something or show the individual something that simply gets their mind away from whatever is causing the stress. It's about managing the emotion.

Examples of distraction may include:

- changing the subject of conversation or asking a question that leads a person to refocus their mind elsewhere
- changing the environment, which may include turning on music or the TV, or relocating to a different room or outside
- changing the activity to an alternative that the person finds engaging, distracting and enjoyable.

In redirection, the focus is redirecting their behaviour to a behaviour or activity that is incompatible with the one we don't desire. If they are doing 'X', they aren't doing 'Y'. It's about managing the behaviour.

For example: if they are painting on paper, they are not painting the walls. If they are doing star jumps, they are not hitting out. If they are organising a tray of pipework at a table, they are not dismantling the sink in their room. If they are out having a walk, they are not harming themselves in their room.

In general, it is about redirecting the situation from one that feels overwhelming and unsafe to one that feels calm and safe.

CASE STUDY 36.7 I WANT MY MUM

Greta is 86 and lives in the dementia unit of a care home.

Manuel, one of the caregivers, discovers Greta on her own in one of the small side lounges looking very distressed. She is trying to move the furniture in the room to block the French doors to the garden.

'Greta, are you okay?' asks Manuel.

'No, they are trying to get in, we need to keep them out!' Greta says agitatedly.

'Okay Greta, you seem really scared. I'm so sorry you don't feel safe,' Manuel responds empathically.

'They want to break in. We must stop them!' Greta is still distressed.

'I understand. How can I help you to feel safer?' Manuel looks to connect and help Greta feel safer.

'Keep them out!' shouts Greta, moving closer to Manuel for comfort.

'Okay, let me check the doors... okay they are locked tight so no one can get in there. Why don't we go and check some of the other doors together and make sure the place is locked up tight?'

'Okay,' replies Greta, now appearing nervous rather than distressed.

As they move out of the room and begin going down the corridor, with Greta walking just behind Manuel's right shoulder, they pass the dining room.

'Shall we check in here Greta – see if it is safe?' 'Okay, it looks safe in here and Sharon is here. Shall we see if we can get a drink and rest for a moment?'

Greta sits with a cup of tea and Sharon sits with her. They begin to chat about the flowers on the table. Manuel carries on with his duties.

Commentary: Notice that at no point did Manuel confirm or deny what Greta was experiencing. He focused on Greta's feeling of being unsafe, which was true, whether the cause was or wasn't real. Once connected, he was able to redirect.

CASE STUDY 36.8 'QUICK! GET YOUR SHOES ON!'

Rashi was absolutely raging. One of his caregivers, Brinda, was at a loss.

Rashi had come from an abusive background, and he would often get stuck emotionally. This can be common – individuals want to reconnect and calm down but they can't let themselves. They especially can't let anyone else calm them, as that involves a willingness to relinquish control (this is not a fully conscious sensation). They perceive other people as unsafe and so letting others have control feels scary, which in turn increases the sensation of anxiety. Rashi was stuck at the top of the roller coaster.

Brinda could see that Rashi was stuck (his meltdowns would often change slightly, so she could see he was now stuck rather than escalating). She could also feel that her own emotions were in danger of taking over, so she needed to calm herself as well.

She used a strategy of distraction.

She mirrored the excitedness of Rashi's voice, saying, 'Quick! Come on, we need to go... Let's get our shoes on, quick, quick... Let's go!'

Rashi showed some curiosity but continued to rant and swear.

Brinda yelled, 'Well, that's all very fine, but... we need to get our shoes on, quick, and follow me!' and she started to walk to the back door.

Rashi didn't get his shoes, but he did follow Brinda, still giving unrelenting verbal abuse, shouting, 'Don't you turn your back on me you b***h.' Brinda was still mirroring his heightened emotions, in a controlled way.

She then started wandering around the garden in a highly agitated state, searching around, saying such things as: 'I can't believe I've lost it. It must be somewhere around here.'

Rashi continued his rant, but it was now interspersed with: 'What the f*** are you doing anyway?' He began to be involved – Brinda had engaged his frontal lobe, his rational, problem-solving brain.

After a while of walking around the garden, Brinda slowly started to calm herself down, slowing her pace and her breathing, saying, 'Oh, it must be here somewhere. I'm so silly. I'm wondering if I lost it when I came out earlier.'

After 10–15 minutes, Rashi began wandering around the garden looking at the ground, saying, 'This is f***ing stupid. I can't help you if you don't tell me what you're looking for.'

So Brinda had allowed him to calm. Well, he'd allowed himself to calm; Brinda had just given him a way to do it by distracting and redirecting him.

So it was a win-win scenario. Once he was calm, she discovered the 'lucky pebble' that she'd been looking for the whole time (a random pebble from the ground), but she made a big fuss about how finding this pebble made her happy.

Rashi told Brinda she was a stupid cow, but by now it was said from a completely different emotional state. Brinda laughed and took Rashi inside to grab a coffee.

So Brinda's aim was not to teach Rashi anything. It wasn't to prevent the behaviour from happening in the first place. It was purely to de-escalate, which is the aim of recognising escalation and responding appropriately.

An interesting follow-up to the story is that the same technique worked with Rashi a number of other times. Every time he began to rage, all Brinda had to say was 'Quick! Get your shoes!', to which Rashi would respond with: 'I'm *not* looking for that bloody pebble again.' And they'd both laugh.

Brinda had generated a close connection with Rashi.*

Commentary: This is more distraction than redirection, but it uses the positive mirroring strategy to engage rather than empathy. Also, creating curiosity was important to redirecting Rashi's behaviour from violence to searching.

ACTIVITIES THAT CAN CALM

In any situation that threatens to escalate, the following techniques can be used to restore and maintain calmness.

Important: Note that, in a state of escalation, the individual may not be acting according to their biological age. It is possible that they will temporarily regress to a more childlike state, and it may be helpful to go along with that.

Regression

CASE STUDY 36.9 REGRESSION

Charlie is in foster care and has been in placement for two years. The foster carers often have babies placed with them for short-term stays. When a new baby arrives in the house, Charlie struggles with the change.

Charlie regresses to a younger age, and behaviours that are assumed to have been grown out of seem to return (emotional tantrums, toileting problems, needing help with eating). Charlie's fears and anxiety of abandonment trigger this regression as an unconscious way to maintain attachment. (When feeling lost, we return to old pathways in the forest.) Rather than trying to fight this behaviour, Charlie's foster parents understand what is going on and allow Charlie to regress, as they know it is only a temporary step back. So, particularly at bedtime, they return to the slightly younger behaviour of reading Charlie a story and tucking him in with a drink... all to show that the nurturing he needs is still there for him.

* Brinda told this story to her friend, Sally, who worked in another place.

Later, Sally told Brinda about finding herself in a similar but even worse predicament. Sally was alone with a raging teenager at the top of some stairs. Sally told Brinda she'd tried the same distraction approach, but it hadn't worked.

Sally had got as far as getting the girl to follow her down the stairs but then broke the curiosity by saying, 'I want you to help me look for something.' At which point the teenager shouted, 'I'm not f***ing helping you to find any f***ing thing. You can just f*** off.'

But the teenager just walked away.

Brinda reckoned that Sally's approach may not have been 100% successful... but look at the outcome: Sally and the girl got away from the dangerous position at the top of the stairs, and the girl had de-escalated enough to walk away rather than become violent. Sometimes that still counts as a success.

Commentary: Regression is common when we feel vulnerable or overwhelmed. Many grown adults would still happily have their mum look after them when ill or feel the need for a cuddle when overwhelmed. ('When we feel lost, we find old paths in the forest...' is reference to 'Case Study 24.1 The Brain Is a Wilderness', page 219.)

Even old bad habits come back when we are stressed, like the businessman who has just been fired buying a pack of cigarettes after quitting smoking for years.

CASE STUDY 36.10 JANET AND JOHN

Alec, who is 25 years old, is autistic. At times, he becomes distressed. An effective way of restoring stability is to use a well-loved book from his childhood – a Janet and John book.

A member of staff stays in the room with him in a safe place and near the door. The caregiver begins reading the book: 'Janet and John had a ball. Janet and John had a big red ball...' And when they reach the end, they start again from the beginning, over and over.

Alec's initial state is great agitation – hitting things and hitting himself. But as the book is being read, he slowly starts to engage with the caregiver who is reading it, and begins to repeat a word (echolalia): 'ball, ball, ball...' The caregiver just carries on reading, and after a while, Alec joins the caregiver on the sofa and looks at the book with them.

Commentary: So what was going on here?

For Alec, the book represented predictability. He knew what was going to happen in that book. It helped him to cope with the unpredictability of the world and the chaos of his own mind by giving him something that was structured and predictable, and he knew what was going to happen.

In turn, that helped him to then regulate.

And that's sometimes why some of us, when feeling a little low, fancy watching a movie we've seen tons of times before – because we know we don't need to pay much attention. We don't need to work hard. We know what's coming. We know what's happening. We know the bits we like; we know the bits that we enjoy.

Part of our response to escalation can include activities that will help the individual to regain calm, bearing in mind the emotional age of the individual.

Breathing Exercises

For example, 'square breathing': first, draw a square. Focus on the top edge and breathe in for four seconds. Focus on the right edge and hold the breath for four seconds. Focus on the bottom edge and exhale for four seconds. Finally, focus on the left edge and hold for four seconds.

This exercise regulates breathing and slows people down.

Strong Sitting/Butterfly Hugs

This includes: hugging yourself; the feeling of a weighted blanket; sitting with a medicine ball on your lap.

Sensory Items

This includes: lights and sensory rooms; toys and fidget spinners; Rubik's cube; anything that will appeal to the senses.

Relaxation Therapy

For example, the spaghetti strategy – a piece of spaghetti is rigid, but it softens as it goes into the water. So, to use the technique, the individual first becomes a stick of spaghetti. They make their body rigid and tense: curl the toes, tense the calves, the knees, the thighs, the abdomen – all the way up.

Then imagine that stick going into the pot and slowly softening from the toes up. Relax the toes. Then the ankles – and wiggle them a little. Then the calves and so on.

This is a grounding technique. It includes mindfulness – they've got to be aware of their own body and it keeps them in the moment, focusing on something other than their issue at the time. It can also help with things like insomnia or whenever stress needs lifting.

Rhythmic Activities

This includes star jumps, skipping, dancing, playing drums, Tai Chi and so on. This type of activity is known as 'bilateral stimulus': two parts of the brain have to work together – in this case, the movement part and the emotional part.

Cosy Corner/Safe Space

This could be a cushion or beanbag potentially complete with weighted blankets, for example. The safe space could even be a tent, so the individual feels enclosed, safer. This should be a place where an individual enjoys spending time that allows a level of sensory input that best suits them and allows them to still feel engaged with other people if need be.

What Strategy When?

Thinking back to the escalation roller coaster, we have mentioned on a number of occasions that the specific tactics that should be implemented to de-escalate will vary depending on where an individual is on their escalation cycle. De-escalation is not an exact science, as there are not clear separations between the levels of escalation an individual can experience. We also need to remind ourselves that we are dealing with complex individuals with different likes, dislikes, personalities and fears, and they all experience the world differently. So a tactic may work with one person but not another; it may work one day but not another. Behaviour and the brain are an ever-changing landscape that we can predict in a similar way to the weather.

'They say that if a butterfly flaps its wings in the Amazonian rainforest, it can change the weather half a world away.' We can have an idea about what the weather might do but anything might change, and so we must be adaptable, flexible and reflective.

The next chapter discusses 'guided scripts' which can be used to indicate appropriate responses depending on a person's level of escalation.

CHAPTER 37

HELP, PROMPT, WAIT, PROTECT

There is a principle of guided scripts that can allow us to gauge to some degree what responses will be most effective depending on where a person is on the roller coaster. We also need to consider factors like safety, which is why the DAPPER approach should be used in all de-escalation situations.

The 'HELP, Prompt, Wait, Protect' strategy aligns with the escalation roller coaster. These tools can be used in succession but do not need to be followed in order if a behaviour rapidly escalates or escalation has occurred before the caregiver is aware. Throughout the stages, caregivers should ensure they:

- are better detectives than judges
- use clear appropriate communication
- use calm body language and voice or positive mirroring
- aim for calm and connection before correction
- allow appropriate wait time for compliance
- reinforce appropriate behaviours
- do not rush; de-escalation takes time
- envision positive outcomes
- demonstrate empathy, alignment and acceptance.

Caregivers should also maintain the DAPPER approach:

Maintain a safe and comfortable *distance* and *attitude*. *Position* and *posture* should signal non-aggression. *Empathise* and *read* the situation to understand feelings, but be aware of situational risks.

HELP STRATEGY (LEARNING/ STIMULUS OR TRIGGER PHASE)

The HELP strategy is used in the early stages of escalation and involves curiosity with or about an individual to understand what can be done to help improve their situation. In this stage, the individual may still have some rational control over their behaviour and be able to recognise their own needs or stressors. This stage requires the individual and the caregiver/s to stop and think about the needs or stressors (*human, emotional/cognitive, location* or *physical*) and then use communication skills to meet needs, reduce stress or explore choices available.

Human

Is someone in the vicinity irritating the individual? Can we remove that person? Is the individual seeking human contact from a particular person? Can we get that person?

Emotional/Cognitive

Is the individual experiencing bad feelings? Negative thoughts? Can we empathise with them? Distract them? Or is it safe to challenge their thoughts? Can we help them to feel safe or understood?

Location

Is there too much or too little going on? Is it too noisy? Can we fix it in any way? Do we need to change location completely?

Physical

Is the individual hungry? In pain? Tired? Can we fix the problem for them? Get them to work with us to fix the problem?

This strategy ideally requires that acceptable choices of alternative behaviours are pre-planned for the individual when they show signs of escalation. For example, leave to get a drink, go outside for a walk, time in or one-to-one activity, etc.

Usually, limited choices should be offered rather than an open choice: 'We can either do A or B – your choice' rather than 'What would you like to do?'

For example, 'You seem really upset and it seems to be making you angry. Now, we can carry on like this, and we're probably not going to get anywhere, or we can go for a walk and we can get ourselves calm, and then we can kind of figure out some solutions in a little bit... Would you like to continue our meeting calmly or would you prefer to stop now and come back tomorrow when things can be more relaxed?'

1. Approach using DAPPER in a non-threatening posture and tone of voice.
2. Notice a sign of escalation and refer to it (verbal attending, e.g., 'I notice you look a little tense – are you okay?').
3. Cue the individual to communicate what they want (or wonder with them).
4. Offer them choices.
5. Encourage them to make a specific request.
6. Allow five to ten seconds to respond.

7. Repeat prompt if necessary.
8. Acknowledge and reinforce an appropriate request ('I need a drink' – 'You need a drink') and then permit the action or meet the need immediately.
9. If they continue to escalate, consider the Prompt, Wait or Protect strategy.

PROMPT STRATEGY (ESCALATION PHASE – LOWER AND HIGHER)

The Prompt strategy involves asking the individual to do something that is incompatible with the actions they are currently doing.

Request and suggest, not command and demand.

1. Identify an incompatible or high-probability behaviour. A high-probability behaviour is something that the person already knows how to do, is simple and can be done right now (e.g., if someone is pacing, request that they sit down; do not tell them to stop pacing!).
2. Use the DAPPER approach, i.e., calm, non-threatening posture.
3. Prompt the desired behaviour in a neutral tone of voice (e.g., 'Please will you sit down'/'I need you to keep your hands still'). We can also use the 'when – if – then' formula here. ('When you sit down, we can find out what's upset you. If you rest your hands still, then I will help you.')
4. Allow five to ten seconds to respond.
5. Repeat prompt if necessary.
6. Reinforce cooperation and follow up with another high-probability behaviour.
7. If prompting does not work, move to the Wait or Protect strategy.

WAIT STRATEGY (HIGHER ESCALATION OR CRISIS PHASE)

The Wait strategy may involve waiting for the behaviour to decrease on its own. In some cases, interacting with the individual may escalate the situation, so it may be best to consider giving them some time and space to keep them safe. If it is not safe for them, or leaving them alone is inappropriate, we may be able to use:

- humour, paradoxical responses, redirection strategies
- time in, where we stay close to the person and allow them to use our calm behaviour and regulated breathing as a source of regulation
- five-step appeal, as described in the bonus chapter 'Tips for Improving Communication', which can be downloaded at https://library.jkp.com/redeem using the code ESGBAKQ.

Consider the following:

- Remove other people and dangerous objects from the area.
- Position yourself to keep you and the individual safe and manage other people/staff.
- Avoid reinforcing the individual's behaviour; minimum communication should be used.
- If there is significant danger to you, the individual or others, the Protect strategy may be required.
- As the individual calms down, consider using the HELP or Prompt strategy.

PROTECT STRATEGY (CRISIS PHASE)

The Protect strategy is a last resort when there is a risk of harm to the individual or others. Immediate intervention is required to either create space or limit movement, and that may require some use of physical force to achieve a safe result.

Consider the following:

- Has de-escalation failed or is it no longer safe to try?
- Can we switch with someone else or safely withdraw to a safe distance?
- Is some use of direct force (holding them or disengaging from their grab) or indirect force (blocking their path) required to manage the risk to them, ourselves or others?
- Is the force necessary? Have all other options been tried or are they unavailable/unsuitable? Is it the last resort?
- Is the force proportionate? What is the risk of the intervention (emotionally, physically and psychologically) versus the risk of not intervening (the level of risk from their actions)? Is the chosen action the least restrictive means or the minimum force we can use to safely manage the risk?
- Follow any pre-planned intervention and/or perform a dynamic risk assessment using APOP: Activity, People, Object, Place (refer to the bonus chapter 'Dynamic Risk Assessments', which can be downloaded at https://library.jkp.com/redeem using the code ESGBAKQ).
- As soon as it's safe, consider using the HELP, Prompt or Wait strategy.

POST-CRISIS

It is important to remember that even on the journey of de-escalation, the individual is still in a heightened state, and if de-escalation is not followed all the way back to a person's baseline (blue), then there is significant likelihood of re-escalation.

The HELP, Prompt, Wait, Protect strategy can be used in reverse as the individual goes back through the stages of escalation.

CASE STUDY 37.1 THE TALK-DOWN SCRIPT

(Wait) 'It's okay Denny, there is no rush. Once you feel calm, we can return to the group.'

(Prompt) 'Okay Denny. Well done for getting calm. I think we can head back to the rest of the group soon if you'd like... To let me know you are ready, can you just take two deep breaths for me? Ready?

'1... 2...

'That's brilliant, thank you.'

(HELP) 'Right, before we go back, is there anything I can do to help you feel better if you feel overwhelmed like that again?'

Commentary: It is important to remember that when we are putting out the fire, we are not trying to stop the fire from happening. When we are *responding*, our aim is never *prevention* in that moment.

Developing prevention strategies and proactive strategies should happen when a person is settled into their blue 'Comfort Zone'. They should be calm and thinking rationally. Prevention strategies should be based on proper post-incident reflection, not caregiver reactions.

As mentioned in Stage 3: Proactive Planning – and this is something that will be explored in Stage 6: Learn from Incident – natural consequences or balanced consequences may be an appropriate opportunity for learning. But if we initiate them during crisis, they are more likely to be perceived as punishment by the individual and others, and that only serves to damage self-esteem and trust.

The next chapter is about planned responses.

CHAPTER 38

PLANNED RESPONSES

So far, we have focused on responding appropriately to an unplanned event that needs to be dynamically managed. We may have little to no information on the triggers, stressors or history of an individual, and so ensuring that caregivers have the skills to manage and de-escalate these situations is vital to ensuring positive outcomes for all.

However, as previously explained, the true aims of the Target system and the 6STM are prevention, proactive management and planned responses, rather than relying on reactive strategies. So although initially we may have to fight the fires as we find them, we should be constantly developing an informed and empathic plan to manage, reduce or change maladaptive behaviours that challenge before they escalate.

The knowledge we have covered so far in Stage 5: Respond Appropriately can be used to develop individual plans but should also be used alongside those plans; i.e., we may have a plan to redirect a person to a preferred activity during the lower escalation stage (yellow), but if a caregiver follows the plan but then doesn't remain calm and empathic, the desired outcome may not be achieved.

Over time, we want to know what works best for any individual, depending on where they are on their escalation cycle. This plan will be developed and adapted over time as we learn more about the person and more about ourselves. By learning through repeated interactions, conversations and reflections, we can develop ever-improving strategies to improve an individual's quality of life, build positive relationships, alter the environment and improve our confidence.

Here is one example of a behavioural plan for Sam. Following Sam's plan, there is a link to the bonus chapter 'Clare and Margaret – Behavioural Plans', which contains behavioural plans for Clare and Margaret. Each one is based on an individual who has been mentioned in the case studies in this book. They are comprehensive and self-explanatory and offer examples of how behavioural plans should be created.

There are some slight adaptions between this example and the others available in the bonus chapter, and some have references to other tools. Each has a brief commentary that explains any elements that may be unclear.

Table 38.1 Sam's Behavioural Plan

Setting	Residential care home for adults with learning disabilities and complex behaviours
Name	Sam
Age/DOB	24
Gender	Male
Physical attributes, e.g., height, weight, etc.	5' 9" and 13 stone
Known medical conditions/diagnosis	Autism (non-verbal) Intellectual disability

Any known history of trauma:

None

Communication/learning skills and abilities:

Sam is described as an affectionate, gentle, kind young man, who displays empathy and compassion towards others; he is helpful, friendly and humorous.

Sam will engage with others but has no verbal communication; he tends to communicate using picture cards and charts. He sometimes communicates using sounds, gestures and signs. Sam has some Makaton skills but prefers pictures.

Sam can understand instructions that he is familiar with.

Sam responds to simple direct instructions given to him one at a time, e.g., Sam stop, Sam come this way.

Sam can focus on a task/activity if it is of interest to him; however, his concentration can be disrupted if other things are happening around him such as a noisy stimulating environment.

Sam can become frustrated and anxious when unable to effectively communicate his wants/needs, especially when emotional or if his cards and charts are not available. This could trigger a change in his behaviour.

Sam has many skills – he can dress himself if clothes are provided, he can bake with support from caregivers, he can make his own bed, tidy his room, hoover, set the dinner table, load the dishwasher, wash dishes.

Sam copes well with transitions away from activities if supported by trusted staff. Sam prefers slow transitions between activities (five-minute warnings).

Sam does like predictable routines, and each morning he likes to know what he is doing that day and who he'll be with.

Preferred activities	Sam likes watching several children's programmes and animal documentaries. He likes to use items/objects that provide stimulation (he has a bag that contains his sensory items) including his favourite head scratcher. Sam has ear defenders but dislikes them most of the time. He likes to put his hand in and out of boxes of Lego. Sam likes animals and can watch animals for long periods. He likes gardening, particularly touching soil and grass. He enjoys messy activities with mud. He loves to have his head massaged, as well as having his hair brushed.

cont.

	He likes to take a shower, especially with 'tingly' shampoo. Sam is very inquisitive and likes to see how things work. He likes to go for long walks (in quieter places with not many people about). He enjoys being in the car. He likes to listen to music. He likes to visit play parks. He likes to go swimming.
Disliked (non-essential) activities	Overly stimulated environments: such as a noisy environment or highly stimulated visual environments. Activities that require concentration. Unfamiliar places. Spicy food, hard fruit like apples. Strong wind that affects going outside (doesn't mind rain).
Preferred conversation topics	Sam likes caregivers talking about Transformers toys, cartoons and films, Sam's family (particularly his parents) and animals. Sam also likes staff saying words with K sounds: 'click clack, clip clop, clinking'.
Disliked conversation topics	None
Preferred people	Sam enjoys interacting with JH and TB, especially in the garden or while watching cartoons. Sam likes having breakfast with staff members John, Simon and Jim. Sam likes going to the park with John but prefers to go in the car with Simon.
Non-preferred people	Sam finds LT triggering due to the noise. Sam struggles with any staff who behave erratically or inconsistently.
Known behaviours that staff should not react to	Sam will often lie on the grass and stay there for 20 minutes or ignore staff when watching animals (unless urgent, Sam should be left). Sam will sometimes walk into a room, see LT and move away if he can't cope with him.
Target behaviours to be promoted	Sam should be encouraged to choose his activities. Sam should be encouraged to engage in activities with others and ones that promote independence (like cooking, personal hygiene, cleaning and laundry). Communicate using his picture charts. Use his sensory items when he is becoming overwhelmed. Re-engage in activities after breaks. To develop resilience during activities so he can complete them. To move to quiet and safe places when feeling agitated.
Potential reinforcers	Head scratcher, tingly shampoo, Lego, Transformers, *PAW Patrol* cartoons, animal documentaries, gardening and mud play, car travel with Simon, swimming, park with John, praise, thank yous.

Behaviours that challenge (maladaptive)	Functions/purpose
Hitting his head Pushing other individuals Ignoring some staff when not wanting to go inside Showing aggression towards staff	To feel in control As a means of communication To escape an activity To avoid people To gain an activity – change what he's doing To reduce anxiety and frustrations To gain something Avoidance Sensory stimulation To escape sensory overload
	Sam has good posture and is alert. He will engage in soft eye contact (he looks at your face), he is often smiling and he laughs randomly or at certain words or behaviours. He will walk around and often moves from room to room. He is happy to sit in a chair or lie on the ground while engaging in passive activities like sensory stimulus, TV. Sam will sometimes zone out when engaging in passive activity (he will stare at what he is watching or close his eyes).

Stressors

Routines: Getting ready in the morning, getting ready for bed, engaging in activities requiring focus.

Setting events: Broken sleep, lots of activities needing completion, transitions without warning, broken routines.

Specific stressors

Human	LT, being pestered when engaged in passive activities, non-planned activities transitions
Emotional/ cognitive	Continuous focus without breaks, when he thinks someone has caused an animal he is watching to run away
Location	Noisy, busy environments, wind
Physical	Tiredness

Strategies – Prevention

Set Sam tasks that are around ten minutes long, then offer a short break.

If Sam has had a bad night's sleep, only request completion of minimal activities, and avoid activities with LT.

Help Sam to set up a day schedule in the morning using a picture board day planner.

Plan garden/outdoor time into each day.

If it's windy, let Sam know by saying 'windy day'; plan other preferred activities.

Allow Sam to do tasks himself; don't take over from him.

Try to give Sam a five-minute warning before transitioning.

Ensure sensory bag with head scratcher, stress balls and picture cards/charts is available at all times.

Avoid environments that may trigger behavioural escalation.

Use simple, clear words when communicating with Sam and use a calm, neutral voice when giving verbal instruction.

Encourage Sam to show/express how he is feeling using pictorials/symbols.

Positive reinforcement and praise.

Don't interrupt Sam when zoned out watching animals, and avoid scaring them away.

Don't interrupt Sam when zoned out lying on grass.

Triggers – unmet needs		Proactive strategies:
Person	To avoid LT, overstimulation	Stimulus change/environmental management. Active listening and calm communication. Offer communication chart. Offer sensory aids. Use of distraction techniques offering alternatives. Apologise and redirect to alternatives if an animal being watched is startled away. If needing to redirect away from zone-out times say 'one minute', wait for two minutes and then redirect with alternative preferred activity before transitioning.
Tangible/ activity	To avoid an activity/ to maintain an activity	
Sensory	To escape noise, to gain head stimulus	
Help	n/a	
Control	To maintain control	

Green zone: Learning Zone Trigger phase	**Looks like:** When Sam is getting overwhelmed during an activity, he will keep pausing and rubbing his head with his hand. When Sam is getting overwhelmed by noise, he will sit and rock and rub his head. When Sam is irritated with someone, he will bare his teeth and thrust his face towards them. When Sam is not happy about a transition, he will sometimes pretend to zone out and stare into space.
Green: Responsive strategies	Offer Sam his communication chart and encourage him to use it. Acknowledge his feelings and meet his need. If Sam cannot engage with his cards, the head scratcher card should be shown and Sam should be redirected to a safe space and given his head scratcher for one minute and then encouraged to return to the activity if needed, or get him to choose a new activity if it isn't important to return. If Sam shows aggression towards someone, that person should give Sam more space by stepping back (DAPPER). If it is another individual, redirect Sam towards you by saying his name firmly and then smile and redirect to a choice of preferred activity. If Sam is pretending to zone out (check he has not spotted something that has caught his attention), say 'One minute' and then wait; after one minute, offer Sam his communication chart or offer a preferred activity.
Yellow to orange zone: Low escalation	**Looks like:** When Sam is getting overwhelmed, he will begin to slap his head with an open hand and show significant distress. When Sam is angry with a person, he will push them if they are too close.
Yellow to orange: Responsive: Prompt to Wait strategies	Staff should redirect Sam to safe space (garden, lounge 2 or bedroom) and give him his head scratcher: 'Sam to the (safe space), thank you.' Use calm and empathy, and then de-escalate and value his calming. If in garden, use redirection, in lounge, use TV, and in bedroom, use music to aid calming. Praise calming.

Red zone: High escalation	**Looks like:** Sam will be violently hitting his head with his hand and will not respond to verbal redirection. Sam can lash out with his fists and headbutt if his aggression becomes directed towards someone and they invade his space.
Red: Wait/Protect strategies to manage behaviour as safely as possible	Sam may respond to a physical non-restrictive guiding technique to be moved to his safe space, where he will continue to bang his head for usually no more than two minutes. If Sam is behaving in an unsafe way to others, follow dynamic risk assessment and either remove the object of his aggression or follow the procedure in Sam's physical intervention plan. Sam does not tend to escalate once held and tends to cooperate.
	Looks like: Sam will sometimes withdraw and not communicate immediately after an episode of head slapping. If Sam has behaved aggressively or had to be held for safety, once released, Sam may cry, and once he has calmed, he will often do the Makaton signal for sorry (this involves rubbing a clenched fist in a circle on his chest) and ask for a drink (sometimes with Makaton – action is like taking a drink, sometimes he will want to use his picture chart).
	If staff managed to intervene and Sam chooses to redirect to his head scratcher all day, Sam gets to use his 'tingly shampoo' in the shower before bed. When Sam is recovering from an emotional episode, he prefers people to stay close but not engage for a few minutes after. If he reached full escalation where he was hitting his head hard, it can be sore and he doesn't like his head scratcher; he will prefer other sensory items and soft lighting. He will often want a drink after and need some quiet time to fully calm. Redirecting to food can also work. If Sam has had to be held, once he has calmed, he will often do the Makaton signal for sorry (this involves rubbing a clenched fist in a circle on his chest). Staff can either say or sign 'okay'.

In Sam's plan, there is mention of his physical intervention plan – this is a document that should include any techniques that are used with Sam, including risk assessments.

Behavioural plans for Margaret and Clare are in the bonus chapter 'Clare and Margaret – Behavioural Plans', which can be downloaded at https://library.jkp.com/redeem using the code ESGBAKQ.

PART 8

THE 6-STAGE TARGET MODEL STAGE 6

Learn from Incident

CHAPTER 39

STAGE 6: LEARN FROM INCIDENT

The last stage of the 6STM is not the end; it is another step. It's a hugely important step for caregivers and individuals to develop and grow, recognise change and make improvements.

> *Mistakes are stepping stones to learning.*

As we move through this chapter, we will be examining a number of different tools and actions that should follow incidents but also underpin the whole process.

- Post-incident actions
- Correction and consequences
- Importance of post-incident recording
- Keeping accurate records: ABC analysis
- Risk assessments
- Monitoring effectiveness of measures taken
- Working with the individual to make change
- Continuing the 6STM

POST-INCIDENT ACTIONS

When an incident of a behaviour that challenges occurs, caregivers have three possible responses: ignore the behaviour, dynamically manage the behaviour or follow existing plans. All cases present opportunities for learning.

Ignoring the behaviour may be chosen because, although a caregiver sees a behaviour that challenges, they decide in the moment that it would be best to not pick a battle at that time. Or the caregiver may decide that paying attention to the behaviour carries a risk of escalation or accidental reinforcement. Nonetheless, there may be information about the incident that should still be examined or at least monitored.

For example, a person who usually likes to get up in the morning wants to stay in bed one day. Caregivers making an issue out of it may create problems and confrontation; maybe it's simply the case that the individual would just like to stay in bed to relax. On the scale of cost versus benefit (from 'Pick Your Battles', Chapter 8, page 77), the behaviour probably wouldn't meet the threshold of maladaptive (depending on what need there may be for them to be up). But if it becomes more regular, we may need to become more curious: 'Are they ill, depressed? Is it apathy or something else?'

So, to reiterate, when we refer to ignoring the behaviour, we are not ignoring the person, we are responding in the appropriate way.

With dynamic situations, we need to record and reflect on the incident to establish what worked, what maybe didn't work so well, what happened and why we think it may have happened.

When we have followed a behavioural plan, we should be reflecting and updating the plan based on incidents and other monitoring factors, such as mood monitoring, positive outcomes, skill and development.

Let's start by exploring actions to be taken immediately post-incident.

The stages below show the process we follow as we move away from the episode.

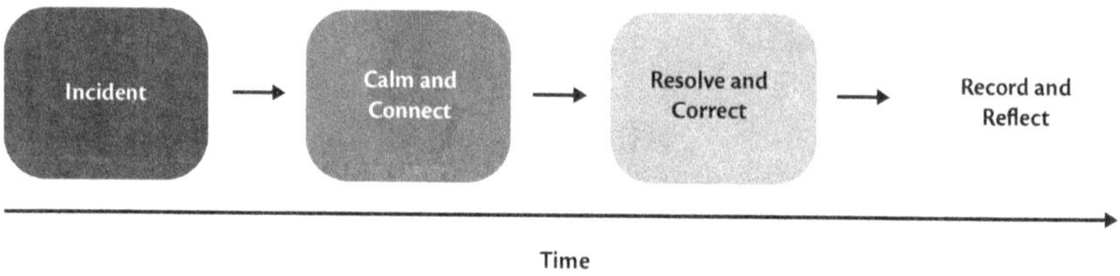

Figure 39.1 Post-Incident Process

First: We must help the person to regulate and calm their fight/flight/freeze responses through calmness and patience; then we should relate and connect with the individual through understanding and empathy.

Second: Once de-escalation occurs, we bring the episode to a resolution, find a solution and correct the situation.

Third: We can then support the individual to reflect, learn, remember, speak about the incident and become self-assured.

CORRECTION AND CONSEQUENCES

In Part 7, we looked at a number of strategies to bring escalation to a resolution or to find a solution and correct the situation for the individual. Sometimes it may be necessary to make a correction of the behaviour. In the section on proactive planning, Chapter 25, the section 'Natural Consequences and Balanced

Consequences' begins to describe how such consequences can be used as a teaching method that differs from punishment (page 242).

After an incident, there may be consequences that the individual may need to experience as a negative outcome to the behaviour to reduce the chances of it happening in the future. It is important to remember that our aim is to promote the positive rather than catch the negative. When initiating any consequence, we also need to be reasonable with our expectations, staying in line with an individual's abilities, history and developmental age.

If a young child breaks an ornament by accident, we may use it as an opportunity to explain a rule or a risk; we probably shouldn't jump to issuing a big consequence for their behaviour, as they are learning. We may give them the benefit of the doubt that it was a mistake. This same principle may need to be applied to an older child or adult, depending on our knowledge about them.

Natural consequences or balanced consequences often revolve around protecting, teaching or improving quality of life for an individual rather than seeking any kind of justice. The aim is not to shame or blame but just to help individuals recognise that actions have consequences. Sometimes the difference between a punishment and a consequence is in the way it is presented rather than the outcome.

For example: 'Right, because you behaved like that and hit another resident, you will not be going to the park now.' This is a punishment – it's a power play of authority: 'Because you did "X" I can take "Y" away from you.'

Alternative: 'Look, I know you've had a tough day, and you seem to be really struggling with your emotions today, but when you hit others, it shows that you can't be safe right now. It's not going to be safe for us to go to the park this morning. If we can work on getting calm and safe, we can try again this afternoon.'

Both of these examples have the same cost to the behaviour but there is no shaming or judgement in the alternative example.

Whether the consequence is natural or balanced, we should never gloat: 'I warned you.' We should recognise it as a mistake or an inability to make safe choices and recognise that it's okay to make mistakes and to find it hard to make safe choices but that these will have an impact on our outcomes. Growth comes from learning from mistakes and improving the choices we make.

Note: Initiating consequences can often increase escalation and emotional distress: 'It's not fair,' or 'You can't do that.' We must maintain our calmness, control our emotions and maintain our boundaries. We can still empathise with these feelings and can use empathic commentary to show understanding. Not getting what we want is not nice, and other people controlling us and our outcomes can feel distressing and hard. However, that's a natural part of life, and people need to learn to cope with frustration and suffering to develop and grow.

Let's revisit an example from earlier in the book to help us to understand why reactions to consequences may occur. It's worth rereading 'Case Study 6.5 "Please Sir, I Want Another Biscuit"', page 58, and the better way to handle the situation in Case Study 34.23, page 344.

If we are supporting individuals who have experienced negative behavioural management in the past, they may perceive a consequence as falling somewhere on the following spectrum. If we are initiating a consequence that either adds pain or removes pleasure, it may trigger an extreme reaction if the person doesn't feel safe. (Reactive, reflex reaction)

Abuse ◄———————— consequence ————————► Neglect

However, another reaction that may occur to an action having a consequence is an intentional behaviour (remember, this is not necessarily consciously) where the individual tries or has even learnt that an emotional reaction to the consequence sometimes works to avoid it: 'If I make a mistake and you impose a consequence but then I get angry or sad, you often take the consequence away.'

This is why, whenever we are either allowing a natural consequence to take place or instigating a balanced consequence, we should empathise with the individual's feelings. However, that doesn't mean we don't maintain the consequence, as long as it is appropriate. Over time, consistency and boundaries help a person to feel safe and build trust.

'I am so sorry we can't let you go to the park. Maybe you are feeling like we are being unfair, but I promise we are only doing that because we want everyone to be safe.'

Natural Consequences

Natural consequences are those things that happen in response to an individual's behaviour without caregiver involvement. These are imposed by nature, society or another person. We do not actually deliver a natural consequence ourselves. Natural consequences require us to not take action rather than take action.

- If a person refuses to eat, they go hungry (if we make them a meal later, there is no consequence).
- If they stay up late, they are tired the next day and may not enjoy activities as much.
- If they break a law, they get into trouble with the police.
- If they break their phone, they can't use their phone.
- If they are mean to someone, that person may not talk to them any more.

Natural consequences may seem like a very simple learning tool, but they have limitations.

- **They may not be safe**: 'If you play with matches, you will get burned' doesn't mean we can let a person play with matches to learn from natural consequences. We can always try to explain what the consequences might be so as to inform the person before it happens, but not every individual learns through explanation – their impulsivity, cognitive ability and core beliefs can get in the way.
- **They may not make the connection**: We cannot assume that because *we* see the connection of a behaviour and an outcome, everyone will make the same connection. Some people may need support to recognise the connection through explanation.

  E.g., 'Why is Billy not talking to me?' Our response might be: 'I think Billy might be upset about what happened yesterday. Sometimes when people feel someone has been mean to them, they feel that they can't be friends with that person for a while.'
- **The consequence may continue to impact on others**: If Jamie breaks the TV, the natural consequence is that he doesn't have a TV to watch anymore; however, that may then impact on everyone else in the setting, which we, as caregivers, may not feel is appropriate.
- **It may affect the person's rights or wellbeing (particularly if the consequence draws out over time)**: People have certain legal rights to such things as basic needs, liberty and safety, and we must uphold those rights if we have a duty of care. If a person smashes up their room, the natural consequence may mean their room stays that way. However, as we will see in 'Balanced Consequences' below, over time, this consequence may drag on and no longer facilitate learning – instead just impacting self-esteem.
- **There may not be a natural consequence, or it may not offer learning**: E.g., if an individual's behaviour only impacts on them and the consequence does not affect the person negatively, it may not add friction to the behaviour.

  If a person broke the TV but they weren't used to having working TVs anyway, they may not experience regret for their behaviour. We may also find that shame shielding (described in Chapter 15, page 140) may impact on a person's ability to accept responsibility for the consequence. (This is why, for some individuals, consequences don't offer opportunity for growth and why we must focus on the positive rather than relying on learning through consequences.)

If there is not a natural consequence available, we may have to use what are called balanced consequences (sometimes called 'logical consequences', as they are logical, not emotional).

Balanced Consequences

Balanced consequences should have the following qualities:

- **Short**: There is no benefit to dragging a consequence out over a long period of time; for individuals who have a limited ability to make connections to the past or the future, a point will be reached where no learning is occurring from the consequence – it will just reduce their quality of life – see the punishment cycle, described on page 238.
- **Immediate**: As above – initiating a consequence days after an incident may have no teaching benefit.
- **Relevant**: Any consequence should relate to the action. This allows individuals to better make connections between the two. If that connection is not obvious, the consequence may not work as a way of teaching.
- **Forgotten**: Once the consequence is acted on, it should not be mentioned in a critical way or dwelt on again. Both caregivers and individuals need to move forwards without any residual feelings they may have about the incident.

Let's look at some examples.

- **Taking back time**: If caregivers have had to take time out of their day to manage a situation, a balanced consequence may be to take time back. This means that we may need to catch up on jobs, activities or breaks, which may mean we don't have time to facilitate something the individual wants. This may need explaining using appropriate language. 'At breakfast time, when you got upset about your cereal not being available, you needed my attention for a while and that put me behind. I have some work I need to catch up on now. This means I'm not going to have time to do "X" with you now, but we can try again tomorrow.'
- **Safety**: If a person is in an emotionally dysregulated state, it may not be safe to take them in a car or for them to interact with certain people.
- **Fixing the mistake**: If we break something, we may have to contribute financially to replacing it, fixing it or tidying it up.

CASE STUDY 39.1 IT WASN'T ME

Anton had come from an environment of trauma, and unfortunately, one of his habitual behaviours involved deflecting through lying.

Anton's foster father, Isaac, came into the lounge and discovered one of the plants had been knocked off the sideboard, and the broken pot, soil and plant were lying on the floor. Anton was the only one home and so Isaac knew who had done it.

Old-Logic Strategy

Isaac: Anton, come here please. Right. What happened here?

Anton: It wasn't me.

Isaac: Anton – you are the only one here. I know it was you.

Anton: It wasn't... maybe it was the wind.

Isaac: There isn't any wind. Look, if you tell me the truth, you won't be in trouble, but if you lie to me, there will be consequences.

Anton explodes: It's always me, it's always my fault, you blame me for everything. I hate you.

Anton storms off.

Commentary: In this example, Anton lies as an intentional reflex to protect himself from abuse, so he lied automatically. When Isaac offered the choice of truth or lie, it is likely that Anton would be mistrusting of the choice, feel shame and feel the need to protect himself from shame by escalating to a meltdown and blaming. Isaac never managed to get Anton to admit it was him.

New-Logic Strategy

Isaac: Anton, come here please. Hey buddy, I have noticed this mess on the floor. We need to get it tidied up. Could you get the dustpan and brush from under the sink for me?

Anton: It wasn't me.

Isaac: I never said it was. We just need to get it tidied up before the girls come home.

Anton: Why do I have to do it – if it wasn't me?

Isaac: I understand that you don't want to do this, but we need to get it tidied. Tell you what – if you get the dustpan, I will get the vacuum and we can tidy it together.

Commentary: The consequence of breaking the pot was to tidy it, not to admit to lying about it. Anton may need to learn that mistakes have consequences but that those consequences are not dangerous for him. Over time, he may feel safe enough to tell the truth.

- **Showing sorry**: If we wrong someone, there is a cultural tradition that we should apologise. But 'sorry' is just a word, and although for many it's enough to make amends, for some it may not have a learning experience, as they have learned to just say the word to appease rather than feeling remorse. On the other hand, for someone who experiences a high level of shame, apologising to someone may be too intense for them emotionally.

  Showing sorry may include doing something nice for a person whom we treated badly or writing them a sorry note expressing our feelings.

There are times when specific consequences may be set in relation to rules, but it is always better to allow a person to be aware of any set consequences before their action to allow them to make a choice. We can then look to support them in improving their ability to make choices that are in their best interests rather than looking to punish mistakes. We will look at rule setting later in the chapter.

Making Mistakes as a Caregiver

It is worth acknowledging that as humans we make mistakes during incidents or even post-incident. We have emotional responses to situations and that may result in a reaction at times. We may raise our voices, behave in ways that escalate a situation or threaten or initiate consequences that are not appropriate or don't follow the SIR rule (short, immediate, relevant). If we realise that we have made a mistake or behaved in a way that was emotive rather than logical, it is important that we amend our mistake. This can feel hard, as it may feel as if we are backing down or showing weakness, but in actuality, we are demonstrating humility and honesty and, as discussed in 'Teaching Technique: Role Modelling', Chapter 25, page 225, these are positive attributes to be modelled rather than negative.

Having the courage to say sorry, and to accept a mistake or a loss of emotional control as steps to learning, should be seen as something to be developed, not as something that makes us bad. We should value such attributes in ourselves and in others.

Reflection

After an incident, there should be opportunity for reflection. As outlined in Figure 39.1, the opportunity for reflection should be taken as the final stage of de-escalation, ideally when everything is calm.

Depending on the individual, the circumstances and the environment, this may be performed at different times for different individuals, and it may not always be appropriate for the individual to be involved.

As mentioned, reflection may be for us to reflect back on *our* behaviour, reactions and emotions to ensure we are doing the best we can.

In some settings after incidents, staff may have an official debrief.

The purpose of the debrief, the *reflection*, is *not* to blame or shame anyone. It is not to criticise or point out mistakes. It is to be non-judgemental and non-critical.

The purpose is:

- to be solution focused: 'Let's not focus on what went wrong, let's look at what we can do to make it better'
- to use any mistakes as a stepping stone to learning
- for caregivers to ask, 'Did we pick the wrong battle?'

- to ask ourselves, 'Did we contribute to the escalation, instead of the goal of de-escalation? If so, do we need to review our behaviour using the 6STM?'
- for the caregiver to ask, 'What have I learned about myself? Why did I behave like that? Why did I choose to have that battle if it wasn't necessary? Did I lose control of my emotions? Did I give up and walk away? Was I scared for my safety?'
- to establish what worked well and what didn't – were things said that should/shouldn't have been said? Be careful not to focus on the negatives – that's easy to do
- to ask, if a de-escalation strategy worked, whether it could have been tried sooner
- for caregivers to ask, 'How do I feel about the individual? How will I cope next time I see them? What self-care strategies will I need?'
- to learn from the incident and move forwards to what would be done differently next time and not repeat the same mistakes.

For the individual, it's a chance for caregivers to learn from them, covering the following points:

- What was wrong for them? How did they feel at the time? What were they trying to achieve? We should also use the skills described in Chapter 32, page 311, and its linked bonus chapters. We want to demonstrate curiosity.
- Find out how the individual feels about what happened. Do they feel anger, shame? Do they feel bad about it?
- To ask the individual if anyone could have done something differently to improve the situation.
- This is often a chance to identify that a certain course of action will produce a certain consequence, but a different action will produce a different consequence. And if a certain outcome is preferred by the individual, we can ask how we can move towards that.

The cycle in Figure 39.2 is for caregivers to work through post-incident.

Straight after the incident, when it is safe, caregivers should record details of what happened. In some settings, this may involve incident reports; in others, perhaps writing in a journal.

Details should always include WWWWH: **What** happened before, during and after, **where** did it happen, **when** did it happen, **who** was there and **how** was it managed?

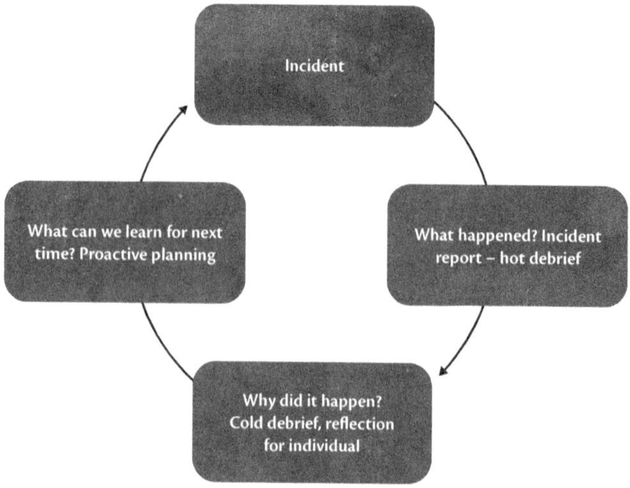

Figure 39.2 The Reflection Cycle

IMPORTANCE OF POST-INCIDENT RECORDING

The Benefit of Recording

We can learn from an incident if it is properly recorded. Documentation can be referred to again and again, whereas people's memories can fade and become distorted.

When there is a series of documents concerning similar incidents, our ability to spot patterns and draw conclusions is greatly increased.

During Stage 1: Identify, it may be decided that incidents involving a particular behaviour may require full Functional Behaviour Analysis using multiple ABC charts to look for patterns or clues to the reason/cause or function/purpose of the behaviour.

The process of recording incidents can also allow us to:

- identify potential future risks
- contribute to effective planning for an individual
- improve risk assessment
- identify training needs.

'Hot' and 'Cold' Debriefs

If an incident has occurred that has been particularly stressful, emotional or even traumatic for the caregiver/s, it can be appropriate to have a 'hot' debrief immediately afterwards. This could be a caregiver talking to a trusted person who will allow the caregiver to express their emotions about what happened, while remaining objective and non-judgemental towards all parties involved.

With emotions possibly still high, there may be blaming and criticism, but these can be a useful way for a person to 'get it out of their system' and de-escalate themselves.

After the incident is logged, usually within 24 to 48 hours of the incident, it is advisable to carry out a 'cold' debrief – to reflect on what happened.

This may just be an informal meeting of the caregivers involved to reflect on the incident – of foster parents or parents sitting together in the evening and having a chat about what happened – or more formal interviews and review by a supervisor.

One of the focuses of incident logging and reflection is to make improvements. This may include environmental improvements and adjustments to behavioural plans, care plans and risk assessments.

KEEPING ACCURATE RECORDS: ABC ANALYSIS

For behaviours that are assessed as maladaptive and in need of management or change, it may be necessary for caregivers to record specific details about those specific behaviours. The information recorded in the ABC analysis can be tracked and analysed – using the principles of 'understanding' as described in this book – to find an individual's motivation for the behaviour. Why this? Why now?

The ABC analysis has four main components:

- **Setting events**: Any known factors that could have impacted on the individual's behaviour (e.g., tiredness, change in routine, etc.).
- **A – Antecedents**:
  - A step-by-step description of exactly what we observed prior to the behaviour. Was anyone else around or had anyone just left? Had a request been made of the person or by them? Had an activity just ended or been cancelled? Where were we and what were we doing?
  - Where did it happen? ('In the dining room.')
  - Who was there? ('Janet (caregiver), Maisie (resident).')
  - When did it happen? ('Breakfast time, 8:15.')
  - Other observations. ('It was quiet that morning, not many people about.')
- **B – Behaviour**: A step-by-step description of exactly what the person did; e.g., 'He ran out of the living room, stood in the kitchen doorway and punched his head with his right hand for approximately one minute.' The action's duration, and any changes in the behaviour, should be detailed.
- **C – Consequences**: What happened after the incident.
  - Step-by-step description of the exact events that occurred immediately after the behaviour. How we responded to the behaviour. How

the person responded to our reaction; e.g., 'When Janet approached to de-escalate, Tim seemed to become more distressed.' How others responded to the behaviour. Did the person's behaviour result in them gaining anything they did not have before; e.g., attention from somebody (positive or negative), an object, food/drink or an escape from an activity or situation?

- Who was there (maybe someone left or someone arrived)?
- How did the incident end? ('Janet managed to calm Tim down by offering him some coffee.')
- When did it end?
- Who else was affected by the incident? ('Maisie became distressed.')
- Other observations.

Here are some examples of very basic ABC reports:

Table 39.1 Example ABC Report 1

Setting events	None
Day and time	Thursday 2pm
Antecedents: Location, people, activity	Jessica was in the dining room at a table by herself. SM was asleep in corner chair. Pete and Gill (staff) were in and out of the room. Gill went over to see if SM wanted a drink.
Behaviour	Jessica vocalised an Urrgghh sound and then started banging her head on the table. She was hitting the table hard enough to shake the table. She continued making a crying-type noise.
Consequences: What happened, how did the person react?	Pete and Gill went over to Jessica. Pete moved the table away. Gill talked to Jessica and firmly stroked Jessica's back. Jessica continued to vocalise for a few moments, then sat back and seemed to calm.
Potential stress and unmet need	Jessica felt distressed or lonely and wanted either attention, help or sensory input.

Table 39.2 Example ABC Report 2

Setting events	None
Day and time	Tuesday 8am
Antecedents: Location, people, activity	Sam was cleaning his room, independently dusting and wiping the sides in his room for five minutes. Isabel (staff) was in the room. Sam started touching his head and making huffing noises.
Behaviour	Sam started hitting his head hard with his hand.
Consequences: What happened, how did the person react?	Isabel took the cleaning material away and gave Sam some space, and after two minutes Sam stopped hitting his head. Sam communicated sorry in Makaton, then asked for a drink. Jessica brought this over.

Potential stress and unmet need	Sam was feeling bored or overwhelmed. He needed sensory input and/or to stop the activity.

Table 39.3 Example ABC Report 3

Setting events	Tim had a disturbed night's sleep
Day and time	Sunday 7.30am
Antecedents: Location, people, activity	Tim was eating his breakfast. Coco Pops. PT came into the room and got himself a bowl of cereal and then left the room. Kayleigh (staff) walked into the room and said 'morning' to Tim.
Behaviour	Tim replied with 'f*** off'. Kayleigh told Tim, 'There was no need for that, I was only saying good morning.' Tim threw his bowl towards (not directly at) Kayleigh. The bowl smashed and cereal/milk went all over the kitchen. Tim then ran out of the kitchen and up to his room.
Consequences: What happened, how did the person react?	Tim stayed in his room for over an hour. Jim (staff) tried to talk to Tim in his room, but Tim refused to respond. Jim could see Tim was upset and needed some time to himself. Jim said he would stay nearby in case Tim needed him. Jim sat on the stairs for a bit until Tim came out and said he was hungry. Jim took Tim downstairs, and they got a snack. Tim still refused to say what was wrong.
Potential stress and unmet need	Tim was feeling, low, angry or depressed. Tim didn't like PT not engaging. Tim wanted to avoid people, gain control.

Table 39.4 Example ABC Report 4

Setting events	None
Day and time	Sunday 11am
Antecedents: Location, people, activity	Margaret was sitting in her room in her chair.
Behaviour	Margaret started to shout the name 'Molly' over and over and seemed distressed. She seemed more agitated when staff asked her what was wrong and seemed to be looking for someone over the staff members' shoulders.
Consequences: What happened, how did the person react?	A staff member brought in a drink for Margaret, and she seemed to settle.
Potential stress and unmet need	Margaret was distressed and upset. Margaret needed a person, 'Molly', or a drink.

The written language used should be plain and free from jargon. The individual who is the subject of the document should ideally be able to read and understand the report, if they wish to.

In turn, these ABC records inform the other stages of the 6STM.

After a plan has been created, we can continue to use ABC charts to examine successes or mistakes in the plan. We are looking to detect improvements such as fewer incidents, lower intensity and shorter duration.

When creating the plan, it is important to manage these expectations. We need to be able to celebrate the little successes and steps in the right direction. These successes should encourage caregivers to focus on the positives for themselves, as well as the individual.

RISK ASSESSMENTS

When there is a risk of violent or hazardous behaviour that could affect the safety of anyone within the setting, a risk assessment should be carried out. Risk assessments are a legal requirement within workplaces, but the process should be followed in all environments to ensure wellbeing and safety. Many people perceive risk assessment as meaning applying 'common sense'. The issue with this is that recognising hazards and risks is an ability that can vary based on experience, cognitive ability, emotional state and sensory abilities and therefore that 'sense' cannot be assumed to be common. We have to assume no common sense and then create a 'common sense' through the risk assessment process. Risk assessments may need to be general to the setting or specific to the individual.

CASE STUDY 39.2 BABY PROOFING

When a family have a child who reaches the age of free movement and is able to move around and get into mischief, steps are often taken to make the environment safe. Cupboards and drawers may have childproof locks added, medication is put out of reach, the pond outside is covered and even ornaments and furniture may be assessed to ensure their suitability.

Over time, the child will be taught what is unsafe and can harm them, and how to navigate the world without such restrictions.

CASE STUDY 39.3 DEMENTIA FRIENDLY

Vera has recently been diagnosed with Alzheimer's disease after her daughter, Anthea, noticed some areas of day-to-day life that Vera seemed to be really struggling with. Vera desperately wanted to stay at home and so Anthea felt some changes needed to be made to help Vera to be safe and happy within her home. After some research, Anthea made some changes.

Anthea started prepping food and placing it in tubs labelled with the day it should be eaten. (One of the issues that flagged Vera's illness was her skipping meals and having a fridge with out-of-date food in it; Vera had contracted food poisoning after eating some 'off' food due to not realising that it smelt 'off'.)

Anthea took photos of the inside of cupboards and wardrobes and placed the photos on the outside of the doors so that Vera could better orientate herself and find things more easily. She also added a red 'T' to the bathroom door to help Vera find the toilet.

Anthea added some labels to the shower and bath clearly showing the hot and cold taps and also turned the boiler down to reduce the risk of Vera burning herself on hot water.

Anthea also increased the brightness of the bulbs around the house to help Vera see, and she put some coloured tape around light switches so that Vera could better find them (white switches on white walls can be hard to see). Vera was struggling with her balance and was at risk of falls, especially in the dark.

CASE STUDY 39.4 COPING WITH HUBERT

Hubert is 15 with learning disabilities and autism and has grown into a big, strong young man. Unfortunately, Hubert, while often a gentle and kind young man, has become unpredictable with his aggression, particularly towards his mum. Recently his mum was badly hurt during an episode where Hubert became overwhelmed and hit her. Social services have become involved.

Hubert's mum is offered support. She receives some training to better understand her son; this includes teaching her behaviour support, de-escalation and some skills to protect herself from strikes and to escape from grabs to increase her confidence if an episode happens again. She is also directed towards some parent support groups that include other victims of child-to-parent abuse and parents of autistic children. It is also decided that Hubert needs more time away from his mum, and so some respite is arranged and plans are made for Hubert to attend a day centre on some weekends to give Hubert's family a break and give Hubert some positive opportunities to gain some independence, make new friends and experience new opportunities.

After the training, Hubert's mum decides to invest in turning the spare room into a sensory space for Hubert to go to reregulate. The space includes beanbags and soft play shapes as well as sensory lights and bubble lamps.

Commentary: In these examples, the people responsible have looked at their environments and assessed the risks to try to make it safe for the people they care about based on their vulnerabilities. Some of the controls are preventative and some are precautionary, but all contribute to improving the situation and reducing risks.

Figure 39.3 shows the typical steps to be followed in any risk assessment.

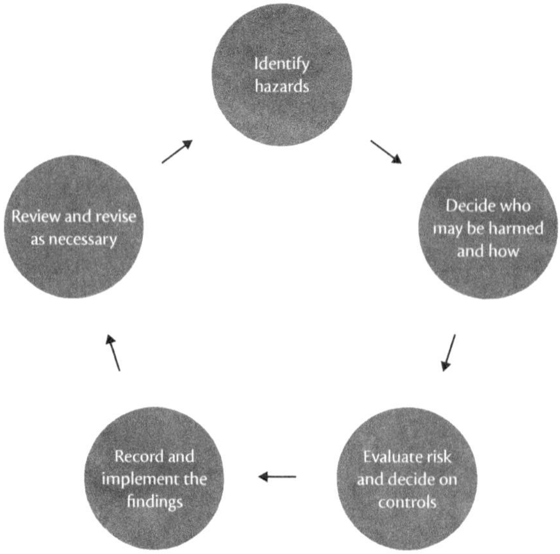

Figure 39.3 Risk Assessment Cycle

1. **Identify hazards**: A hazard is anything that could cause harm; this may include situations where violence could occur or be based on any behaviour that could cause harm.
2. **Decide who may be harmed and how**: This would include the individuals themselves, caregivers and anyone else within the setting. Factors that might affect the risk would depend on multiple elements ranging from mobility to sensory abilities, cognitive abilities and vulnerabilities (e.g., vulnerable to sexualised behaviour due to past experiences). For caregivers, it may include caregiver-to-individual ratios, the nature of activities and experience.
3. **Evaluate risk and decide on controls**: How likely is the possible event to occur, and what would be the likely severity if it did? This may be low, medium or high. Low risk may be considered an acceptable risk but medium to high would mean that control measures should be explored to reduce the risk to a reasonable level.

   It is neither possible nor necessarily desirable to achieve 100% 'no risk'. But risks should not cause significant harm.

   Once risks are recognised, we then can decide what controls and/or actions would be needed to reduce the risk. We would need to assess whether the controls are reasonably practicable – that the cost, effort and time required is in proportion to the risk it is preventing (e.g., we wouldn't spend thousands to prevent a stubbed toe, but we would to save a life) and also socially valid (see 'Testing the Social Validity of Interventions', Chapter 26, page 254). For example, Hubert's mum would never be trained in applying handcuffs to Hubert in a meltdown to protect herself from being hit.

4. **Record and implement the findings**: Writing this down allows everyone in the setting to be aware of the risks and controls, but this must be a living document that is updated and adapted based on changes.
5. **Review and revise as necessary**: People change, environments change, circumstances change or we may need to review after any incident that shows the current controls are not adequate.

Hierarchy of Controls

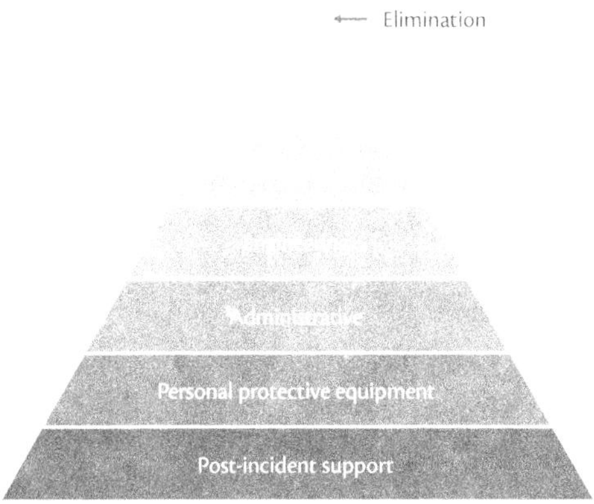

Figure 39.4 Hierarchy of Controls

- **Elimination**: The most effective way to reduce a risk is to remove it. Elimination of some behaviours is not always possible or at least may take time, but elimination may include actions that remove items that could be used in harmful ways; e.g., removing ligature points or ligature material to prevent suicide or removing batteries for someone who eats batteries to self-harm. It may also include removal of particular triggers from a setting to reduce distress (whether that be a person, object or activity).
- **Substitution**: If elimination is not available, we may have to substitute the hazard for an alternative; e.g., choosing an item that would make a less effective weapon or would not cause harm if used with intent on themselves or others, or in 'Case Study 39.3 Dementia Friendly' above, substitution of lightbulbs and labelled meals to make the environment safer.
- **Isolation**: This doesn't necessarily mean isolation of the person, although sometimes the safest way to manage an incident of violent behaviour may be to give the individual some space. It may include

removing the audience or even ensuring the environment is safe before initiating an activity that we know may cause escalation; e.g., if we need to inform Tom that his family is not coming, we should do this in the second lounge rather than his bedroom because caregivers will have more room to give him space and there are usually no other individuals in that space.

- **Engineering**: This might include adjusting the environment to reduce risks, like ligature-proof door handles and picture frames being screwed rather than hung on the walls. It may also include how a room is laid out; e.g., providing more than one exit, providing more space or installing alarm systems, nurse-call systems and CCTV.
- **Administrative**: This control measure introduces the caregiver to the process. It requires people to follow the risk assessment and follow plans and procedures. We have to consider that people make mistakes, and therefore, once we reach this control measure, the effectiveness of it will depend on consistency and boundaries.

  Examples here may include reviewing the caregiver-to-individual ratio for safety or caregivers following specific processes in regard to specific activities or how they manage engagement with a specific individual. Knowledge about how to fulfil their role safely and competently may require training. However, training does not make people safer or better at their role... it is only the application of that training that improves outcomes. That may mean that part of this control measure should include ensuring that the training is being applied. This control measure may include all policies, documentation and review processes.
- **PPE**: This includes PPE such as bite-proof jackets, scratch-proof gauntlets and hats to prevent hair grabs. PPE only works as a control if it is used correctly and appropriately, and it only protects the person who is using it. Ideally, other controls will take away the need for such things, but as a last resort it may be necessary.

CASE STUDY 39.5 USE OF PPE

In some settings, complaints have occurred as some caregivers have claimed that bite-proof jackets don't work. Their reasoning has been that 'by the time the incident happens, there's no time to put on the jacket'. This is not how PPE works.

Take the example of a building site: a worker is not going see a falling brick and decide, 'Now's the time to put on my hard hat.' As the risk is unpredictable, the PPE is worn whenever there's *potential* for a problem, not when the problem occurs.

- **Post-incident support**: Part of the risk assessment should include what to do if something still occurs. This is equivalent to having first aiders (first aiders don't prevent the risk but they still act to reduce the severity if a hazard occurs), so in relation to behaviour post-incident, topics such as psychological support, supervision, caregiver wellbeing programmes and ensuring self-care strategies are used can be considered.

MONITORING EFFECTIVENESS OF MEASURES TAKEN

No setting always gets it right first time. As long as the aim is growth and improvement, we know we are on the path to improving outcomes.

Monitoring the effectiveness of the behavioural plans, risk assessments and strategies is important for not only analysing strategies but also the psychological benefit of seeing positive results.

In many situations, caregivers can get caught up in the perceived failures of strategies rather than seeing the successes. As has been discussed throughout the book, humans innately tend to focus on the negative. Sometimes, when you are so close to a situation you can't see the wood for the trees, it can feel like no progress is happening.

Think of the example of losing weight. A person on a diet looking at themselves in a mirror every day may see no change and feel they are not getting anywhere and be at the point of giving up. But then they meet up with a friend whom they haven't seen for a few months and their friend is blown away by how much weight they have lost.

If the dieter had taken body measurements every week and logged them, they would clearly see the inches/centimetres disappearing and the step-by-step improvements.

We can apply this same principle to behaviour. When creating the plan, we should have an idea about what we want our outcome to be. We then want to measure:

- any increase in target behaviours
- any decrease in frequency, intensity or duration of any maladaptive behaviours.

We have included all three aspects of the maladaptive behaviours, as any reduction in any of these is success. Suppose, for example, an individual's meltdowns used to happen every day, be a significant danger to themselves and others and typically last 30 minutes. Improvement would include: 'Meltdowns tend to now be de-escalated in 15 minutes and a caregiver is now safe to stay in the room with them, even though meltdowns are still occurring every day.' This doesn't mean the journey is complete, but acknowledging the improvement can give hope to everyone involved.

Let's think back to 'Case Study 20.5 Tania, the Survivor', page 185, about

Tania, who self-harms. Initially, she may be cutting every day, so even if that behaviour reduces to every other day, we have made progress. Over time, the gap between the behaviours increases, and the hope is that we reach a period where we can't remember the last time she self-harmed.

If we continue with Tania's monitoring, we may find that it seems that going for a run (one of the steps in her strategy instead of self-harm) works best at reducing her distress. So the caregivers can discuss with Tania whether she would be interested in joining a running club and begin to support her in making running a regular hobby rather than just a strategy.

By exploring through evidence (records) what works and what doesn't work, outcomes can be improved by adapting the plan.

Mood Monitoring

Mood monitoring is a process in which caregivers, and/or an individual, regularly monitor the individual's emotional state during each day over a period of time.

This can be used as part of introspection work in Chapter 31, page 300.

The following categories can be used to separate the levels and types of emotions:

1. **Blue**: Happy, calm, relaxed.
2. **Green**: Uncomfortable, nervous, excited, agitated, restless.
3. **Yellow**: Anxious, sad, disappointed, annoyed.
4. **Orange**: Angry, frustrated, irritated, cross, stressed.
5. **Red**: Rage, frightened, overwhelmed, hyper.
6. **Purple**: Low, shutdown, empty, nothing, disconnected.

The goal, of course, is for an individual to mostly be 'blue'. If these colours can be added to a chart, the amount of 'blue' and 'not blue' can easily be seen. The 'not blues' can then be analysed.

Mood monitoring can be used for psychoeducation (teaching individuals about feelings). The aim is to raise self-awareness; from there we can help individuals to improve their self-management.

We can also use it as a tool to help individuals with self-regulation by getting them to explore the range of possible emotions a person can have in response to situations.

For example, let's look at the use of a word like 'anger'. If we say a situation makes us angry, it denotes one reaction or behavioural response. However, if we explore the scope of emotions that are similar to anger – frustration, irritation, annoyance, fury – it can allow us to view emotions as a spectrum and range of feelings that can be managed or expressed differently.

CASE STUDY 39.6 CEREAL WOES, AT A PUSH

Jomo was doing some reflection with a trusted caregiver at his weekly review.

Jomo's emotions chart showed that he had experienced a couple of red episodes (rage) through the week.

One was triggered by his favourite cereal not being available that day.

The other was when Jomo was pushed by someone.

The caregiver used these two examples to help Jomo examine the difference in severity of the two incidents and then look at how these maybe deserved different emotional responses.

If Jomo feels emotional if his favourite cereal is not available, rather than triggering a 'red' rage, could Jomo recognise his emotion and dial it back to 'yellow – disappointed'?

We can also use mood monitoring as a way of gauging positive outcomes for individuals. Is the individual feeling happier generally on a day-to-day or week-to-week basis? We can use it alongside incident reports to learn stressors and triggers for emotional responses and patterns of moods.

WORKING WITH THE INDIVIDUAL TO MAKE CHANGE

As explored in various sections of the book, the individual should be at the centre of their care and should be included as much as is practicable in the process of improving their outcomes and quality of life. Encouraging them to reflect on experiences is an important aspect of independence and autonomy. Working in collaboration to explore what they would like in life and what skills and changes they may need to work on to help that to happen is an opportunity that every individual should receive.

Helping individuals see how their choices and behaviour impact on their outcomes, and improving their self-esteem through successes, achievements and improvements, is the main philosophy of the whole process.

We need to be gentle; change for anyone can be stressful and difficult. Being open to change and opportunity can seem scary and uncomfortable and is a journey with no distinct end. The importance of trusted helpers is vital. For many of us, these trusted helpers have been parents, friends and role models, but for many people in care, this has not always been available or in some situations is no longer available. This may be due to early circumstances or life experiences. For many, through no one's fault, the needs, challenges or complexities of the individual's condition, disorders, illness or disabilities mean that the individual hasn't been or is no longer understood.

Whether a child with autism, an adult with mental health concerns or an adult living with dementia, everyone needs people to step into their world and support them as they navigate this maze called life – sharing in successes, supporting in mistakes, showing good paths while accepting that wrong paths may need to be tested but providing the tools, aids and skills to get through.

Collective Negotiation Technique

This technique is a process of exploring a conflict between the behaviour of the caregivers and the behaviour of the individual.

This often includes situations where caregivers are trying to support positive choices for an individual but the strategy seems to be making things worse rather than better, and it's becoming a battle of wills rather than a collaborative endeavour.

At least two people will be involved when using the technique – the individual and a caregiver. But other people who are affected by the situation can be invited, with the individual's approval.

The problem is defined and agreed by all. Both parties explain their point of view of what they find difficult.

For example:

1. Individual: 'I don't like being made to have a bath every day.'
1. Caregivers: 'We are sorry if you are feeling like we make you; we don't want you to feel like we are forcing you to have a bath. We just want to ensure that you are clean and comfortable for your health; but also, smelling nice can encourage people to want to spend time with you.'
2. Individual: 'I don't want to get up so early.'
2. Caregivers: 'We don't like having to rush you to get to college, so we want you up early to give us plenty of time.'
3. Caregivers: 'We don't like it when we have to ask you multiple times to do your chores.'
3. Individual: 'I want to do my own thing and play on my Xbox without being nagged.'

These examples are only a few ideas of potential points of view. The individual should be encouraged to express their feelings about an issue and the caregiver should be mindful to remain non-critical and rational. Or the caregiver can raise a concern and allow the individual to express their own point of view.

We may try to explore any reasons why the individual feels the way they do to see if there are underlying issues (e.g., what don't they like about bathing every day, how do they feel when asked to have a bath?) but otherwise we move on to the next step.

From this point, everyone brainstorms possible solutions to the problem and these are written down for all to see. There should be no constraints on the orthodoxy of proposals... it's a wide-open field, and even out-of-the-box ideas may spark a good solution.

If we take number 1:

- Bath once a day (a caregiver suggests)
- Shower every day instead
- Never bath or shower (the individual's suggestion, which should be recorded with no disagreement)
- Bath every two days
- Shower every other day and strip wash every day
- And so on

Once a number of proposals have been recorded, each person in the discussion gives a 'plus' or 'minus' vote that is marked on the list against the solution. 'Plus' means 'Okay, I could live with that'. 'Minus' means 'No way'.

The votes for each proposal are summed. It is to be hoped that at least one proposal will score positively. Even if the individual has scored such a proposal with a 'minus', the individual can see from other scores that their voice has been heard.

So, the most positively scored proposal(s) can be a way forwards. For example:

- Bath once a day + + -
- Shower every day instead + + -
- Never bath or shower - - +
- Bath every two days + - -
- Shower every other day and strip wash every day + + +

From this solution, we create an agreement and plan to try the solution for a set time to see if it suits everyone better. Reinforcements or consequences may be added to the choice of following the agreement or not following the agreement and, if appropriate, it is written into the individual's care or support plan for everyone to follow.

Setting Rules

Part of the planning process may involve setting certain rules, boundaries or consequences that are needed to improve a person's outcomes. Sometimes when we are looking at long-term benefits, we may be supporting a person to learn skills such as responsibility, independence, delaying gratification or making good decisions. It may be appropriate to set boundaries and rules to help a person develop these skills.

So, if we feel a rule is needed, we should set the rule and the consequences of following or not following the set rule.

During a calm discussion we should:

- explain the reasoning for a rule
- set clear, reasonable expectations
- outline the consequence of following or not following the rule.

Then we instigate the rule.

- Allow them to make their choice.
- Follow through with consequence if required.
- Allow them to make the mistake – no criticism, gloating or shaming is required.

Example: 'So we have been thinking about the rules around your iPad. Sometimes when we ask you to come off your iPad, we feel ignored or sometimes you get irritated with us. Being able to use electronics sensibly is a sign of maturity, and when you don't come off when we ask, it indicates that you may not be mature enough to use electronics yet so we need to set a rule. When we ask you to come off your iPad, we will give you five minutes to save what you need to save and come off. If you can't do that, maybe the maturity isn't there yet. So if you don't come off, you will not be allowed your iPad for the rest of the day.'

'I see you have made the choice to not come off, so you understand the consequences.'

'I can see you're upset and maybe feel like you have made the wrong choice, and that's okay, we can try again tomorrow.'

Example: 'We are worried that you are using your PRN medication too much. The medication could make you poorly if you use it too much, but we understand that you sometimes feel that you need it to cope when you are anxious. We want to help you find other ways to cope with your feelings and see if we can reduce the number of times you need your PRN. So when you ask for your PRN, we want you to try three things on your activity list that also help you to feel better. If after doing the three things you still need your medication, you can have it. Is that fair?'

Later: 'PRN!'

'Okay Theo, let's first try doing the first thing on your list and see if that helps.'

'I want PRN.'

'I understand, but we need to try the first thing on your list before you can have it.'

In this example, the three things were chosen from a list of positive activities that Theo loved. Examples included a shower, going in the garden, hand massage, one-to-one time with Sylvia and jigsaw puzzles. Theo often still wanted his PRN after the three things, but the delay meant that he was still using his PRN fewer times through the day.

Challenging Negative Thoughts and Limiting Beliefs

In the 'Challenging' section on responding appropriately, Chapter 35, page 357, there is a section on challenging. Challenging involves gently questioning whether a person's thoughts and way of seeing the world are helpful or may actually inhibit their wellbeing and outcomes.

If a person thinks that they 'always fail anyway so what's the point in trying...?', it can seem obvious to a person on the outside that this thought process is a) untrue and b) self-limiting. However, although it can be easy to hold that judgement when viewed from the outside, when a person feels they are not good enough, such thoughts can feel very real and very true.

Changing these thoughts is part of the metabolisation process described in 'Metabolisation (Biological Change) and Integration', Chapter 21, page 190. As changing them involves changing the way a person may see the world and themselves within it, in turn, this can change the way they feel and think.

As described above, this can feel uncomfortable for the individual. This is because people often believe that the way they think and feel protects them from pain. But this is without being able to see the costs of this thinking pattern.

'When I say I don't care about something, they don't make me do it, therefore I don't fail at it and don't feel bad when I fail and that way I haven't let myself or anyone else down.'

The potential perceived benefit from this type of thinking is easily seen. This is why we must build a person's trust in themselves and in others before we start to directly challenge their way of thinking.

The reason this section is included in this stage of the 6STM is because challenging may be done in post-incident reflection to help explore and manage future incidents, but negative thoughts and limiting beliefs should also be explored with the caregivers. Caregivers can fall into exactly the same thought traps as any individual, and these thought processes and false beliefs can lead to damaged relationships, stigmatisation of individuals and blocked care (where a caregiver disengages from the therapeutic relationship).

Automatic Negative Thoughts and Negative Thinking Patterns

We can all experience automatic negative thoughts. The negative voice in everyone's head engages in some of the examples below at some points in our life, but when these perpetually fall into people's narratives and become a pattern in people's view of the world, they can become extremely toxic to the person's wellbeing.

Below are a few types of negative thoughts, and they are followed by some examples of each. This was put together by Tim Sharp of the Happiness Institute.

Examples of Automatic Negative Thoughts (ANTs)[83]

One of the basic assumptions of the cognitive model that underlies much of the broader positive psychology model is that the way we think about things is important in determining how we feel. Further, there are times when are thoughts are unhelpfully negative. Recognising these ANTs is the first step in learning to change them. Here are some of the more common types of negative thoughts.

1. **Overgeneralisation:** Coming to a general conclusion based on a single event or one piece of evidence. If something bad happens once, you expect it to happen again and again. Such thoughts often include the words 'always' and 'never'.

   For example: I forgot to finish that project on time I never do things right. He didn't want to go out with me. I'll always be lonely.
2. **Filtering (selective abstraction):** Concentrating on the negatives while ignoring the positives. Ignoring important information that contradicts your (negative) view of the situation.

   For example: I know he [my boss] said most of my submission was great but he also said there were a number of mistakes that had to be corrected...he must think I'm really hopeless.
3. **All or nothing thinking (dichotomous reasoning):** Thinking in black and white terms (e.g., things are right or wrong, good or bad). A tendency to view things at the extremes with no middle ground.

   For example: I made so many mistakes. If I can't do it perfectly, I might as well not bother. I won't be able to get all of this done, so I may as well not start it. This job is so bad...there's nothing good about it at all.
4. **Personalising:** Taking responsibility for something that's not your fault. Thinking that what people say or do is some kind of reaction to you, or is in some way related to you.

   For example: John's in a terrible mood. It must have been something I did. It's obvious she doesn't like me, otherwise she would've said hello.
5. **Catastrophising:** Overestimating the chances of disaster. Expecting something unbearable or intolerable to happen.

   For example: I'm going to make a fool of myself and people will laugh at me.

   What if I haven't turned the iron off and the house burns down.

If I don't perform well, I'll get the sack.

6. **Emotional reasoning:** Mistaking feelings for facts. Negative things you feel about yourself are held to be true because they feel true.
   For example: I feel like a failure, therefore I am a failure.
   I feel ugly, therefore I must be ugly.
   I feel hopeless, therefore my situation must be hopeless.
7. **Mind reading:** Making assumptions about other people's thoughts, feelings and behaviours without checking the evidence.
   For example: John's talking to Molly so he must like her more than me.
   I could tell he thought I was stupid in the interview.
8. **Fortune telling error:** Anticipating an outcome and assuming your prediction is an established fact. These negative expectations can be self-fulfilling: predicting what we would do on the basis of past behaviour may prevent the possibility of change.
   For example: I've always been like this; I'll never be able to change.
   It's not going to work out so there's not much point even trying. This relationship is sure to fail.
9. **Should statements:** Using 'should', 'ought', or 'must' statements can set up unrealistic expectations of yourself and others. It involves operating by rigid rules and not allowing for flexibility.
   For example: I shouldn't get angry. People should be nice to me all the time.
10. **Magnification/minimisation:** A tendency to exaggerate the importance of negative information or experiences, while trivialising or reducing the significance of positive information or experiences.
    For example: He noticed I spilled something on my shirt. I know he said he will go out with me again, but I bet he doesn't call.
    Supporting my friend when her mother died still doesn't make up for that time I got angry at her last year.

Challenging Negative Thoughts and Negative Core Beliefs

These questions from PositivePsychology.com challenge negative outlooks.[84]

Remember: Challenging of any description is best done by someone a person trusts.

- What facts support this thought? What existing evidence contradicts it?
- What would the worst possible outcome be if this thought were true?
- Is a past experience being used to overgeneralise?
- Is there any way this might be viewed in a positive way?
- Will this matter one day from now? What about in one week or one month? How?
- What are some ways this scenario has been dealt with before?

- What advice would a counsellor or therapist give about this situation?
- What is ready to be accepted about this event or person?
- Are the thoughts helpful for dealing with this scenario? Or are they aggravating the situation?
- Can this genuinely be controlled?
- Besides ourselves, what else might be affecting this situation?
- Is 'I must', 'I have to' or 'I should' thinking being used here? Is it truly necessary?
- What advice would we give a friend in this scenario?

CONTINUING THE 6STM

The whole philosophy of the 6STM is that it is a journey – a journey whose end may never be reached. If things don't work out as planned, and/or an individual's behaviour changes, we must go back and review our strategy, our hypothesis, our responses. We will be constantly making adjustments and, hopefully, improvements.

And always remember that if we spend all our time looking for 'the answer' to an individual's behaviour, we may never find it. Meanwhile, we are missing the opportunities for building connections and enjoying the good times.

It's the journey that counts.

SUMMARY

Sometimes We Get it Wrong

We learn through our mistakes.

By admitting our mistakes, we demonstrate humility.

Our mindset should be: 'Okay, I made a mistake. I'll try again tomorrow.'

To encourage others: 'Okay, I made a mistake. I'll try again tomorrow, just as you will.'

Even better: 'Okay, I made a mistake. Let's learn from that, reset, and I'll try again tomorrow, just as you will.'

Keep a Growth Mindset

Don't say, 'I can't.'

This is limiting.

'I can't juggle.'

'I won't even pick up the beanbags.'

Instead, say, 'I'm finding it difficult.'

This is open.

'I find juggling difficult.'
'I'll find a YouTube video to instruct me and keep practising.'

Miracles Happen Every Day

Don't give up on somebody too easily.

Sometimes, trying to guide an individual through their problems is like throwing pebbles in a lake. Our efforts disappear without a trace.

But over time, those pebbles accumulate on the lake floor. One day, the pile will break the surface.

All that effort can eventually yield its rewards.

We get a phone call from a child we cared for: 'I've just been accepted for university.'

An individual we bonded with in a care home moves to independent living.

We learn that a person with dementia we cared for has had a peaceful and happy death.

If our philosophy is 'Positive outcomes for all', we can only try the very best we can.

That will either work or it won't.

That is the nature of care.

APPENDIX 1

How Angry Do You Get?

Answer each question with a, b or c. Check your scores at the end to find out how your anger levels may be affecting you.

a = Untroubled, b = Annoyed, c = Angry

1. Somebody insists on arguing with you about something they know nothing about.
2. You step on chewing gum.
3. Someone bumps into you and doesn't say sorry.
4. At the last moment someone cancels a long-standing arrangement with you.
5. The car parking machine steals your last change.
6. A cold-caller refuses to take no for an answer.
7. Your partner fails to understand the point you have just carefully made.
8. You get reprimanded for something that was someone else's fault.
9. Someone interrupts you while you are talking to a friend.
10. An authority figure fails to recognise your achievements.
11. A pen leaks on your new clothes.
12. Your car fails its MOT and you thought it was fine.
13. A hotel tries to charge you extra for something you thought was inclusive.
14. You lend someone an important object and they fail to return it.
15. You are kept waiting at a shop counter as the assistant is on the phone.
16. You are kept on hold and only hear automated messages when you call a company.
17. Someone you have done many favours for fails to help you out.
18. You are kept waiting by the doctor.
19. At the end of a busy day, just when you are trying to relax, the phone rings.
20. Someone doesn't return your call/text.

Scores: a = 0, b = 3, c = 5.

Now add your scores up.

91–100: Your emotions are largely out of control. You are openly hostile and vengeful.

81–90: Try to improve your communication to enhance your relationships.

71–80: Despite your many abilities, your temper could be holding you back.

61–70: Your anger is easily raised.

51–60: You deal with provocation by openly asserting yourself.

41–50: You appear angry but have learned to keep your composure.

31–40: You can be irritable, particularly with friends and family.

21–30: You see the positive side in people. You don't get angry or even.

11–20: You have more friends than others but are less likely to stick to your principles.

0–10: Your calmness may be at the expense of passion.

APPENDIX 2

The Adverse Childhood Experiences (ACE) Study

The following is a summary of the findings from: Felitti, V. J., Anda, R. F., Nordenberg, D., Williamson, D. F., et al. (1998) 'Relationship of childhood abuse and household dysfunction to many of the leading causes of death in adults. The Adverse Childhood Experiences (ACE) Study.' American Journal of Preventive Medicine 14, 4, 245–258.

The CDC-Kaiser Permanente Adverse Childhood Experiences (ACE) Study is one of the largest investigations of childhood abuse, neglect, household challenges and later-life health and wellbeing.

This study reviewed rates of adverse childhood experiences and the effect these had during a person's lifetime. Negative experiences included suffering abuse, witnessing abuse, neglect, loss of a caregiver, abuse from an incarceration of caregiver, substance abuse in the home and so on. Instances of negative experiences contributed to a 'score'.

It was found that the higher a person's score, the more likelihood there was of a negative long-term effect – not just on their psychological wellbeing, but also on their physical wellbeing. It was also found that negative experiences happening during critical and sensitive developmental periods (particularly under the age of five, when the brain is still at its most plastic, or even in the womb, with the mother experiencing high levels of stress during pregnancy) contributed significantly to problems in later life.

Problems that developed included higher than normal incidences of chronic disorders, such as fibromyalgia, diabetes and dementia, and psychiatric disorders, such as schizophrenia, personality disorders, depression and anxiety, and impaired cognition. As a result, learning disabilities were increased, there was a higher risk of behavioural problems at school and school attendance tended to be lower.

There were high rates of inappropriate relationships with food and higher rates of substance misuse and alcoholism. Other findings showed increased risk-taking behaviour from activities such as engaging in inappropriate sexualised behaviour, stealing and other crimes.

Sufferers were not just at higher risk of being involved in crime, they were also at higher risk of being the victims of crime, especially crimes such as domestic abuse and sexual abuse.

An intergenerational effect was also found, where there is a 'knock-on' effect from a compromised mother to her children, who inherit the mother's symptoms.

An interesting outcome of the study was the possibility that children have been incorrectly diagnosed as having ADHD or as autistic, when in fact the cause of their problems could be early-life trauma that affected the development of the brain. High levels of trauma and amygdala hijacking reduce blood flow to certain parts of the brain and also induce higher than normal levels of cortisol.

Put simply: if a child is subject to high stress, or has a biological predisposition to experiencing high stress, the alarm bell in the child's brain will keep going off. If there is a lack of adequate external help to effectively turn off the alarm, there will be repeated occasions where there is a reduction in blood flow to, and activation of, the still-developing cerebral cortex. This can seriously affect brain development.

The ACE Study is summarised in the following diagram.

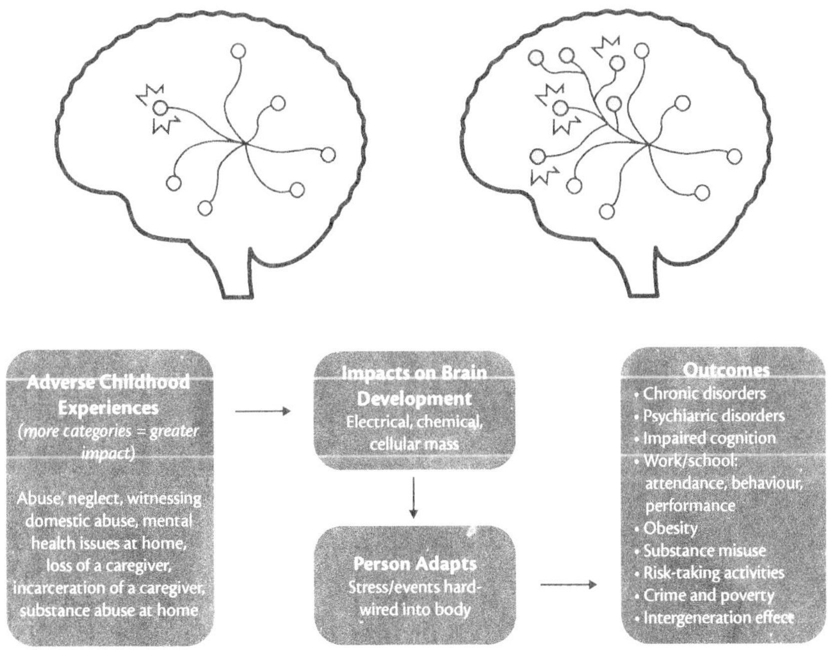

Figure A.1 Lifetime Impacts of Adverse Childhood Experiences

References

1 New Scientist (n.d.) 'Introduction: The Human Brain.' *New Scientist*. https://www.newscientist.com/article/dn9969-introduction-the-human-brain.

2 Enmarker, I., Olsen, R. and Hellzen, O. (2011) 'Management of person with dementia with aggressive and violent behaviour: A systematic literature review.' *International Journal of Older People Nursing* 6, 153–162.

3 Maslow, A. H. (1943) 'A theory of human motivation.' *Psychological Review* 50, 4, 370–396.

4 Kitwood, T. (1997) 'The experience of dementia.' *Aging & Mental Health* 1, 13–22.

5 Sackmann, S. A. (1991) 'The "Iceberg" model of organisational culture', 'Uncovering culture in organizations.' *Journal of Applied Behavioral Science* 27, 3, 295–317. See also Braithwaite, J. (2011) 'A lasting legacy from Tony Blair? NHS culture change.' *Journal of the Royal Society of Medicine* 104, 2, 87–89.

6 Alexander, B. K., Beyerstein, B. L., Hadaway, B. F. and Coombs, R. B. (1981) 'Effect of early and later colony housing on oral ingestion of morphine in rats.' *Pharmacology, Biochemistry, and Behavior* 15, 4, 571–576.

7 Milgram, S. (1963) 'Behavioral study of obedience.' *Journal of Abnormal and Social Psychology* 67, 4, 371–378.

8 Zimbardo, P. (2007) *The Lucifer Effect: How Good People Turn Evil*. New York: Random House.

9 Thorndike, E. L. (1898) 'Animal intelligence: An experimental study of the associative processes in animals.' *Psychological Monographs: General and Applied* 2, 4, i–109.

10 Skinner, B. F. (1938) *The Behavior of Organisms: An Experimental Analysis*. New York: Appleton-Century.

11 Thompson, G. (2000) *The Elephant and the Twig: The Art of Positive Thinking*. Chichester: Summersdale.

12 Kirkova, D. (2013) 'Stunning new EastEnders actress Kierston Wareing confesses she was beaten to a pulp by TWO ex-boyfriends who made her feel "worthless".' *Mail Online*, 15 January.

13 Farnam Street (2024) Brené Brown on The Difference Between Guilt and Shame. https://fs.blog/brene-brown-guilt-shame.

14 Brown, B. (2010) *The Gifts of Imperfection*. Center City, MN: Hazelden Information & Educational Services.

15 Eagleman, D. (2016) *The Brain: The Story of You*. Edinburgh: Canongate Books.

16 Daniel Hughes (n.d.) *Dyadic Developmental Psychotherapy: Attachment Focused Treatment for Childhood Trauma & Abuse*. www.danielhughes.org/about.html.

17 Williams, R. in Shadyac, T. (dir.) *Patch Adams* (1998) Universal Pictures.

18 Adapted from: Research findings of Streissguth, C. *et al.* Diane Malbin 1994, cited at www.come-over.to/FAS/timeline.htm

19 The State of Queensland (2022) *Brain Map Frontal Lobes*. Queensland Health. https://www.health.qld.gov.au/abios/asp/bfrontal.

20 Low, K. (2023) *What are the effects of impaired executive functions?* Verywell Mind. https://www.verywellmind.com/what-are-executive-functions-20463.

21 Queensland Brain Institute (n.d.) *The limbic system*. The University of Queensland. https://qbi.uq.edu.au/brain/brain-anatomy/limbic-system.

22 Demetriou, A., Christou, C., Spanoudis, G. and Platsidou, M. (2002) 'The development of

mental processing: Efficiency, working memory, and thinking.' *Monographs of the Society for Research in Child Development* 67, 268.

23 Giedd, J.N. (2024) 'The amazing teen brain.' Scientific American. https://www.scientificamerican.com/article/the-amazing-teen-brain.

24 Raising Children Network (2024) *Brain development in pre-teens and teenagers.* https://raisingchildren.net.au/pre-teens/development/understanding-your-pre-teen/brain-development-teens#basics.

25 Beyer, A. and Lazzara, J. (2020) *Chapter 7: Adolescence, Psychology Through the Lifespan.* Maricopa. https://open.maricopa.edu/psy240mm/chapter/chapter-7-adolescence-2.

26 Hoose, N.A.-V. (2020) *Adolescent Psychology*. Lumen Learning. https://courses.lumenlearning.com/adolescent/chapter/brain-changes.

27 Jones, T. (n.d.) *Brain Development During Adolescence*. Lumen Learning. https://courses.lumenlearning.com/wm-lifespandevelopment/chapter/brain-development-during-adolescence.

28 Salim, R. (2024) *An Introduction to the Sympathetic and Parasympathetic Nervous System.* iMotions. https://imotions.com/blog/learning/research-fundamentals/nervous-system.

29 Goleman, D. (1996) *Emotional Intelligence: Why it can matter more than IQ*. London: Bloomsbury.

30 Unyye (2018) What is Trauma? https://integratedlistening.com/blog/what-is-trauma.

31 Mind (n.d.) *What is complex PTSD?* https://www.mind.org.uk/information-support/types-of-mental-health-problems/post-traumatic-stress-disorder-ptsd-and-complex-ptsd/complex-ptsd.

32 Adapted from Fry, B. (2019) *The Invisible Lion: Flatpack Instructions for Life*. Independently published.

33 Adapted from Fahlberg, V. (2012) *A Child's Journey through Placement*. London: Jessica Kingsley Publishers.

34 Child Welfare Information Gateway (n.d.) *Parenting your adopted school-age child.* https://health.uconn.edu/adoption-assistance/wp-content/uploads/sites/68/2016/07/Parenting-Your-Adopted-School-Age-Chil.pdf.

35 Davies, D. and Troy, M.F. (2020) *Child Development: A Practitioner's Guide, Fourth Edition.* New York: Guilford Press.

36 Porges, S. W. (2011) *The Polyvagal Theory: Neurophysiological Foundations of Emotions, Attachment, Communication, and Self-Regulation.* New York: W. W. Norton & Co.

37 Samsel, M. (n.d.) 'Finding feeling and purpose.' Social Engagement System. https://reichandlowentherapy.org/Content/Vegetative/ventral_shift.html.

38 Walker, P. (n.d.) *The 4Fs: A Trauma Typology in Complex PTSD.* https://pete-walker.com/fourFs_TraumaTypologyComplexPTSD.htm.

39 Peters, S. (2018) *My Hidden Chimp*. London: Studio Press. Peters, S. (2012) *The Chimp Paradox*. London: Vermilion.

40 Alzheimer's Society (2023) *Dementia Friends.* www.dementiafriends.org.uk.

41 Jones, E. and Nisbett, R. (1987) *The Actor and the Observer: Divergent Perceptions of the Causes of Behavior*. In E. E. Jones, D. E. Kanouse, H. H. Kelley, R. E. Nisbett, S. Valins, & B. Weiner (Eds.), Attribution: *Perceiving the causes of behavior* (pp. 79–94). Lawrence Erlbaum Associates, Inc.

42 Clear, J. (2018) *Atomic Habits*. London: Random House Business Books.

43 Clear, J. (2018) *Atomic Habits*. London: Random House Business Books.

44 Cuncic, A. (2023) The Psychology of Shame. Verywell Mind. www.verywellmind.com/what-is-shame-5115076.

45 Farnam Street (2024) Brené Brown on The Difference Between Guilt and Shame. https://fs.blog/brene-brown-guilt-shame.

46 Adapted from Golding, K.S. and Hughes, D. (2012) *Creating Loving Attachments: Parenting with PACE to Nurture Confidence and Security in the Troubled Child.* London: Jessica Kingsley Publishers.

47 International Institute for Restorative Practices. www.iirp.edu.

48 Brown, B. (2018) *Dare to Lead: Brave Work. Tough Conversations. Whole Hearts.* London: Vermilion, p. 193.

49 Gatchel, R. J., Peng, Y. B., Peters, M. L., Fuchs, P. N. and Turk, D. C. (2007) 'The biopsychosocial

approach to chronic pain: Scientific advances and future directions.' *Psychological Bulletin* 133, 4, 581–624.

50 Center on the Developing Child at Harvard University (2020) *What is Epigenetics? The Answer to the Nature vs. Nurture Debate.* https://developingchild.harvard.edu/resources/what-is-epigenetics-and-how-does-it-relate-to-child-development.

51 Kitwood, T. (1997) *Dementia Reconsidered: The Person Comes First.* Buckingham: Open University Press.

52 Naish, S., Dillon, S. and Mitchell, J. (2019) *Therapeutic Parenting Essentials: Moving from Trauma to Trust.* London: Jessica Kingsley Publishers.

53 Rathbone, C. J., Moulin, C. J. and Conway, M. A. (2008) 'Self-centered memories: The reminiscence bump and the self.' *Memory and Cognition* 36, 8, 1403–1414.

54 Clear, J. (2018) *Atomic Habits.* London: Random House Business Books.

55 Adapted from Greater Good In Education (2024) *SEL for Students: Self-Awareness and Self-Management.* https://ggie.berkeley.edu/student-well-being/sel-for-students-self-awareness-and-self-management.

56 Adapted from Tudor, K. (1996) *Mental Health Promotion: Paradigms and Practice: First Edition.* Routledge. https://doi.org/10.4324/9781315812670.

57 Mencap (2007) *Death by Indifference: Following Up the Treat Me Right! Report.* London: Mencap. www.mencap.org.uk/sites/default/files/2016-07/DBIreport.pdf.

58 Lally, P., van Jaarsveld, C. H. M., Potts, H. W. W. and Wardle, J. (2009) 'How are habits formed? Modelling habit formation in the real world.' *European Journal of Social Psychology* 40, 6, 998–1009.

59 Clear, J. (2018) *Atomic Habits.* London: Random House Business Books.

60 Reproduced with permission from Prochaska, J. O. and DiClemente, C. C. (1983) 'Stages and processes of self-change of smoking: Toward an integrative model of change.' *Journal of Consulting and Clinical Psychology* 51, 3, 390–395.

61 Bandura, A. (1977) *Social Learning Theory*. Englewood Cliffs, NJ: Prentice Hall.

62 McLeod, S. A. (2014) 'Bobo doll experiment.' *Simply Psychology*. www.simplypsychology.org/bobo-doll.html.

63 Goleman, D. (2008) 'Hot to Help.' *Greater Good Magazine.* https://greatergood.berkeley.edu/article/item/hot_to_help

64 Dweck, C. (2016) *Mindset: The New Psychology of Success*. New York: Ballantine Books. There are also several TED talk videos available on YouTube.

65 Badia, P., Harsh, J. and Abbott, B. (1979) 'Choosing between predictable and unpredictable shock conditions: Data and theory.' *Psychological Bulletin* 86, 1107–1131.

66 Alcaraz, K. I., Eddens, K. S., Blase, J. L., Diver, W. R. *et al.* (2019) 'Social isolation and mortality in US black and white men and women.' *American Journal of Epidemiology* 188, 1, 102–109.

67 Novotney, A. (2019) The Risks of Social Isolation. *Monitor on Psychology*. https://www.apa.org/monitor/2019/05/ce-corner-isolation.

68 Carnegie, D. (2009) *How to Win Friends and Influence People.* New York: Simon & Schuster, p. 113.

69 Vaynerchuk, G. (2017) *Being Selfless by Being Selfish.* www.garyvaynerchuk.com/being-selfless-by-being-selfish.

70 Vaynerchuk, G. (2017) Being Selfless by Being Selfish. www.garyvaynerchuk.com/being-selfless-by-being-selfish..

71 Adapted from Edgell-Horvath, T. (2023) 'Building Your Resilience with Self-Care.' *LifeWorks.* https://totalhealth.cat.com/content/dam/totalhealth/a-z/taking-time-for-you/self-care/Building-Your-Resilience-With-Self-Care.pdf

72 Official U.S. Marine Corps (2016) Combat and Operational Stress Control (COSC) (MCTP 3-30E/NTTP 1-15M). Quantico, VA: Marine Corps Combat Development Command. http://www.marines.mil/News/Publications/MCPEL/Electronic-Library-Display/Article/899535/mcrp-6-11c.

73 This list and the STAMP acronym are reproduced under a Creative Commons License from YouthAOD Toolbox (n.d.) '5. Recognising the warning signs for potential aggressive behaviour & violence.' *YouthAOD Toolbox.* https://www.youthaodtoolbox.org.au/5-recognising-warning-signs-potential-aggressive-behaviour-violence.

74 The National Council of Juvenile and Family Court Judges (n.d.) De-escalation Skills. https://www.ncjfcj.org/wp-content/uploads/2022/03/ten_critical_deescalation_skills.pdf.

75 Student Support Services, Department for Education (n.d.) Regulation Scale (HSP432). Developed by Michelle McAuley, Behaviour Support Coach, https://www.education.sa.gov.au/docs/support-and-inclusion/disability-advice-and-research/hsp432a-regulation-scale-guide.pdf. Reproduced under Creative Commons 4.0 https://creativecommons.org/licenses/by-sa/4.0/legalcode.

76 Egan, G. (1990) *The skilled helper: A systematic approach to effective helping.* Pacific Grove, CA: Brooks/Cole Pub. Co.

77 Adapted from Skolnik-Acker, E. (n.d.) *Verbal De-Escalation Techniques for Defusing or Talking.* https://ppsfba.weebly.com/uploads/2/5/0/7/25071730/verbal_de-escalation.pdf.

78 Goleman, D. (2008) 'Hot to Help.' *Greater Good Magazine.* https://greatergood.berkeley.edu/article/item/hot_to_help.

79 University of Kent (n.d.) Dr Damian Milton. www.kent.ac.uk/social-policy-sociology-social-research/people/1419/milton-damian.

80 Elliott, A. (2013) *Why Can't My Child Behave? Empathic Parenting Strategies That Work for Adoptive and Foster Families.* London: Jessica Kingsley Publishers.

81 Reproduced with permission from Elliott, A. (2013) *Why Can't My Child Behave? Empathic Parenting Strategies That Work for Adoptive and Foster Families.* London: Jessica Kingsley Publishers.

82 Cherry, K. (2024) 'How Does Reverse Psychology Work?' *Verywell Mind.* https://www.verywellmind.com/what-is-reverse-psychology-5115635.

83 Sharpe, T. (2002) *Examples of Automatic Negative Thoughts (ANTs).* The Happiness Institute. https://courses.thebehaviourinstitute.com/wp-content/uploads/2020/04/Automatic-Thoughts.pdf.

84 Selva, J. (2018) *Questions For Challenging Thoughts.* PositivePsychology.com. https://positive.b-cdn.net/wp-content/uploads/Questions-For-Challenging-Thoughts.pdf.

Index